AUDIOLOGY
FIFTH EDITION

HAYES A. NEWBY
University of Maryland

GERALD R. POPELKA
Central Institute for the Deaf

PRENTICE-HALL, INC., Englewood Cliffs, N.J. 07632

Library of Congress Cataloging in Publication Data

NEWBY, HAYES A.
  Audiology.

  Includes bibliographies and indexes.
    1. Audiology. 2. Hearing disorders. I. Popelka, Gerald R.
II. Title. [DNLM: 1. Hearing. WV 270 N535a]
RF290.N47 1985   617.8'9   84–17958
ISBN 0-13-050865-9

RF290
N47
1985

Editorial/production supervision: Colleen Brosnan
Cover design: Ben Santora
Manufacturing buyer: Barbara Kelly Kittle

Printed in the United States of America

10 9 8 7 6 5 4 3 2 1

ISBN 0-13-050865-9   01

Prentice-Hall International, Inc., *London*
Prentice-Hall of Australia Pty. Limited, *Sydney*
Editora Prentice-Hall do Brasil, Ltda., *Rio de Janeiro*
Prentice-Hall Canada Inc., *Toronto*
Prentice-Hall Hispanoamericano, S. A., *Mexico*
Prentice-Hall of India Private Limited, *New Delhi*
Prentice-Hall of Japan, Inc., *Tokyo*
Prentice-Hall of Southeast Asia Pte. Ltd., *Singapore*
Whitehall Books Limited, *Wellington, New Zealand*

CONTENTS

12
REHABILITATING THE HARD-OF-HEARING ADULT

13
THE PROFESSION OF AUDIOLOGY

APPENDIX: MATERIALS FOR SPEECH AUDIOMETRY

INDEX

PREFACE

In 1958, when the first edition of this book was published, I had no idea that some 27 years later I would be writing a preface for a fifth edition. I am most grateful to all those instructors and students whose loyalty has inspired me to revise and update the book every six to seven years.

While I was active in the field as a teacher and clinician, I felt capable of keeping myself and the book reasonably up-to-date. Since my retirement from the University of Maryland in 1979, I have not attempted to keep active in the field of audiology. There are so many interesting activities competing for my time that I have felt no need or inclination to maintain any professional involvement. Thus, as the time approached when another revision of this book became necessary, I realized that I needed help. Fortunately, help was available in the person of Dr. Gerald R. Popelka, Head of Audiology at Central Institute for the Deaf and Associate Professor of Audiology at Washington University in Saint Louis. Since receiving his Ph.D. from the University of Wisconsin in 1974, Dr. Popelka has been associated with New York University, UCLA School of Medicine, and California State University at Los Angeles before affiliating with Central Institute and Washington University. By training and experience, he is eminently qualified to be co-author of this book. He has been almost solely responsible for the preparation of this fifth edition.

As I have stated in prefaces to previous editions, this book is designed as a textbook for beginning courses in audiology at either an advanced undergraduate or graduate level. In beginning survey courses, I recommend that the instructor omit or cover only superficially Chapters 5, 6, 7, 8, and possibly 9. In beginning courses that emphasize testing or the evaluation of hearing, Chapters 5, 6, and 8 should be retained. Chapters 5, 6, and 8 can also serve as the nucleus for a second course specifically in basic hearing measurements; Chapter 7 can lay the foundation for a course in advanced hearing measurements; and Chapter 9 can serve a similar function for a course in industrial audiology.

While this book is designed primarily for students, I hope that it will prove useful to other professionals who need to have at least a nodding acquaintance with the field of audiology, and to hearing-impaired individuals and their families.

I suggest that instructors supplement this book with assignments in other books and in professional journals. One book I especially recommend is a workbook or study guide, *Principles of Audiology: A Study Guide* (Baltimore: University Park Press, 1984), prepared by Dr. Frederick N. Martin to be used in conjunction with this book and two other books used as texts in beginning courses in audiology: Martin's *Introduction to Audiology,* 2nd edition (Englewood Cliffs, N.J.: Prentice-Hall, 1981), and Hallowell Davis and S. Richard Silverman's *Hearing and Deafness,* 4th edition (New York: Holt, Rinehart and Winston, 1978).

Finally, I want to express once again my appreciation to all those individuals who have contributed to this book during the past quarter-century. They are so numerous I hesitate to try to name them for fear I might inadvertently omit one or more.

Hayes A. Newby
Punta Gorda, Florida

ACKNOWLEDGMENTS

I would like to thank Mary M. Sicking, Librarian at Central Institute for the Deaf, for helping in the preparation of the manuscript for the fifth edition. Her attention to detail and willingness to undertake even the most tedious tasks are appreciated greatly.

The following reviewers selected by the publisher aided the revision process: Gary J. Beeby, Oklahoma State University; William D. Chapman, Indiana University of Pennsylvania; Allan O. Diefendorf, University of Tennessee, Hal A. Dorsey, Central Connecticut State College; and Phillip A. Yantis, University of Washington.

I especially would like to thank Dr. Newby for asking me to help write the fifth edition. I am honored to be associated with him and hope that my contribution will continue the tradition of his fine work.

Gerald R. Popelka
St. Louis, Missouri

CHAPTER ONE
THE LINEAGE
OF AUDIOLOGY

Audiology refers to the study of hearing and hearing disorders. The field of audiology is a broad one that can be approached from many aspects and to which varied specialists contribute their knowledge and skills. So far as these specialists make contributions to this field, they are properly designated as audiologists, even though audiology may be their secondary interest. Generally, however, the term *audiologist* is reserved for the individual whose primary interest is in the identification and measurement of hearing loss and the rehabilitation of those with hearing impairments. Usually, the training has been academic rather than medical, although there are a few notable exceptions. Most audiologists are products of university graduate-training programs in speech and hearing, and many have Ph.D. degrees in this field.

Speaking figuratively, audiology is the offspring of two parents: speech pathology and otology. Speech pathology deals with the diagnosis and treatment of individuals who suffer from disorders in oral language. Otology is concerned with the diagnosis and treatment of individuals who have an ear disease or disorders of the peripheral mechanism of hearing. Speech pathology is primarily a nonmedical specialty, whereas otology is purely a medical specialty, one division of otorhinolaryngology (ear, nose, and throat). The two fields—speech pathology and otology—were wedded in World War II in the so-called aural rehabilitation centers established by the armed forces for the benefit of hearing-impaired service personnel. The care and rehabilitation of these people required the closest teamwork between medical and non-medical specialists. Some nonmedical persons recruited for work in the aural rehabilitation centers were former teachers of the deaf, but for the most part they were people whose training and experience had been in the field of speech pathology and speech correction. For years, speech correctionists had assumed responsibility for working with the speech problems of hard-of-hearing children and adults. Now in the aural rehabilitation centers, they extended their responsibilities to the development of tests of hearing function, selection of hearing aids, and development of various rehabilitative techniques that extended far beyond speech correction. Thus, through the cooperative efforts of the two specialties of speech pathology and otology, a new field of specialization was created. Although there had been notable examples of individuals who devoted themselves to working with the hard of hearing before the 1940s, the professional field of audiology did not exist until World War II.

As a matter of fact, the word *audiology* did not come into general use until 1945, when Carhart, a speech pathologist recruited for the Army aural rehabilitation work, and Canfield, an otologist who was serving as consultant to the War Department, applied the term to the field that had been created through the joint efforts of the two fields of specialization that these men represented.[1] The identity of the person who coined the word *audiology* has been disputed by representatives of the hearing-aid industry and others. Trainor and Hargrave claim to have originated the word in 1939, and they report that as early as 1940 news items appeared with the words *audiology*, *audiologist*, and *audiological*.[2] Whatever the true origin of the word, it is nevertheless a fact that *audiology* as a popular term dates from the time that Carhart and Canfield "coined" it, and *audiologist* has come to designate the professional rather than the commercial worker in the field. The origins of the field of audiology will be discussed more fully in Chapter 13.

If the mother and father of audiology are speech pathology and otology, there are many living relatives on both the medical and nonmedical sides of the family. Among the medical relatives are pediatrics, gerontology, psychiatry, and neurology. Pediatricians and gerontologists represent extremes in ages of patients, yet both are concerned with problems of impaired hearing as they affect the health and adjustment of their patients. Because a hearing impairment frequently does produce maladjustment, the psychiatrist, too, has an interest in audiology. Because some "auditory" disorders may involve pathology of the central nervous system, the neurologist on occasion is also vitally interested in audiology.

[1]George E. Shambaugh, Jr., and Raymond Carhart, "Contributions of Audiology to Fenestration Surgery," *A.M.A. Archives of Otolaryngology* 54 (December 1951):699.

[2]M. E. Trainor and Willard Hargrave, "Audiology," *The Auricle* 3 (May 1963):3.

Among the nonmedical relatives of audiology are psychology, physics, and education. Clinical psychologists formed an important unit in the team approach so successfully developed in the military aural rehabilitation programs. Since the war, clinical psychologists have assumed an important role in such activities as assessing the aurally handicapped individual's potential and in counseling the deaf and hard of hearing and their families. In addition, psychologists have shed light on an important and puzzling problem in audiology—the question of nonorganic or functional hearing loss in children and adults.

Two branches of the field of physics are importantly related to audiology: acoustics and electronics. Because hearing disorders represent an inability to respond normally to acoustic stimulation, the audiologist must have some knowledge of the physical properties of sound stimuli. The measurement of hearing loss requires accurate and dependable instrumentation, as does the "correction" of hearing loss by means of amplification. It is becoming increasingly important for the audiologist, regardless of basic orientation, to develop some knowledge and understanding of electronics as it is applied to problems of diagnosing and rehabilitating those with auditory impairments. The audiologist must become, to some extent, an acoustics and electronics engineer.

Audiology is related to education, particularly in matters concerning the training of deaf and hard-of-hearing children. Considerable emphasis is now being placed on training of the preschool deaf child, and nursery schools for such children are developing as part of the program of hearing centers or as separate entities. The audiologist who works with these children must be grounded in nursery-school teaching principles and methods and must have a specialized knowledge of the training of the deaf and the hard of hearing. Rehabilitation of older children should be integrated with their regular schoolwork, and the audiologist must cooperate closely with the classroom teacher. To work effectively with the school-age child, therefore, the audiologist should have some acquaintance with the work of the classroom teacher.

Thus, we see that audiology is not a strictly delimited field but one that springs from many sources and draws on a variety of skills and backgrounds. The "compleat" audiologist would be a combination of speech pathologist, otorhinolaryngologist, pediatrician, gerontologist, psychiatrist, psychologist, physicist, electronics engineer, and educator. This list includes only the clinical aspects of the field. Actually, what might be called experimental audiology is a highly important branch; out of information gained experimentally come improved techniques for clinical application. In the consideration of experimental work and research, the work of the physiologist must receive recognition. In audiology the physiologist is concerned with problems in how we hear. The work is based on the principles of medical and surgical care of individuals with hearing impairment and also the principles of preventive medicine, or hearing conservation. In addition to the physiologist, the experimental psychologist contributes to the field of audiology through research in the psychological processes of hearing and in psychoacoustics. And, of course, all the specialists mentioned in connection with clinical audiology are concerned also with research and experimentation in the areas of their principal orientation.

It can be seen, therefore, that no one individual can be expected to be the "compleat" audiologist. Every clinical audiologist, however, should have some awareness of the complexities of the field and respect for the array of talents and backgrounds presented by coworkers of various specialties. It is the hearing-handicapped patient who benefits from this concentration of professional interests in the field of audiology.

REFERENCES

CANFIELD, NORTON. *Audiology, the Science of Hearing, a Developing Professional Specialty.* Springfield, Ill.: Charles C Thomas, 1949.
DAVIS, HALLOWELL, and SILVERMAN, S. RICHARD, eds. *Hearing and Deafness,* 4th ed. Chap. 1. New York: Holt, Rinehart and Winston, 1978.
FELDMANN, HAROLD. "A History of Audiology." *Translations of the Beltone Institute for Hearing Research,* no. 22 (January 1970).

CHAPTER TWO
WHAT AND HOW WE HEAR

Because audiology is concerned with the response of the human ear to auditory stimuli, it is necessary for the audiologist to know something of the physical nature of sound (the tools of the trade, so to speak) and also of the structure and functioning of the body's hearing mechanism. No attempt will be made here to go into great detail on either subject. The serious student of audiology will naturally want to pursue these subjects in a more thorough way, and a number of excellent books are mentioned at the end of this chapter.

THE PHYSICS OF HEARING

The Propagation of Sound

Sound is created when some force sets an object into vibration, to the extent that molecular movement of the medium in which the object is situated occurs, and a "sound wave" is propagated. Sound is "heard" when the characteristics of the wave propagated fall within the limitations of the human ear and nervous system. The essentials for sound to be created and heard, then, are a vibrator of some sort, a force to set the vibrator into vibration, a medium to convey the wave motion originating at the vibrator, and a hearing mechanism that can receive and perceive the energy of the propagated wave.

Sound sources may be of various kinds: reeds (as in woodwind instruments), strings (as in the piano and other stringed instruments), membranes (as in drums), and columns of air (as in the pipe organ), to mention just a few. The force to set the vibrator in motion may originate in nature (as the wind causing a shutter to rattle, for example) or may be produced by human contrivance. Most sound with which audiologists are concerned is of human origin. In our modern civilization, the most important sounds are those communicating information, primarily the sounds of spoken language. The way in which sound may originate can be illustrated by describing how the human voice is produced. The source of the voice is the vibrating vocal folds in the larynx. By muscular action, the vocal folds are brought together, thus blocking the free airway through the larynx. The motive power for voice is provided by air pressure built up below the vocal folds by the muscles of exhalation. When the air pressure below the larynx overcomes the muscular tension of the vocal folds, the folds are separated momentarily. When conditions of muscular tension and air pressure are almost in balance, the vocal folds are set into vibration. The original vibrations of the vocal folds are then transmitted to columns of air in the throat, mouth, and nose, which act as resonators to reinforce and selectively amplify the vibrations produced by the vocal folds.

The transmission of sound from a vibrating source to a receptor requires some kind of medium. It cannot be transmitted through a vacuum. The medium may be a gas (such as air), a fluid (such as water), or a solid (such as steel). Most sound with which we are concerned is airborne. The sound is transmitted from its source to the ear by movements of the molecules of air. These movements of the air particles are called a *sound wave.*

In the production of a sound wave, the air particles adjacent to the vibrating source are set in motion by the movements of the sound source. The moving particles next to the sound source in turn set the particles adjacent to them in motion. Thus, the motion of each particle affects the position of the particle next to it, and a wave of particle movement emanates in all directions from the vibrating sound source, proceeding outward in concentric spheres at a set velocity that is determined by the temperature and density of the air. Under "standard" conditions of temperature and density as defined by engineers, this wave of particle displacement proceeds at a velocity of about 1100 feet per second.

Actually, there are two parts to a sound wave: *compression* and *rarefaction.* The sound source "oscillates," or vibrates, in simple or complex movement. A sound medium, such as air, is characterized by elasticity; that is, the particles of the medium can move in any direction in which force is applied, and when that force is removed they tend to return to their former positions. In reality, the particles oscillate also. When they are compressed, pressure is built up that forces them to "rebound" when that pressure is removed, so that the particles actually "overshoot" their former positions when compression ceases. Thus, in the compression cycle of the wave, the particles force against each other; in the rarefaction phase, they separate from each other. However, as they separate, another compression is initiated by the oscillating action of the sound source. Alternate compressions and rarefactions, then, characterize the sound wave, and each compression and rarefaction proceeds outward from the sound source at a steady velocity.

A visible illustration of this invisible phenomenon can be cited. Visualize a line of men waiting to get into a mess hall. Along comes a practical joker who gives the last man in line a shove forward. This man pushes into the man ahead of him, and so on, until finally the poor fellow at the head of the line gets his head banged into the door. A wave of compression has passed down the line of men, and an interval of time has been required for the man at the head of the line to feel the effects of this compression. Now what happens? As soon as the man at the rear of the line can regain his balance, he reacts to having been pushed forward by moving back. Each man in turn regains his balance and moves back until finally the fellow at the head of the line can pull his head away from the door. Thus, a wave of rarefaction has passed down the line of men. Now assume that the joker continued to shove the last man in line at regular intervals. Successive waves of compression and rarefaction passing down the line of men would be visible to the observer, and the man at the head of the line would alternately bang his head into the door and withdraw it. At any one time along the line of men, several points of compression and rarefaction would be visible. The longer the line, the more such points could be seen. In this illustration, the joker would be the sound source; the line of men, the particles affected by the vibration of the sound source; and the door, the ear receiving the vibrations.

Because in a sound wave the direction of particle movement is the same as the direction of wave propagation, we say that sound travels in *longitudinal* waves. Although, as we have said, sound waves proceed outward from the source in constantly expanding spheres, if we could visualize just one radius of the sphere, we would see the particles oscillating along that radius. Other types of energy are propagated in *transverse* waves, for example, electromagnetic radiation, including light. Such waves are called transverse because fluctuations in the magnitude of their electric and magnetic fields (corresponding to particle movement in sound waves) occur at right angles to the beam of radiation. Incidentally, electromagnetic waves, unlike sound waves, do not require a medium. They can be transmitted through a vacuum.

The repetitive back-and-forth motion or oscillation of a pendulum is called *simple harmonic motion*. This is the same kind of motion characteristic of a vibrating tuning fork—and of the particles of a medium set into motion by the vibrating tuning fork. If a pen were attached to a swinging pendulum so that it inscribed the pendulum's motion on a roll of paper moving at a constant velocity, it would generate a series of curves such as those in Figure 2–1. The

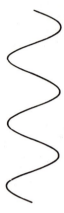

FIGURE 2-1.
Curves representing simple
harmonic motion of a swinging
pendulum.

shape of the curves defining simple harmonic motion is the same obtained from graphing the trigonometric sines of angles from 0 to 360 degrees. The graph of a single sine wave is shown in Figure 2–2.

The harmonic motion described by an oscillating particle of a medium set in motion by a vibrator, such as a tuning fork, can be graphed as a sine wave, also called a *sinusoidal* wave. When used to graph particle motion, the ordinate (vertical dimension) of the graph represents degree of displacement of the particle. Thus, the zero point on the ordinate represents the position of the particle at rest. Compression—or movement of the particle toward its outside neighbor—is represented by designations on the ordinate above the zero point, or in a positive direction; rarefaction is represented by designations below the zero point, or in a negative direction. The ordinate may also be labeled as pressure exerted on a particle—positive pressure occurring during compression, and negative pressure occurring during rarefaction. The zero point on the ordinate represents no pressure. The abscissa (horizontal dimension) of the graph of the sinusoidal wave representing particle motion indicates time, or the period of the sound being graphed. (See the following section for the definition of *period*.)

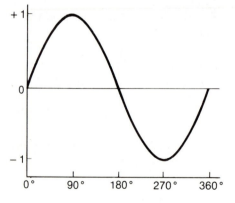

FIGURE 2-2.
Graph of sines of angles.

Just as with light waves, sound waves will reflect from a nonabsorbent surface and be subject to refraction. Of course, there is a great deal of difference between light waves and sound waves in their velocity of propagation. Light waves travel at about 186,000 miles per second in contrast to the comparatively slow speed of sound. The difference between the velocity of light and of sound causes some interesting phenomena that we all have observed in some form. In the days before diesel engines replaced steam locomotives, we could see the column of steam escaping from the train's whistle sometimes several seconds before hearing the sound of the whistle, depending, of course, on how far away the train was. Another common experience is the time that frequently elapses between observing a streak of lightning and hearing the sound of the thunder. We can obtain an approximate measure of the distance of the lightning by counting the number of seconds until we hear the thunder. If we multiply the number of seconds by 1100 feet, we will have the distance.

So far we have been talking about the behavior of sound waves in air. As we mentioned previously, sound can also be propagated in liquids and in solids. In these media, the velocity of sound differs somewhat from its speed in air. In salt water of a standard temperature and density, for example, sound will travel at the rate of about 5000 feet per second; in steel, the velocity of sound is about 15,000 feet per second. Thus, an approaching train can be heard more quickly if an ear is placed on the rail.

Attributes of a Sound Wave

We have discussed the origin and method of propagation of a sound wave. Sound has several measurable attributes that are of importance to the audiologist in the analysis of hearing impairment. The ones with which we shall be concerned are *frequency, amplitude,* and *spectrum.*

Frequency.   Most sounds are characterized by periodicity; that is, the sound wave consists of repetitions of compressions and rarefactions that occur at the same rate over a period of time. One successive compression and rarefaction constitute one *cycle* of a sound wave. The frequency of a sound wave is the number of cycles that occur in a second's time. The unit for expressing frequency is the *cycle per second,* abbreviated c.p.s., c/s, or most commonly cps. Thus, if in a second's time a sound produces 1000 compressions and rarefactions, that sound has a frequency of 1000 cps.

The length of time required for one cycle to occur is called the *period* of the sound. Thus, for a sound with a frequency of 1000 cps, the period is 1/1000 second. If 1000 cycles occur in one second's time, each cycle lasts just 1/1000 second. The period of a sound is the reciprocal of the frequency (one divided by the frequency). Since 1960, following a recommendation of an international congress on weights and measures, the term *hertz,* abbreviated *Hz,* has been employed increasingly as a substitute for cycle per second. The new term honors the memory of a famous physicist, Heinrich Hertz. Thus, today we usually speak of a 1000-cps tone as a 1000-Hz tone. The term *kilocycle*, abbreviated *kc*, means 1000 cycles per second, and so *kilohertz*, abbreviated *kHz*, means the same thing. We may speak of a tone as having a frequency, for example, of either 4000 Hz or of 4 kHz; the terms are used interchangeably. In keeping with the present trend, we shall refer to frequency in this book in terms of hertz instead of cycles per second.

Related to frequency is wavelength. Because sound in air travels at a fixed velocity of about 1100 feet per second, the wavelength of 1 cycle of a sound wave is equal to the frequency of the wave divided into 1100 feet. Thus, for a sound of the frequency of 1000 Hz, the wavelength is 1.1 feet. In other words, each cycle (one compression and one rarefaction) occupies the space of 1.1 feet. It can be seen that frequency and wavelength are inversely related. As the frequency of a sound increases, the wavelength must decrease, as there are then more cycles to fit into the space of 1100 feet. Thus, in formula form, $W = V/F$, where W = wavelength, V = velocity, and F = frequency. If we desire to solve for frequency instead of wavelength, the formula would be written $F = V/W$. Because for sounds of higher frequency the wavelength may be expressed in inches, we must remember to convert wavelength into a fraction of a foot before solving for frequency. Suppose, for example, we want to know the frequency of a sound that has a wavelength of three inches. The formula should be written $F = 1100/0.25$, and not $F = 1100/3$. In this example, $F = 4400$ Hz.

The human ear has certain limitations in the frequencies that it can perceive. Although there is a wide range of individual differences, it can be generalized that the young adult with normal hearing can perceive frequencies from about 20 to 20,000 Hz. We call this the *audible range* of frequencies. Moreover, the ear is not equally sensitive to all frequencies within this range. The ear is most sensitive to the frequencies from 500 through 8000 Hz. Sounds of frequencies below 500 Hz and above 8000 Hz must be made more intense in order to be perceived.

Sounds outside the frequency range of the human ear are referred to as *ultrasonic*, if they are above the human limits, or *infrasonic*, if they are below. Dogs appear to have more sensitivity to higher frequencies than do humans. Several years ago, dog whistles of ultrasonic frequency (for human beings) appeared on the market. They enable dog owners to summon their pets without disturbing the neighborhood (except for other dogs). Dogs are frequently seen to react to train whistles and to sirens as if the sounds pained them. It is possible that the dogs are receiving very high frequencies of strong intensity, which are not even perceived by us. Ultrasonic frequencies are of interest to engineers and physicists and are being put to industrial and medical use, but as of the present time, at least, they do not concern the audiologist. Our concern is with audible frequencies.

The physical attribute of frequency of an audible wave is primarily responsible for the psychological sensation of *pitch*. As the frequency of a sound increases, the pitch of the sound as heard becomes higher. Scales of pitch are based on the assumption that as frequency is doubled (intensity remaining constant), pitch is raised one octave, and as frequency is halved, pitch is lowered one octave. The relationship between frequency and pitch scales is thus logarithmic to the base 2. The logarithm to the base 2 of a number is the power to which 2 must be raised—that is, the number of times that 2 must be multiplied by itself—to equal the number. Thus, the logarithm to the base 2 of the number 16 is 4, because 2^4 $(2 \times 2 \times 2 \times 2) = 16$. Similarly, the number that has a logarithm to the base 2 of 6 is 64, because 2^6 $(2 \times 2 \times 2 \times 2 \times 2 \times 2) = 64$.

For scientific work, an arbitrary scale has been devised in which 256 Hz equals middle C. In such a scale, 1 Hz would also be equal to C. It can be seen that this scale offers mathematical conveniences. Successive octaves of C would be 1, 2, 4, 8, 16, 32, 64, 128, 256, 512, 1024, 2048, 4096, 8192, 16,384, 32,768, and so on. Of course, the first four frequencies in this series would be infrasonic, and the last frequency would be ultrasonic. The otologist's tuning forks are in octaves of C on the scientific scale, and the early audiometers also were calibrated in octaves and mid-octaves of C on the scientific scale. However, for the convenience of audiometrists and others dealing with hearing-test results, all current audiometers have been calibrated in round numbers of hertz instead of in octaves of C. Thus, modern audiometers generate the following frequencies: 125, 250, 500, 750, 1000, 1500, 2000, 3000, 4000, 6000, and 8000 Hz. It is interesting to note that for musical purposes a scale in which A equals 440 Hz has been adopted. In the concert scale, middle C equals 261.6 Hz.

The term *octave* is misleading because an octave has six main divisions, not eight. In other words, an octave consists of six *tones*, or twelve *semitones*. To find the number of hertz for the frequency that is one tone higher in pitch than a given frequency, multiply the lower frequency by the sixth root of 2 ($\sqrt[6]{2}$), which equals 1.1224. Thus, the frequency that is one tone higher in pitch than 1000 Hz is 1122.4 Hz. To find the frequency of the next higher tone, multiply 1122.4 by $\sqrt[6]{2}$ (1.1224). Continuing this process yields the frequencies of successively higher tones, until the result of the sixth such multiplication equals 2000 Hz.

The frequency values of semitones can be computed in similar fashion by using the twelfth root of 2 ($\sqrt[12]{2}$), or 1.059, as the multiplier. Because frequency is a logarithmic function, the number of hertz in an octave interval is different from octave to octave, and the same is true, of course, for tonal and semitonal intervals. Thus, the octave from 500 to 1000 Hz spans a range of 500 Hz, but the octave from 4000 to 8000 Hz covers a range of 4000 Hz. Once the frequency values of tonal and semitonal intervals have been computed for one octave, they can be determined for the next higher octave by multiplying them by two, or for the next lower octave by dividing them by two.

Striking each key on a piano in succession, whether white or black, produces a series of semitones. Thus, in an octave we would have the following musical designations of semitones: C, C#, D, D#, E, F, F#, G, G#, A, A#, and B. Table 2–1 gives the semitonal values in hertz for a span of three octaves for both the scientific and concert scales.

Amplitude.   The amplitude of a sound, or the strength of a sound, is related to how far the particles are displaced. The amplitude is directly proportional to the magnitude of particle displacement, which depends on many factors, including the energy in and distance from the sound source. A given sound source may be made to vibrate at a single frequency at high or low amplitudes, depending on the amount of force that sets it into vibration and the distance over which the source is moving back and forth. For example, a tuning fork may be struck lightly or strongly. The resulting energy in the sound source is emitted as an ever enlarging spherical sound wave with the energy spread over the entire surface of the sphere. As the distance from the sound source increases, the sphere increases in diameter, and thus the energy per unit of area decreases. It is very difficult to measure sound energy since measurements would have to be made over an area of the curved surface of the sphere. At any point on the sphere, however, sound pressure can be measured easily. Sound energy per area is proportional to the square of sound pressure. If the amplitude of a sound is expressed in terms of sound energy per area, the term *intensity* is used. If the amplitude is expressed in terms of sound pressure, a term employing the word *pressure* is used. In practical usage, however, the term *intensity* often is used for both sound intensity and sound pressure. We will use the term *intensity* to refer to the amplitude of a sound, whether it is expressed in sound intensity or sound pressure.

Amplitude is usually measured in terms of relative pressure, using an in-

TABLE 2–1.   Approximate frequency values in hertz for semitones in two pitch scales*

	Scientific	Concert	Scientific	Concert	Scientific	Concert
C	128.0	130.8	256.0	261.6	512.0	523.2
C#	135.6	138.5	271.2	277.0	542.4	554.0
D	143.6	146.8	287.2	293.6	574.4	587.2
D#	152.0	155.5	304.0	311.0	608.0	622.0
E	160.8	164.8	321.6	329.6	643.2	659.2
F	170.4	174.6	340.8	349.2	681.6	698.4
F#	180.4	184.9	360.8	369.8	721.6	739.6
G	191.2	196.0	382.4	392.0	764.8	784.0
G#	202.4	207.6	404.8	415.2	809.6	830.4
A	214.4	220.0	428.8	440.0	857.6	880.0
A#	227.2	233.0	454.4	466.0	908.8	932.0
B	240.8	247.0	481.6	494.0	963.2	988.0

* Because of rounding errors, the values of each semitone will differ depending on the starting point of the computations. The computations for the scientific scale were made for the octave 32–64 Hz and extended to the higher octaves by simple multiplication. The computations for the concert scale were made for the octave 110–220 Hz.

strument called a sound-level meter (Chapter 9). Absolute pressure is expressed in microbars (μbars), dynes per square centimeter (dynes/cm²), newtons per square meter (N/m²), or pascals (Pa). Intensity may also be expressed as power in watts per square centimeter (watts/cm²).

A microbar is one-millionth of a bar. Standard atmospheric pressure, 14.7 pounds per square inch, is 1,013,250 μbars, or slightly more than 1 bar.[1] One newton per square meter is equal to 10 μbars, or put another way, 1 μbar equals 0.1 N/m². Microbars and dynes per square centimeter are synonymous, as are pascals and newtons per square meter.

The normal human ear is sensitive to a wide range of amplitudes, from 10^{-16} watt/cm² (0.000,000,000,000,000,1 watt/cm²) to 10^{-2} watt/cm² (0.01 watt/cm²) expressed in units of power per area, or from 0.0002 dyne/cm² (2×10^{-4} dyne/cm²) to 2000 dynes/cm² (2×10^3 dynes/cm²) expressed in units of pressure. The least amplitude corresponds to the threshold of the average normal ear, and the highest amplitude represents the point at which, on the average, sound produces a sensation of pain.

Because of the difficulty of dealing with the absolute units of power or pressure, it is customary to convert units of amplitude to a ratio between a given sound power, or sound pressure, and a standard reference power, or pressure that for audiologic convenience approximates the threshold of the normal ear. The use of a logarithmic scale to the base 10 for expressing this ratio results in a greatly simplified means of referring to amplitude. The logarithm to the base 10 ($\log_{10}$) of a number is the power to which 10 must be raised (the exponent of 10) to equal the number. Thus, the logarithm to the base 10 of the number 1000 is 3, because 10^3 ($10 \times 10 \times 10$) = 1000. The exponent of 10—in this case 3—is the logarithm of the number obtained when 10 is raised to the third power. The logarithm of any number that is an integer power of 10 can be determined simply by counting the number of zeros after the 1. Thus, 1 followed by six zeros (1,000,000) has a logarithm of 6. The logarithm of the number 1 is zero because there are no zeros following the 1. Put another way, $10^0 = 1$.

The logarithm of a number less than 1 is the negative power to which 10 is raised in order to equal the number, or the reciprocal of the number of times 10 is multiplied by itself. Thus, the logarithm of .001 is -3 because 10^{-3} ($1/10 \times 10 \times 10$) = 1/1000 or .001. Similarly, the number that has a logarithm of -6 is .000001 because 10^{-6} ($1/10 \times 10 \times 10 \times 10 \times 10$) = 1/1,000,000 or .000001. The logarithm of any number that is a negative integer power of 10 can be determined by simply counting the number of places to the right of the decimal. Thus, the logarithm of .0001 is -4.

A convenience in using logarithms is that numbers can be multiplied by adding their logarithms, or divided by subtracting their logarithms. For exam-

[1] Arnold P. G. Peterson and Erwin E. Gross, Jr., *Handbook of Noise Measurement* (Concord, Mass.: General Radio Company, 1972), p. 3.

ple, to multiply 100 by 10,000, one needs only to add their logarithms (2 + 4), yielding a logarithm of 6 or 1,000,000. To divide 10,000,000 by 1000, subtract the logarithm of the divisor (3) from the logarithm of the dividend (7) to obtain a logarithm of 4, or 10,000. When the divisor is a negative logarithm, one must remember the rule that in subtracting a negative number, the sign changes to a plus. Thus, subtracting a -10 [$-(-10)$] results in a $+10$. For example, dividing 100 by .0001 is accomplished by subtracting the logarithm -4 from the logarithm 2, resulting actually in adding 4 to 2, giving a logarithm of 6 for the quotient, or 1,000,000.

In the foregoing examples, we have used numbers that are integer powers of 10. The logarithms of such numbers can be determined by inspection, as we have seen. In using numbers that are not integer powers of 10, it is necessary to consult a table of logarithms or a calculator to determine the power to which 10 must be raised to equal the number. The principle is the same as we have illustrated; it is just that the logarithm cannot be determined by simply counting the number of zeros or the number of places to the right of the decimal.

The reference for *intensity level* (IL) is 10^{-16} watt/cm² (ten to the minus sixteen watt per square centimeter) and for *sound-pressure level* (SPL) is 0.0002 dyne/cm² or μbar (two ten-thousandths, or point triple-zero-two, dyne per square centimeter or microbar), 20 μN/m² (twenty micronewtons per square meter), or 20μPa (twenty micropascals). *Sound-power level* (PWL) refers to a reference power of 10^{-12} watt (ten to the minus twelve watt). Alternate ways of abbreviating the terms *intensity level, sound-pressure level,* and *sound-power level* are L_I, L_p, and L_w, respectively.[2]

The ratio between two powers is computed from the formula $\log_{10}(I_1/I_0)$, where I_1 equals the greater power and I_0 equals the lesser power. The formula yields the logarithm of the ratio, which is also the number of *bels,* named for Alexander Graham Bell, between the two powers. Because the bel is too gross a unit for practical use, it is subdivided into ten parts, each of which is called a *decibel,* abbreviated dB. The formula for determining the decibel ratio between two powers then becomes $N_{dB} = 10 \log_{10}(I_1/I_0)$. When I_0 is the standard reference level of 10^{-16} watt/cm², the formula yields the intensity level of the higher power in decibels. Although tables are readily available to convert various ratios into their decibel equivalents, ratios that are powers of ten may be easily determined by counting the number of zeros and multiplying by ten. Thus, a power ratio of 10 to 1 is an increase of 10 dB; 100 to 1 is 20 dB; and 1000 to 1 is 30 dB.

Pressure is proportional to the square root of power, or, put another way, power is proportional to the square of pressure. The ratio between two pressures can thus be expressed by the formula $N_{dB} = 10 \log_{10}(p_1^2/p_0^2)$, where

[2] Lewis S. Goodfriend, "Terminology, Definitions, and Usage," *Sound and Vibration* 2 (June 1968):9.

p_1 is the higher pressure and p_0 is the lower pressure. Because, with logarithms, doubling is the equivalent of squaring real numbers, the formula can be more simply written $N_{dB} = 20 \log_{10} (p_1/p_0)$. When p_0 is the standard reference level of 0.0002 dyne/cm², 0.0002 μbar, 20 μN/m², or 20 μPa, the formula yields the sound pressure level in dB. Because the formula for pressure utilizes a multiple that is twice that used for power, the rapid method for determining the number of decibels between pressure ratios in powers of ten is to count the number of zeros and multiply by twenty. Thus, a pressure ratio of 10 to 1 is equal to an increase of 20 dB; 100 to 1, to 40 dB; and 1000 to 1, to 60 dB. Table 2–2 gives decibel equivalents of various power and pressure ratios.

One advantage of logarithms, as we pointed out earlier, is that multiplication is accomplished by simple addition of the logarithms of the numbers to be multiplied, and division is accomplished by subtraction of the corresponding logarithms. Thus, in Table 2–2 we can see that the ratio of 20 equals a dB (logarithmic) equivalent of 13.0 for power and 26.0 for pressure. Now, because a ratio of 20 is the same as a ratio of 10 × 2, we should be able to arrive at the same dB equivalents by adding those dB values corresponding to ratios of 10 and 2. In terms of power, this means adding 10.0 dB and 3.0 dB for a total of 13.0 dB; and in terms of pressure, adding 20.0 dB and 6.0 dB for a

TABLE 2–2.   Ratios in decibels of power and pressure

Ratio	Power (dB)	Pressure (dB)
1	0	0
2	3.0	6.0
3	4.8	9.5
5	7.0	14.0
7	8.5	16.9
9	9.5	19.1
10	10.0	20.0
11	10.4	20.8
13	11.1	22.2
17	12.3	24.6
19	12.8	25.6
20	13.0	26.0
30	14.8	29.6
40	16.0	32.0
50	17.0	34.0
60	17.8	35.6
70	18.4	36.9
80	19.0	38.0
90	19.5	39.0
100	20.0	40.0
1000	30.0	60.0
10000	40.0	80.0
100000	50.0	100.0
1000000	60.0	120.0
10000000	70.0	140.0

total of 26.0 dB. It can be seen, therefore, that the decibel equivalents are the same regardless of how the ratio is expressed.

By multiplying the appropriate ratios and adding the corresponding dB values for these ratios, dB values can be obtained for ratios not contained in Table 2–2. For example, to determine the dB equivalents in power and pressure for a ratio of 39, add the dB values for ratios of 13 and 3, yielding values of 15.9 dB (11.1 + 4.8) for a power ratio of 39 to 1, and 31.7 (22.2 + 9.5) for a pressure ratio of 39 to 1. Incidentally, the reason that the pressure value is not exactly twice the power value in this example is that for purposes of simplification the dB values in Table 2–2 have been rounded to the nearest tenth of a decibel.[3]

Just as there are limitations in the frequency response of the human ear, so there is a definable range of intensities to which it will respond. The psychological sensation of loudness is closely related to intensity of the sound wave. The greater the intensity of vibration, the louder the sound appears to the listener. It has already been mentioned that a sound pressure level of 0.0002 dyne/cm² corresponds closely to the least sound pressure to which the normal ear can respond. A sound pressure 140 dB greater produces the sensation of pain in the average normal ear.

As was stated in the preceding section of this chapter, the ear is not equally sensitive to all frequencies. In other words, to reach the threshold of the human ear, greater intensities are required at the lower and higher end of the frequency scale than for the medium frequencies (500 through 8000 Hz, roughly). Figure 2–3 shows the limits of the human ear both for frequency and for intensity. The two lower curves represent the minimum levels of intensity to which the ear can respond in two different types of listening situations. *Minimum audible field* (MAF) describes the minimum intensities that can be detected when the listener is placed before a loudspeaker at a prescribed distance in a room specially constructed to eliminate all reflections or reverberations. Such a room is called an *anechoic* chamber, which attempts to duplicate listening conditions in a large outdoor space far removed from any natural or man-made reflecting surfaces. Under such circumstances, we say sound is propagated in a *free field,* in which the inverse-square law of sound propagation obtains; this law states that the intensity of a sound decreases in inverse proportion to the square of the distance of the observer from the sound source. At a distance of four feet from the source, the intensity will be 1/16 of that at the source; at six feet, the intensity will be 1/36; and so forth.

Because it is difficult to imitate nature's free field, we describe the listening conditions in an anechoic chamber, or in a "soundproof" audiometric test room, as a *sound field* instead of a free field. In sound-field listening, usually

---

[3] For clarification of the concept of the decibel and applications of the concept for solving simple problems involving increases and decreases of power and pressure, the reader is referred to a programmed text entitled *Elements of Hearing Science* by Arnold M. Small (New York, NY, John Wiley and Sons, 1978).

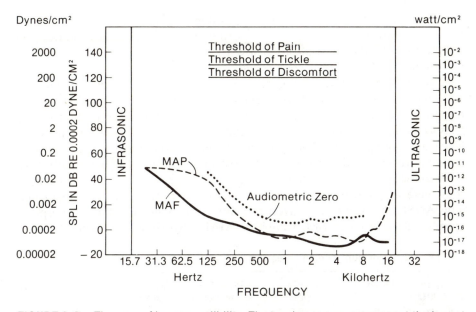

FIGURE 2-3.   The area of human audibility. The two lower curves represent the lowest (best) thresholds of hearing of young adults. The solid curve is the minimum audible field (MAF) and the dashed curve is minimum audible pressure (MAP). (See text for explanation of these terms and Tables 2–3 and 2–4 for data points.) The dotted curve is the current standard for audiometric zero (ANSI-1969). The upper three curves represent averages for sensations of discomfort, tickle, and pain. The ordinates define intensity in terms of pressure in dynes/cm2, sound pressure level in dB, and power flow in watt/cm2.

both the subject's ears are stimulated simultaneously by the loudspeaker sound source. In contrast to sound-field measurements, *minimum audible pressure (MAP)* measurements are taken while the subject wears a headset and only one ear at a time is stimulated by a signal coming from an earphone. Naturally, one's hearing sensitivity is greater when using both ears in a sound field than when listening with only one ear under an earphone. It is difficult to compare the two listening situations, however, because of such factors as the diffraction of sound around the head in a sound field and the different resonance characteristics of the ear.

The MAP and MAF curves in Figure 2–3 represent points that are two standard deviations below the mean; in other words, the curves represent the minimum intensities detected by approximately 2.5 percent of a population of young adults (sixteen to twenty-five years of age) determined by examination and history to be otologically normal. The MAP and MAF curves of Figure 2–3 were taken from data reported in two separate studies performed approximately four years apart at the National Physical Laboratory in Great Britain. The data were not obtained with the same observers, therefore, and the crossing of the MAP and MAF curves at two points in Figure 2–3 may be a function of differences between the two groups of subjects. Tables 2–3 and 2–4 present the means and standard deviations reported in these two studies and the data points (two standard deviations below the means) on which the MAP and MAF curves of Figure 2–3 were based.

The dotted curve of Figure 2–3 represents the intensities defining audiometric zero at each of the standard frequencies on a pure-tone audiometer. These intensity values were agreed on by scientists from many countries as being representative of the average minimum audible sound-pressure levels for young adult ears and have been incorporated in standards for audiometric calibration throughout most of the world. In this country, we refer to these values for audiometric zero as the ANSI-1969 standard because they were adopted in 1969 by the American National Standards Institute.[4] The ANSI-1969 values are given in Table 2–3. Note that they correspond closely with the mean SPL values for MAP, also shown in Table 2–3. See

TABLE 2–3.   Minimum audible pressure

Freq. in Hz & kHz	Mean SPL in dB	σ in dB	SPL at 2 σ below mean	ANSI-1969
80 Hz	61.0	8.0	45.0	
125	45.5	6.8	31.9	45.5
250	28.0	7.3	13.4	24.5
500	12.5	6.5	−0.5	11.0
1 kHz	5.5	5.7	−5.9	6.5
1.5	8.5	6.1	−3.7	6.5
2	10.5	6.1	−1.7	8.5
3	7.0	5.9	−4.8	7.5
4	9.5	6.9	−4.3	9.0
6	10.5	9.1	−7.7	8.0
8	9.0	8.7	−8.4	9.5
10	17.0	9.0	−1.0	
12	20.5	9.6	1.3	
15	39.0	10.7	17.6	
18	74.0	21.9*	30.2	

* Calculated from reported standard error of the mean.

Data on mean sound pressure levels and standard deviations (σ) for 80 Hz through 15 kHz taken from R. S. Dadson and J. H. King, "A Determination of the Normal Threshold of Hearing and its Relation to the Standardization of Audiometers," *Journal of Laryngology and Otology* 66 (1952): 366–78, as reproduced in *Forty Germinal Papers in Human Hearing*, ed. J. Donald Harris (Groton, Conn.: The Journal of Auditory Research, 1969), pp. 48–58. The data for 18 kHz were taken from J. Donald Harris and C. K. Myers, "Tentative Audiometric Hearing Threshold Level Standards from 8 through 18 Kilohertz," *Journal of the Acoustical Society of America* 49 (February 1971): 600–601.

[4]*American National Standard Specifications for Audiometers,* ANSI S3.6-1969 (New York: American National Standards Institute, 1970).

TABLE 2–4.   Minimum audible field

Freq. in Hz & kHz	Mean SPL in dB	σ in dB	SPL at 2 σ below mean
25 Hz	63.5	8.0	47.5
50	43.0	6.5	30.0
100	25.0	5.0	15.0
200	15.0	4.5	6.0
500	5.5	4.5	−3.5
1 kHz	4.5	4.5	−4.5
2	0.5	5.0	−9.5
3	−1.5	6.0	−13.5
4	−5.0	8.0	−21.0
6	4.5	8.5	−12.5
8	13.5	8.5	−3.5
10	16.5	11.5	−6.5
12	13.0	11.5	−10.0
15	24.5	17.0	−9.5

Data on mean sound pressure levels and standard deviations (σ) taken from D. W. Robinson and R. S. Dadson, "A Re-determination of the Equal-Loudness Relations for Pure Tones," *British Journal of Applied Physics* 7 (1956): 166–81, as reproduced in *Forty Germinal Papers in Human Hearing,* ed. Harris, pp. 185–200.

Chapter 5 for a discussion of the ANSI-1969 standard and audiometric calibration.

Before leaving Figure 2–3, we should make some additional observations. Note that the intensity of any point on the figure can be described in three different ways: pressure in dynes/cm^2, power flow in watt/cm^2, and sound pressure level in dB re 0.0002 dyne/cm^2. Actually, we could also have labeled the sound-pressure level ordinate sound-intensity level re 10^{-16} watt/cm^2. In practice, however, we usually speak of sound-pressure levels instead of sound-intensity levels because we commonly measure intensities with a sound-level meter, which measures pressure rather than power. The point to be made, however, is that the ear has the same range in decibels above the standard reference points of 0.0002 dyne/cm^2 and 10^{-16} watt/cm^2 regardless of whether we are concerned with pressure or power. Because a given ratio of pressures results in a decibel equivalent that is twice the decibel equivalent of the same ratio of powers, as was shown in Table 2–2, it is not easy to understand that we can use the same scale for graphing sound-pressure level and sound-intensity level. By comparing the two outside ordinates of Figure 2–3 with the ordinate scaled in decibels, we can see that a 20-dB step represents a hundredfold increase in power but only a tenfold increase in pressure. A sound of a given dB level has the same loudness for a listener, however, whether we measure its ratio with a reference point in pressure or in power.

Finally, mention should be made of the three upper curves of Figure 2–3, labeled thresholds of discomfort, tickle, and pain. As sound intensity is steadily increased above the point where it can first be detected, it eventually causes the listener to experience physiological discomfort. Increasing the intensity further will produce a sensation in the ear described as a tickle. The listener feels like putting a finger in the ear canal to scratch. An additional increase in intensity causes the listener to experience pain and induces an immediate avoidance reaction analogous to withdrawing one's hand from a hot stove. Just as audiometric zero represents a statistical average of MAP for young adult ears, and normal hearing includes a range of values above and below the mean or median, so the thresholds of 120, 130, and 140 dB for discomfort, tickle, and pain, graphed in Figure 2-3, are average values, also characterized by a range above and below the average. These average values were determined in a study performed at the Central Institute for the Deaf.[5] These thresholds were essentially the same for normal-hearing and hearing-impaired subjects.

An audiometer is an electronic instrument for measuring an individual's hearing sensitivity. A considerable part of this book is devoted to hearing testing, and we will not discuss the audiometer here, except to mention that measurements obtained with an audiometer are called *hearing levels,* and they are expressed in decibels re audiometric zero. Previously, the term *hearing loss* was used to refer to audiometric measurements, but because it is contradictory to speak of a 5 or 10 dB hearing loss when such audiometric measurements are well within the limits of normal hearing, the term *hearing level* was substituted. As we have seen in Figure 2-3 and Table 2-3, audiometric zero is defined by national and international standards as so many dB of sound-pressure level for each of the audiometric frequencies. For example, audiometric zero at 1000 Hz is an SPL of 6.5 dB. This is the SPL that corresponds with the average threshold of audibility at this frequency for normal, young adult ears as agreed on by the scientists from laboratories throughout much of the world who contributed to the writing of the standards. Now, if an individual patient can just barely detect the presence of a 1000-Hz tone when the audiometer reads 50 dB, we say that the threshold is at a hearing level of 50 dB. If we want to convert this hearing level (HL) to SPL, we need to add 6.5 dB to the HL of 50 dB, resulting in an SPL of 56.5 dB. In other words, to convert HLs to SPLs we must add the number of dB separating audiometric zero from 0dBSPL at each frequency to the HL corresponding to threshold at each frequency. If, however, an individual's threshold at a given frequency is expressed in SPL and we wish to convert it to HL, we must subtract the difference between 0dBSPL and audiometric zero at that frequency from the threshold that was expressed in SPL. For example, if an individual has a threshold at 500 Hz of 41 dB expressed in SPL, we must subtract 11.0 dB—the SPL of audiometric zero for 500 Hz—which tells us that the individual's

    [5] S. Richard Silverman, "Tolerances for Pure Tones and Speech in Normal and Defective Hearing," *Annals of Otology, Rhinology, and Laryngology* 56 (September 1947):658–77.

threshold in HL (as measured with an audiometer) is 30 dB. We must remember that SPL and HL have different reference points or baselines. A review of Figure 2–3 will help us to see the relationships between the two reference points.

Another term frequently employed in psychophysical measurement is *sensation level* (SL). Sensation level is ". . . the pressure level of the sound in decibels above its threshold of audibility for the individual subject or for a specific group of subjects."[6] Most frequently, the term refers to the individual subject's threshold. Thus, if a stimulus is presented at a level of 30 dB above an individual's threshold for that sound, we say the sound was presented at an SL of 30 dB. Sensation level does not give us any information directly concerning the physical intensity of the stimulus. Before we can tell what the SPL or the HL of the stimulus is, we must first know what the listener's threshold is in terms of either SPL or HL. For example, assume that an individual's threshold of audibility at 2000 Hz is 45 dB HL and we wish to present a stimulus at this frequency at an SL of 20 dB. The HL of the stimulus is thus 65 dB (the person's HL at threshold plus 20 dB). The SPL of the stimulus is 73.5 dB because audiometric zero at 2000 Hz is defined as an SPL of 8.5 dB. A *suprathreshold* stimulus, then, can be described in terms of SPL (with a reference of 0.0002 dyne/cm²), HL (with a reference of audiometric zero), or SL (with a reference of the individual's own threshold).

In graphing a sound wave, amplitude is indicated by the height of the waveform. As we said earlier in discussing Figure 2–2, the ordinate of the graph represents displacement of an individual particle of the medium. The greater the intensity of the vibration of the source, the greater the amplitude of the particle displacement. Figure 2–4 shows three waves of the same frequency but of different amplitude, representing three different intensities.

FIGURE 2–4.
Three waves of the same frequency but of different amplitude.

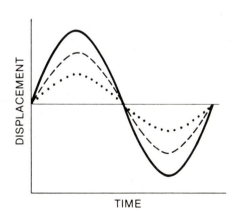

DISPLACEMENT

TIME

[6]*American National Standard Psychoacoustical Terminology*, ANSI S3.20-1973 (New York: American National Standards Institute), p. 45.

The sensation of loudness is related to the amplitude of the stimulus, but loudness does not grow equally at all frequencies as amplitude is increased above threshold. Equal-loudness contours are curves connecting SPL points of equal loudness for a number of frequencies as judged by observers. These curves are also called *phon curves*. A *phon* is a unit of loudness level that, at the frequency of 1000 Hz, is equated to the decibel. Phon curves are constructed by asking subjects to judge when tones of various frequencies are equal in loudness to a 1000-Hz tone of a specified SPL. Although phon curves can be plotted while a subject listens with one ear to stimuli presented through an earphone, the official definition of the phon specifies binaural (two-ear) listening to stimuli presented in a sound field.[7] Figure 2–5 presents equal-loudness contours at steps of 10 phons. The MAF curve shown in dashes is based on the data presented in Table 2–4. The reference base for SPL in Figure 2–5, although expressed in different units, is the same as 0.0002 dyne/cm².

FIGURE 2-5. Equal-loudness contours. (Based on data from Robinson and Dadson, "A Re-determination of the Equal-Loudness Relations," as presented in Arnold P. G. Peterson and Ervin E. Gross, Jr., *Handbook of Noise Measurement,* Concord, Mass.: General Radio Company, 1972, p. 21. Reproduced by permission.)

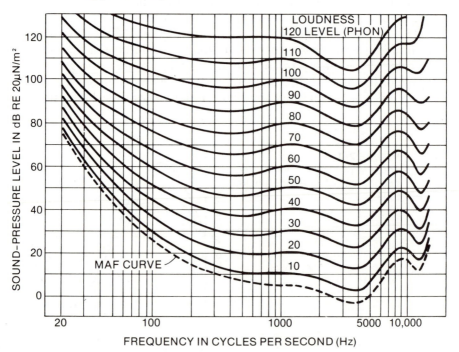

[7] *American National Standard Psychoacoustical Terminology*, p. 25.

Spectrum. The simplest form of sound is a *pure tone,* a single frequency. Such a sound can be adequately described in terms of only its frequency and intensity. Pure tones outside the laboratory, however, are exceedingly rare. Most sounds in nature are *complex,* consisting of a number of frequencies with various intensities. Figure 2–6 shows a complex wave resulting from the combination of three pure tones of different frequency and one of different intensity. The complex wave is not itself sinusoidal, although it is composed of three sinusoidal waves. Component (b) has three times the frequency of component (c), and component (a) has five times the frequency of component (c). The resultant complex wave (d) contains all three component frequencies, (a), (b), and (c). With appropriate instrumentation, any complex wave can be analyzed into its component frequencies and intensities in the form of a *tonal spectrum.* Figure 2–7 is the spectrum of the complex wave (d) of Figure 2–6.

All sounds can be placed on a continuum between musical sounds and noise. Musical sounds are those that have *periodicity*—the waveform is repeated with the frequency of the lowest component, termed the *fundamental.* In addition to the fundamental, a complex wave consists of higher frequencies, or *overtones,* which, when their frequencies are multiples of the fundamental, are termed *harmonics.* The process of breaking down a complex

FIGURE 2-6.
A complex wave (d) resulting from the combination of three pure tones (a), (b), and (c). (From *The Speech Chain* by Peter B. Denes and Elliot N. Pinson. Copyright © 1963 by Bell Telephone Laboratories, Inc. Reproduced by permission of Doubleday & Company, Inc.)

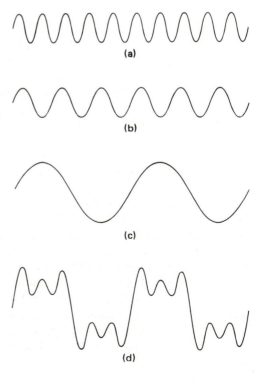

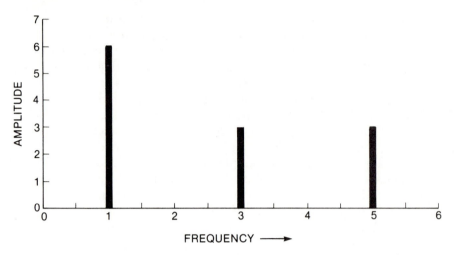

FIGURE 2-7. The tonal spectrum of complex wave (d) of Figure 2-6. The ordinate is relative amplitude in arbitrary units, and the abscissa is relative frequency. (From *The Speech Chain* by Peter B. Denes and Elliot N. Pinson. Copyright © 1963 by Bell Telephone Laboratories, Inc. Reproduced by permission of Doubleday & Company, Inc.)

wave into its component frequencies and intensities to obtain a tonal spectrum is termed *harmonic analysis,* or Fourier analysis after the French mathematician who first proved that such an analysis of complex waves was possible. The fundamental is the first harmonic. The components with two and three times the frequency of the fundamental are the second and third harmonics, and so forth. Noise is *aperiodic*; that is, although it may be analyzed into its component frequencies and intensities, the waveform cannot be described as having repeatable cycles, or a frequency the same as the frequency of the fundamental. Figure 2–8 compares two speech sounds—one a vowel that has periodicity and therefore is a musical sound, and the other a fricative consonant that has no periodicity and thus is noise. Note that for the vowel the sample waveform shown contains almost four complete cycles, but the consonant has no cycles that can be identified by inspection.

With musical tones, it is not necessary for the fundamental frequency to be present for the ear to identify it. The missing fundamental will be perceived, provided that the harmonic structure is presented. Higher harmonics are multiples of the fundamental frequency. Thus, the higher harmonics for a fundamental frequency of 500 Hz would be 1000, 1500, 2000, 2500, 3000, and so on. If a filter introduced into a communication system were to filter out all frequencies below 1000 Hz, a complex tone with the previous harmonic structure would still be recognized as having a fundamental frequency of 500 Hz, because that specific structure could exist only for a fundamental frequency of 500 Hz—the highest frequency that will divide evenly into all the higher harmonics.

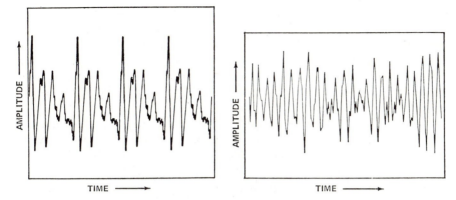

FIGURE 2-8.   Comparison of a periodic and an aperiodic speech sound. The waveform to the left is for the vowel *ah,* and the waveform to the right is for the fricative consonant *sh.* (From *The Speech Chain* by Peter B. Denes and Elliot N. Pinson. Copyright © 1963 by Bell Telephone Laboratories, Inc. Reproduced by permission of Doubleday & Company, Inc.)

The perception of missing fundamental frequencies simplifies considerably the problem of communication systems. The average adult male voice has a fundamental frequency between 120 and 150 Hz, and the average adult female voice has a fundamental frequency between 210 and 240 Hz; yet we usually have no difficulty in distinguishing between male and female voices over the telephone, although the telephone does not carry frequencies lower than about 300 Hz. This may be true in part because we are able to perceive the fundamental frequency that is missing from the signal coming through the receiver.

The spectrum of a sound affects the psychological sensation of quality. We recognize the difference between a saxophone and a trumpet playing the same note because of the differences in spectra, which in turn are a function of both the complexities of vibration of the sound source and the selective characteristics of the resonators provided for the sound source. Likewise, we recognize differences among the various speech sounds because of differences in the spectra of the sounds. People's voices are recognizable, even over the telephone, because of differences in the spectra of their sounds.

Other Characteristics of Sound

Phase.   *Phase* refers to the time relationship between two or more pure tones occurring simultaneously. In the case of pressure phase, if two tones of the same frequency and intensity are produced so that their periods of compression and rarefaction agree exactly, they will combine into a tone with twice the amplitude of either one alone. These tones are said to be "in phase." On the other hand, if the tones are separated by half a cycle, so that one wave is in compression while the other is in rarefaction, the two tones will cancel each other, and amplitude will be zero. These tones are in "opposite phase," or 180 degrees "out of phase." The cancellation effect of tones in opposite phase can be observed in some auditoriums or theaters that are of poor acoustic design. In such rooms, there are seats so located that the auditor simultaneously receives both original and reflected waves originating from the stage, but with sufficient time lag between the original and reflected waves for them to tend to cancel each other.

Phase differences account for an interesting acoustic phenomenon referred to as *beats*. If the ear receives simultaneously two tones of slightly different frequency, the sensation of beats, or pulsations, will be heard. The ear will hear as many beats per second as there are cycles of difference between the two tones in frequency. Thus, if tones of 500 and 505 Hz are presented simultaneously, five beats per second will be heard. The beats result from phase differences between the two tones. The wavelength of the tone of 505 Hz is slightly less than that of the 500 Hz tone. For that reason, the periods of compression and rarefaction of the two waves occur at slightly different times. Their phase relationships are constantly changing. Five times a second, however, the two waves will be in phase for one cycle and 180 degrees out of phase for the space of one cycle. When they are in phase, or approaching an in-phase relationship, their amplitudes are additive, so that the ear transmits a sensation of increasing loudness. When they are out of phase, or approaching an out-of-phase relationship, the ear transmits a decreasing loudness. This swelling to a peak and diminishing to zero of the sound pressure five times a second produces the sensation of beats.

If the two frequencies are more than 15 to 20 Hz apart, the beats will occur so rapidly that the ear will not be aware of them but will hear two separate tones. If the tones are far enough apart and of sufficient intensity, a *difference tone* will be perceived, equal in frequency to the difference in Hz between the two stimulus tones. Thus, if tones of 1500 and 2000 Hz are presented simultaneously at high intensity, the ear will hear, in addition to these two tones, a fainter tone of 500 Hz.

Another manifestation of phase differences between tones occurs in *standing waves*. When a pure-tone sound wave is introduced into a closed pipe of the same length as the wavelength of the tone, a wave is reflected back from the closed end of the pipe 180 degrees out of phase with the original wave. Thus there is a cancellation effect, and no audible sound results, as with the "dead spots" in auditoriums. We shall see later how such standing waves may affect hearing-test results at certain frequencies.

Masking.   When noise or sound of any kind interferes with the audibility of another sound, masking has occurred. Masking is a common auditory experience. We all know how futile it is to try to converse while a train is passing close by, and probably we have all been frustrated in movies or plays when the audience's noise prevents our hearing the actors' lines. Considerable research on the subject of masking has been undertaken. Much has been conducted by experimental psychologists in the laboratory, but some has been directed at practical problems of improving the audibility of speech in the presence of noise, as, for example, in military communications.

In audiometric work, it is frequently desirable to employ a masking tone or noise in one ear while the other is being tested. When there is a great difference in sensitivity of hearing between an individual's two ears, it is necessary to rule out the participation of the better ear while the poorer ear is being tested. This is done by the introduction of masking into the better ear. Such masking may be in the form of a pure tone (of the same frequency as the test tone), amplified "sixty-cycle hum," saw-tooth (complex) noise, white noise, or narrow-band noise. More will be said about the audiometric use of masking in later chapters.

Reflection, refraction, and diffraction.   When a sound wave strikes a hard, nonabsorbent surface, a *reflection* occurs, just as light waves are reflected from a mirror. When the reflecting surface is at some distance from the sound source, the reflected wave will be heard as a separate and distinct sound after the original sound has ended. Such reflections are termed *echoes.* Thus, in a hard-walled canyon, we can shout "hello" and moments later hear our own greeting returning to us, perhaps several times as our voice waves bounce or echo back and forth between the canyon walls. In enclosed spaces, reflections may interfere with our understanding of speech, the reflected waves serving to mask the original ones. The persistence of multiple reflections in an enclosed space is called *reverberation,* which may be reduced or controlled by the use of sound-absorbing materials on the walls, ceilings, and floors of rooms. The control of reverberation may be effected by installing acoustic tiles on the walls and ceiling of a room. These tiles are made of sound-absorbent materials, usually with a rough rather than smooth surface, and sometimes containing many drilled holes. The purpose of the rough texture and holes is to increase the absorbent area for the sound waves to strike. Other means of reducing reverberation are draperies of coarse material and rugs or carpets with heavy piling.

Some degree of reverberation in auditoriums, lecture rooms, and concert halls is aesthetically desirable. Too much sound absorption produces a "deadness" of sound that is aesthetically displeasing and makes the listener uncomfortable. The challenge to the acoustical engineer or architect is to provide enough acoustic treatment to prevent interference with speech without destroying the desirable aspects of reverberation, which produce a "live" quality to speech or music. In planning acoustic treatment, the engineer or architect must take into account the fact that the human body and its clothing will also absorb sound. The reverberation characteristics of an auditorium will thus be different, depending on whether or not an audience is present. Multipurpose auditoriums may require variable "tuning" in the form of removable panels of sound-absorbing material, so that the most desirable level of reverberation may be achieved for the particular performance. Architectural acoustics is both a science and an art.

Reflection of sound is used in the guidance systems of some animals, for example, the bat, which emits very high-frequency squeals, beyond the frequency range of human ears. A bat can avoid obstructions—or zero in on an insect target—by making use of the reflected squeals which the bat, with its extended frequency range of hearing, can perceive. This same principle is employed in radar systems, using ultra high radio frequencies that travel at the velocity of light instead of sound. Some blind people can be guided by the use of an acoustic "flashlight" that emits high-frequency audible "beeps." With practice, the blind person learns to differentiate echoes from reflecting surfaces and to identify various objects in the environment. The higher the frequency, the better it can be beamed or focused like a flashlight, which is why guidance systems employ the highest frequencies possible.

Echo-ranging with ultrasonic beams is used in antisubmarine warfare. Ships are equipped with movable sound transducers, attached to the hull, that serve both as transmitters and receivers. Ultrasonic frequencies are emitted from the transducer in brief bursts. If the ultrasonic beam strikes a reflecting object, an echo will be produced that is received by the transducer acting as a receiver. The distance of the reflecting object, or its range, is computed by timing the interval between the emission and the reception of the echo. The interval of time is a function, of course, of the velocity of sound in water. The operator of the echo-ranging equipment—called *sonar* in the Navy—sweeps 360 degrees around the ship by moving the transducer a few degrees at a time, listening for echoes following each emission. Because ultrasonic frequencies are used to obtain narrow beaming, the operator cannot hear these frequencies. By using two ultrasonic frequencies simultaneously that differ by a fixed number of Hz, say 1000 Hz, a different tone is produced that is audible to the operator. The skilled sonar operator learns to differentiate echoes from various undersea objects, so that a submarine can be distinguished from a whale or from other inanimate objects.

The operator can also determine whether the ship is approaching the target (closing the range) or moving away from the target (opening the range) by noting whether the echo differs in pitch from the emitted sound, thus making use of what is called the *Doppler* effect. If the pitch of the echo is higher than the emitted sound (up-Doppler) the range is closing; if the pitch of the echo is lower (down-Doppler) the range is opening. If the range remains constant, there will be no difference in pitch between the emission and the echo, or in other words, no Doppler effect will occur. If there is no Doppler effect, it is evident that the reflecting object is moving at the same speed and on the same course as the ship. The Doppler effect is based on the relationship between frequency and wavelength. As wavelength increases, frequency is lowered; as wavelength decreases, frequency is raised. A common illustration of the Doppler effect is the difference in the pitch of a train when it is approaching and when it is receding, particularly if the locomotive is sounding its whistle as it passes. When the train is approaching, its speed shortens the wavelength of the sound it emits. When the train is moving away, its speed lengthens the wavelength. The contrast between the wavelength of the approaching and receding train causes a distinct lowering of the pitch as the locomotive speeds past. Similarly, the wavelength of a reflected sonar signal from an approaching target will be shorter than the wavelength of the original emission, resulting in an echo that is higher pitched. The greatest contrast between the pitch of the emission and the echo occurs when the ship and target are both moving directly toward each other or in exactly opposite directions from each other.

Refraction refers to the bending of sound waves because of differences in the medium—primarily temperature differences. The velocity of sound waves changes with temperature. In warmer air, the velocity is greater than in cooler air. This relationship accounts for the observation that sound can be heard further at certain times of the day than at other times. When the sun is well above the horizon, the air nearest the earth is warmer than air at higher altitudes. Thus, the part of the sound wave next to the earth will travel farther in a given amount of time than the part of the wave higher above the earth. The effect of the differing velocities of the lower and upper parts of the wave is to produce a bending of the wave away from the earth as the wave pivots around its upper (slower) part. Shortly before sunrise and after sunset, however, the usual temperature gradient of the air is reversed. The sun below the horizon warms the upper air while the earth remains cool. At these times of day, the upper part of the sound wave travels faster than the lower part, bending the wave toward the earth as the wave pivots around its lower (slower) part. The result is that before sunrise and after sunset sound can be heard at greater distances than at midday, because of the bending, or refraction, of the sound wave toward the earth. The energy of the sound wave, instead of being dissipated in the upper atmosphere, is thus concentrated on the earth's surface. The phenomenon is enhanced when sound is propagated over a still body of water, because the water surface will produce reflection of the refracted sound wave, enabling it to travel even further on the earth's surface.

Although light waves will reflect and refract, and thus are similar to sound waves in these respects, they are limited in their capacity to bend around obstructions, or to *diffract*. Sound waves, however, can pass around obstructions and thus are capable of diffraction. A darkroom for photographic work can be kept lightproof by using a series of baffles instead of a door. One can enter the room by walking around the baffles, but the outside light is excluded because it cannot bend around them. On the other hand, one can converse with someone in the darkroom from outside because sound waves will diffract around the baffles. The smaller the obstruction in relation to the wavelength of the sound, the greater the degree of diffraction that occurs.

Thus, in general, low frequencies (with long wavelengths) will diffract more completely than high frequencies (with short wavelengths).

THE HUMAN MECHANISM OF HEARING

Sound waves are received by the ear and transmitted to the brain, where meaning is attached to them. In the following sections of this chapter, we shall examine in some detail the three principal parts of the hearing mechanism: the outer ear, the middle ear, and the inner ear. The ear is encased in the temporal bone of the skull. The innermost part of the canal of the outer ear and the middle ear are in the *mastoid* part of the temporal bone, and the inner ear is within the *petrous* portion of the bone. Figure 2–9 is a coronal section of the right ear. The labeled parts of this figure will be discussed in the following sections.

The Outer Ear

The outer ear consists of the *pinna,* or *auricle,* and the *external auditory meatus,* or *canal.* Of all the parts of the ear, the pinna is the most prominent and the least useful. It serves the purpose of directing sound waves into the external meatus in a more concentrated fashion than would otherwise be possible. The function of the pinna in relation to the external canal can be likened to that of cupping the hand behind the ear in a difficult listening situation.

The *helix* is the name given to the outer edge of the pinna that consists of folded tissue extending in almost a complete circle from just above the *tragus,* the small projection just ahead of the opening of the external meatus, to the *lobule,* which is the point at which an earring is attached. The *anthelix* is a ridge that is concentric with the helix, and the *antitragus* is the point opposite the tragus, posterior and slightly inferior to the opening of the meatus. The cavity bounded by the anthelix, the tragus, and the antitragus is called the *concha.* The opening of the external meatus is within the concha. These and other landmarks of the pinna are identified in Figure 2–10.

In many animals, the pinna serves the useful purpose of providing more acute hearing and more precise sound localization. This is accomplished when the animal moves the pinna by muscular action until it is operating most efficiently and is directed toward the source of the sound. We have all observed a dog "prick up" its ears and listen intently until it has identified the source of a faint sound. In more primitive days, when humankind's existence depended on the acuity of the senses, it may have been possible to manipulate one's pinnae or "prick up" one's ears. Now that accomplishment is limited to a few talented individuals who are thus able to amuse children and attain some distinction in "parlor tricks." In modern society, the pinna is almost purely ornamental, inappropriate though the word may seem, applied to something as homely as the ear.

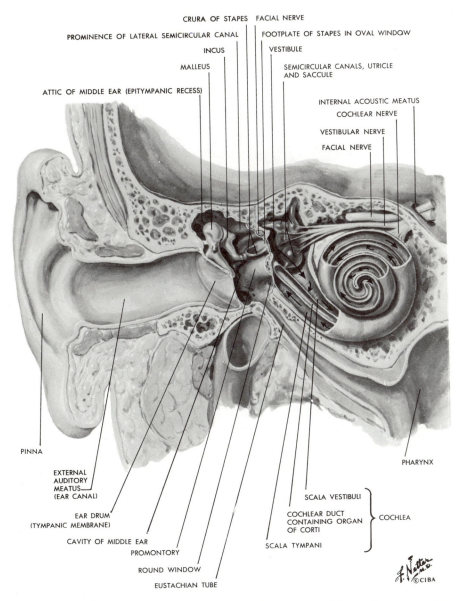

CRURA OF STAPES   FACIAL NERVE

PROMINENCE OF LATERAL SEMICIRCULAR CANAL

INCUS

MALLEUS

ATTIC OF MIDDLE EAR (EPITYMPANIC RECESS)

FOOTPLATE OF STAPES IN OVAL WINDOW

VESTIBULE

SEMICIRCULAR CANALS, UTRICLE AND SACCULE

INTERNAL ACOUSTIC MEATUS

COCHLEAR NERVE

VESTIBULAR NERVE

FACIAL NERVE

PINNA

EXTERNAL AUDITORY MEATUS (EAR CANAL)

EAR DRUM (TYMPANIC MEMBRANE)

CAVITY OF MIDDLE EAR

PROMONTORY

ROUND WINDOW

EUSTACHIAN TUBE

PHARYNX

SCALA VESTIBULI

COCHLEAR DUCT CONTAINING ORGAN OF CORTI   } COCHLEA

SCALA TYMPANI

FIGURE 2-9.   Coronal section of the right ear. (Copyright © 1970 CIBA Pharmaceutical Company, Division of CIBA-GEIGY Corporation. Reproduced with permission from *Clinical Symposia,* illustrated by Frank H. Netter, M.D.)

The external meatus is a roughly cylindrical passage about a quarter of an inch in diameter and a little over an inch long. Its resonant frequency is between 3500 and 4000 Hz. The outer half of the meatus is cartilaginous; the inner half is encased in the mastoid portion of the temporal bone. At the junc-

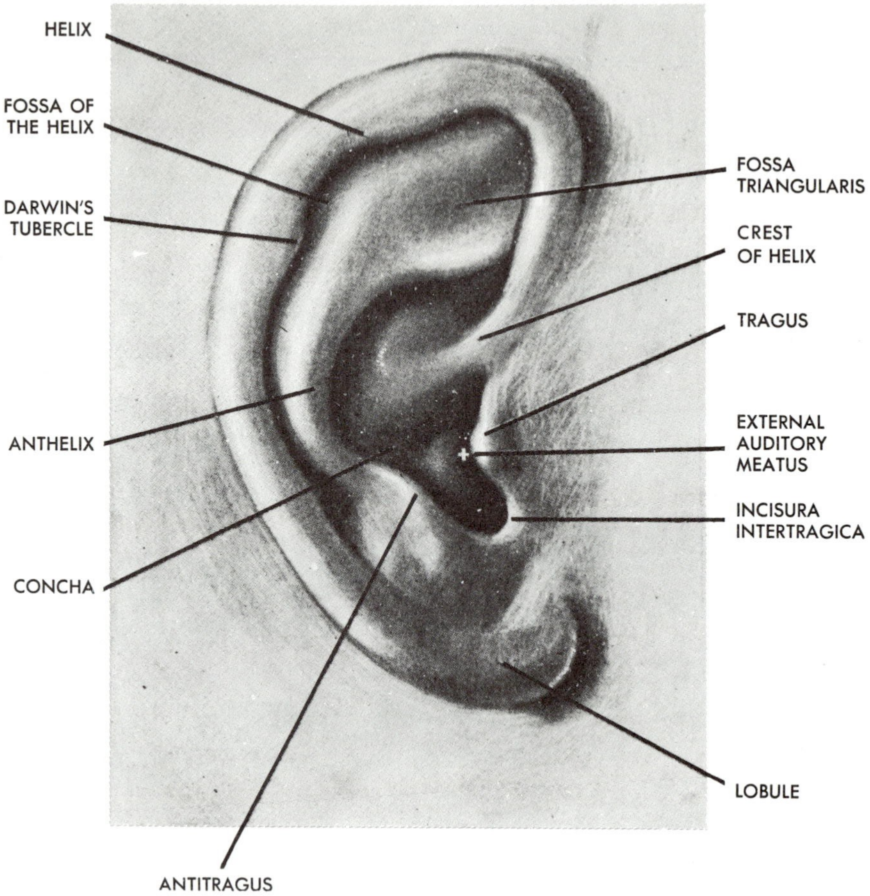

HELIX

FOSSA OF
THE HELIX

DARWIN'S
TUBERCLE

ANTHELIX

CONCHA

FOSSA
TRIANGULARIS

CREST
OF HELIX

TRAGUS

EXTERNAL
AUDITORY
MEATUS

INCISURA
INTERTRAGICA

LOBULE

ANTITRAGUS

FIGURE 2-10. Landmarks of the pinna. (From Francis L. Lederer and Abraham R. Hollender, *Textbook of the Ear, Nose, and Throat,* Philadelphia: F. A. Davis Company, 1947. Reproduced by permission of the publishers.)

ture of the cartilaginous and bony portions of the meatus, there is a narrowing of the passage. This point, where the diameter of the meatus is the smallest, is called the *isthmus.* Generally, there is sufficient bend in the meatus so that it is not possible to see the eardrum membrane by simply looking into the opening of the meatus. When the otologist examines the eardrum membrane, a funnel-shaped instrument called a *speculum* is introduced into the canal, which, in combination with pulling the pinna up and back, has the effect of straightening the canal and, with proper illumination, bringing the membrane into view. For examining the drum membrane, the otologist either reflects light from a naked bulb with a head mirror into a hand-held speculum or uses an *otoscope,* an instrument containing a light source and batteries and having an attached speculum. The external meatus is lined with epithelium (skin) containing hairs and wax-producing glands, which serve to protect the drum membrane from the penetration of dirt and insects. In many people, the glands produce too much wax, or *cerumen*, with the result that the excess must be removed at regular intervals to prevent blockage of the canal.

The external meatus ends at the eardrum membrane, or *tympanic membrane*, which is the external boundary of the second part of the hearing mechanism, the middle ear. The drum membrane is a thin diaphragm that completely closes the canal.

The Middle Ear

The space between the drum membrane and the bony capsule of the inner ear is called the middle ear, or *tympanum*, so named because it resembles a musician's drum. Technically, the term *eardrum* is synonymous with tympanum, that is, the whole middle ear, although popularly "eardrum" refers only to the "drumhead," or membrane. In line with popular practice, *eardrum* will be used in this book to refer only to the membrane that separates the middle ear from the outer ear.

The middle-ear cavity is between 1 and 2 cubic centimeters in volume. It is about 15 millimeters high but only from 2 to 4 millimeters wide. The cavity is lined with mucous membrane that is continuous with the mucous membrane lining of the nasal cavities. In fact, the middle ear is actually an extension of the *nasopharynx* by way of the *Eustachian tube*. Connecting the eardrum and an opening in the bony wall of the inner ear is a bridge of three tiny bones that is called the *ossicular chain*. These bones, the *ossicles*, are the tiniest bones in the body. They are named the *hammer*, or *malleus*; the *anvil*, or *incus*; and the *stirrup*, or *stapes*. The malleus is secured to the eardrum; the footplate of the stapes is set in the opening in the inner ear that is called the *oval window* and held in place by an *annular ligament* around its perimeter; and the incus connects the malleus and the stapes. Figure 2–11 shows the ossicles separately and identifies their various landmarks.

As can be seen in Figure 2–9, the head of the malleus and the body of the incus are in the uppermost part of the middle-ear cavity, called the *attic*, or the *epitympanic recess*. There is an opening through the posterior wall of the epitympanic recess, the *tympanic aditus*, which connects the middle-ear cavity with a sinus called the *tympanic antrum*. The antrum connects with the air cells of the mastoid part of the temporal bone. These air cells, interconnected and lined with the same mucous membrane that lines the middle-ear cavity, thus communicate with the middle-ear cavity. It is possible, therefore, for infection within the middle ear to spread to the mastoid air cells. The "roof" of the middle-ear cavity, called the *tegmen tympani*, separates the cavity and the antrum from the cranial space and the *meninges* covering the brain.

The eardrum is roughly circular in shape, semitransparent, slightly coned inward toward the middle-ear cavity, and pearly gray in color. It completely closes the end of the external meatus. The eardrum consists of a large

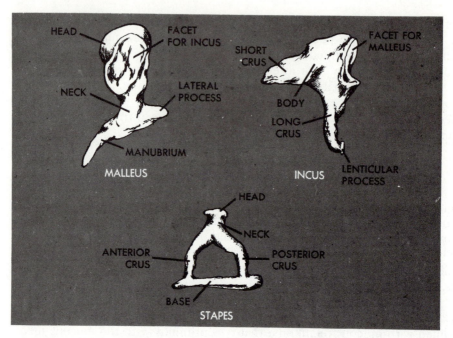

FIGURE 2-11. The ossicles. (From Harold M. Kaplan, *Anatomy and Physiology of Speech.* Copyright, 1960. McGraw-Hill Book Company, Inc. Used by permission.)

area called the *pars tensa* and a smaller area called the *pars flaccida,* or Shrapnell's membrane. The pars tensa is composed of three layers of tissue. The outer layer is a continuation of the skin lining the external canal; the inner layer is a continuation of the mucous membrane lining the cavity of the middle ear; and the middle layer is connective tissue. The pars flaccida does not contain the middle layer of connective tissue. Near the center of the eardrum is its most depressed point, corresponding to the tip of the *manubrium,* the long process of the malleus. This point is referred to as the *umbo.* In Figure 2–12, the manubrium may be seen through the eardrum, corresponding to the eleven o'clock position of the hour hand on a clock. In a right ear, the manubrium of the malleus would be seen in the one o'clock position. The *cone of light* is seen as a reflection from the eardrum of the external light source used by an examiner looking down the external canal. For convenience, the eardrum may be divided into quadrants, as shown in Figure 2–13.

The Eustachian tube provides a means of ventilating the middle-ear cavity. It serves as an air-pressure equalizer because oxygen is constantly being absorbed. In addition, it enables the middle ear to compensate for changes in outside air pressure, as in crossing mountains or in flying. Without the action of the Eustachian tube to equalize air pressure in the middle ear with that outside it, the eardrum would be subject to considerable stress, being forced out-

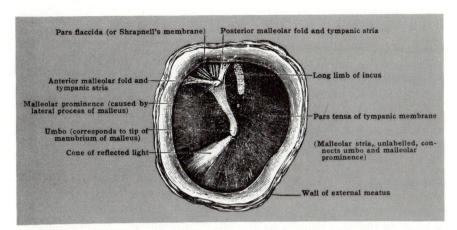

FIGURE 2-12. The left eardrum. (From J. Parsons Schaeffer, ed., *Morris' Human Anatomy,* 10th ed. Copyright, 1942. Blakiston Div., McGraw-Hill. Used by permission.)

ward when the outside pressure became less (increasing altitude) and inward when the outside pressure became greater (decreasing altitude). Normally, the Eustachian tube is in a collapsed state, so that an individual's voice and breathing sounds are not directly transmitted to the ear. It is opened only under the stress of air-pressure changes or by action of certain of the pharyngeal muscles during the act of swallowing or yawning.

The ossicular chain is suspended within the middle-ear cavity by means of ligaments that extend from the roof and walls of the cavity to the malleus and incus. Two muscles act on the ossicular chain: the *tensor tympani* and the *stapedius*. Both these muscles are encased in bony canals. The tensor tympani, the larger of the two muscles, runs in a canal parallel to the Eustachian tube. The muscle originates in the cartilaginous part of the Eustachian tube. Its tendon emerges from the *cochleariform process*, the termination of the muscle canal, and attaches to the neck of the malleus. The muscle is innervated by a

FIGURE 2-13. The quadrants of the eardrum. (From *Speech and Hearing Science,* 2nd ed., by Willard R. Zemlin, copyright © 1981. Reprinted by permission of Prentice-Hall, Inc.)

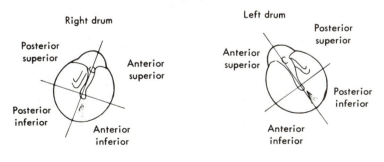

branch of the Vth cranial nerve, the trigeminal. When it contracts, the tension of the eardrum is increased. The tensor tympani muscle is shown in Figure 2–14.

The stapedius muscle originates in the posterior wall of the middle-ear cavity and runs in a canal approximately parallel to the facial nerve canal. Its tendon attaches to the neck of the stapes. The stapedius is innervated by a branch of the facial nerve, the VIIth cranial nerve. When the muscle contracts, the stapes is pulled posteriorly, thus impeding its movement in the oval window. The stapedius muscle is diagrammed in Figure 2–15.

The tensor tympani and the stapedius muscles, referred to together as the *intra-aural muscles,* contract reflexively in response to an auditory stimulus of high intensity. The muscles of both ears contract even though the stimulus is introduced to only one ear. The action of these muscles serves to brake the movement of the ossicular chain and thus reduce the energy transmitted through the oval window into the inner ear. More will be said about the protective function of the intra-aural muscles in a later section of this chapter.

Just below the oval window is another connection between the middle and inner ears, the membrane-covered *round window.* Between the oval and

FIGURE 2-14. The tensor tympani muscle. (From *Speech and Hearing Science,* 2nd ed., by Willard R. Zemlin, copyright © 1981. Reprinted by permission of Prentice-Hall, Inc.)

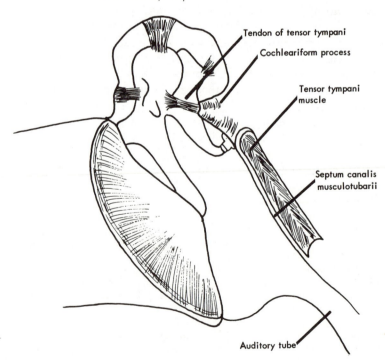

Tendon of tensor tympani

Cochleariform process

Tensor tympani muscle

Septum canalis musculotubarii

Auditory tube

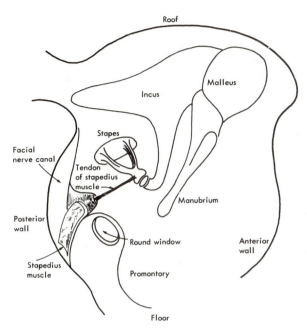

Roof

Malleus

Incus

Stapes

Facial
nerve canal

Tendon
of stapedius
muscle

Manubrium

Posterior
wall

Round window

Anterior
wall

Stapedius
muscle

Promontory

Floor

FIGURE 2–15. The stapedius muscle as seen from the middle-ear cavity looking toward
the eardrum. (From *Speech and Hearing Science,* 2nd ed., by Willard R.
Zemlin, copyright © 1981. Reprinted by permission of Prentice-Hall, Inc.)

round windows is a rounded projection of bone, formed by the basal turn of
the cochlea, that is called the *promontory*. Just above the oval window is the
canal that encases the facial nerve. These landmarks can be seen in Figure 2–9
and in greater detail in Figure 2–16.

A branch of the facial nerve, called the *chorda tympani,* courses through
the middle-ear cavity just behind the eardrum. It can be seen in Figure 2–17.
The chorda tympani, together with a branch of the trigeminal nerve, carries
taste sensation from the anterior two-thirds of the tongue.

The oval and round windows communicate with different parts of the
inner-ear mechanism, as we shall see in the following section.

The Inner Ear

The inner ear is more than an end organ for hearing; it is also the sensory
organ for balance. Both these important end organs are encased in the same
bony capsule, both have the same fluid systems, and both send their impulses
along the same cranial nerve. Together, they are known as the inner ear,
although only one of them is actually concerned with hearing. The close
association of the end organs of hearing and balance, however, has important
implications for the otologist, as we shall see in the next chapter.

The balance part of the inner ear, usually referred to as the *vestibular ap-*

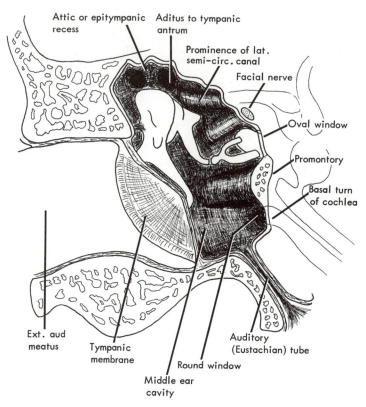

Attic or epitympanic recess

Aditus to tympanic antrum

Prominence of lat. semi-circ. canal

Facial nerve

Oval window

Promontory

Basal turn of cochlea

Auditory (Eustachian) tube

Round window

Middle ear cavity

Tympanic membrane

Ext. aud meatus

FIGURE 2-16. Schematic of the middle ear. (From *Speech and Hearing Science,* 2nd ed., by Willard R. Zemlin, copyright © 1981. Reprinted by permission of Prentice-Hall, Inc.)

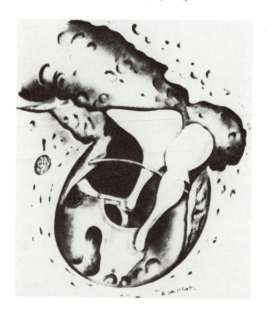

FIGURE 2-17.
A view into the middle ear with the eardrum removed. The chorda tympani passes behind the manubrium of the malleus and in front of the long crus of the incus. (From David D. DeWeese and William H. Saunders, *Textbook of Otolaryngology,* 5th ed. St. Louis: C. V. Mosby Co., 1977. Reprinted by permission.)

paratus, consists of the *utricle,* the *saccule,* and the three *semicircular canals:* the superior (or anterior vertical), the posterior (or posterior vertical), and the lateral (or horizontal) canals. These canals are located in planes that are at right angles to each other—analogous to the floor and two side walls of a corner of a room—and together with the utricle and the saccule they help maintain our equilibrium regardless of the position of our head in space. The ends of the semicircular canals connect with the utricle. One end of each canal is enlarged into an *ampulla* that contains an end organ consisting of ciliated sensory cells called the *crista ampullaris* and a gelatinous substance, in which the cilia are imbedded, called the *cupula.* Similar end organs are situated in the utricle and the saccule and are called *maculae* (plural of *macula*). The smaller ends of the two vertical canals are joined together in a *common crus* before connecting with the utricle. Nerve fibers from the end organs of the semicircular canals and the utricle and the saccule join together to form the *vestibular* portion of the VIIIth cranial nerve.

The hearing part of the inner ear is the *cochlea,* which resembles a snail shell in appearance. The basal end of the cochlea is nearest the middle ear, the apical end is farthest from the middle ear. The cochlea and the semicircular canals meet in a common area designated the *vestibule.* It is in the bony wall of the vestibule that the oval window is located, and it is within the vestibule that the utricle and saccule are found.

Sometimes, the inner ear is referred to as the *labyrinth,* because of its intricate construction. The outer hard shell of the inner ear is called the bony labyrinth, and the inner, membranous portion of the apparatus is called the membranous labyrinth. The entire inner ear is filled with fluid. The membranous labyrinth is protected from the bony labyrinth by a fluid called *perilymph,* which is apparently cerebrospinal fluid supplied from the ventricles of the brain through the *cochlear aqueduct* that links the cochlea with the subarachnoid space—the space between the middle covering (*arachnoid*) and the innermost covering (*pia mater*) of the brain—which is filled with cerebrospinal fluid. Inside the membranous labyrinth is found another fluid called *endolymph.* The endolymphatic system is apparently entirely separate from the perilymphatic system. Whereas the perilymph cushions the membranous labyrinth throughout the inner ear, the endolymph is a closed system, with the cochlear portion and vestibular portions connected by a narrow passage called the *ductus reuniens.* Perilymph and endolymph both contain sodium and potassium, but in differing amounts. Perilymph is high in sodium and low in potassium, whereas endolymph is high in potassium and low in sodium. Endolymph is thought to be secreted by the *stria vascularis* (identified in later illustrations showing the details of cochlear anatomy). Figures 2–18 through 2–21 show various views of the bony (osseous) and membranous labyrinths and the connections between the vestibular and cochlear portions of the inner ear.

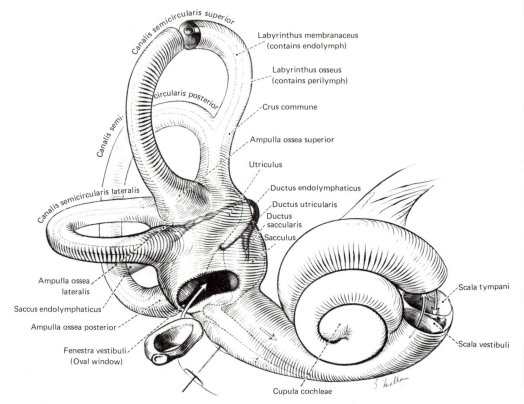

Labyrinthus membranaceus
(contains endolymph)

Labyrinthus osseus
(contains perilymph)

Crus commune

Ampulla ossea superior

Utriculus

Ductus endolymphaticus

Ductus utricularis

Ductus saccularis

Sacculus

Canalis semicircularis superior

circularis posterior

Canalis semi.

Canalis semicircularis lateralis

Ampulla ossea lateralis

Saccus endolymphaticus

Ampulla ossea posterior

Fenestra vestibuli
(Oval window)

Scala tympani

Scala vestibuli

Cupula cochleae

FIGURE 2–18.   The bony (osseous) labyrinth. Note the oval window into the vestibule from which the stapes has been removed. The membranous utricle and saccule are connected by the *utriculo-saccular duct,* consisting of two branches of the *endolymphatic duct* (ductus endolymphaticus), which is shown in light shading to terminate in the *endolymphatic sac* (saccus endolymphaticus) under the *dura mater,* the outermost covering of the brain. (Reproduced with permission from "The Internal Ear," *What's New,* North Chicago: Abbott Laboratories, Spring 1957.)

The membranous cochlea consists of a closed passage, the *cochlear duct,* or *scala media* (*ductus cochlearis* in Figure 2–22), running the length of the two-and-three-quarters turns of the spiraling cochlea. The cochlear duct, occupying the central portion of the interior of the cochlea, separates its peri-lymphatic spaces into two so-called *galleries,* or *scalae:* the *scala vestibuli,* separated from the cochlear duct by the *vestibular membrane of Reissner,* and the *scala tympani,* separated from the cochlear duct by the *basilar membrane.* At the apex of the cochlea, these two perilymphatic spaces are connected by the *helicotrema.* The scala vestibuli communicates with the middle ear by

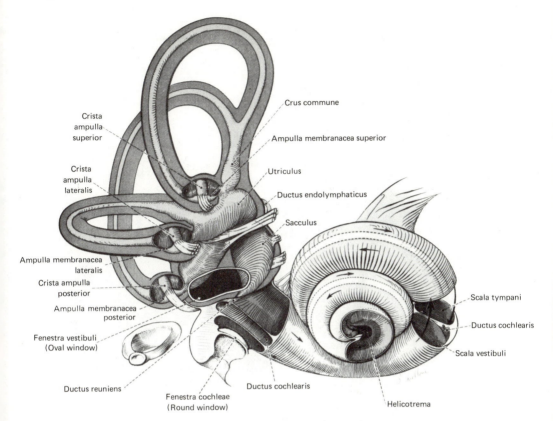

Crus commune

Crista
ampulla
superior

Ampulla membranacea superior

Crista
ampulla
lateralis

Utriculus

Ductus endolymphaticus

Sacculus

Ampulla membranacea
lateralis

Crista ampulla
posterior

Scala tympani

Ampulla membranacea
posterior

Ductus cochlearis

Fenestra vestibuli
(Oval window)

Scala vestibuli

Ductus reuniens

Ductus cochlearis

Fenestra cochleae
(Round window)

Helicotrema

FIGURE 2-19. The membranous semicircular canals showing the cristae within the ampullae. (Reproduced with permission from "The Internal Ear," *What's New,* North Chicago: Abbott Laboratories, Spring 1957.)

means of the oval window, situated in the vestibule, and the scala tympani is connected to the middle ear by the round window (see Figure 2–19).

Figure 2–23 shows an enlarged view of the cochlear duct (scala media), which contains endolymph. The basilar membrane, which separates the cochlear duct from the scala tympani, extends from the bony *spiral lamina,* a shelf from the central core of the cochlea called the *modiolus,* to the *spiral ligament* (see also Figure 2–22). Situated on the basilar membrane is the end organ of hearing, the *organ of Corti.* The *arch of Corti* separates a single row of from 3000 to 3500 *inner hair cells* and three or sometimes four rows of from 9000 to 12,000 *outer hair cells*—or even more according to some authorities. The inner and outer hair cells run in parallel rows along the basilar membrane from the base to the apex of the cochlea. Many hairs, or *cilia,* project from each of the

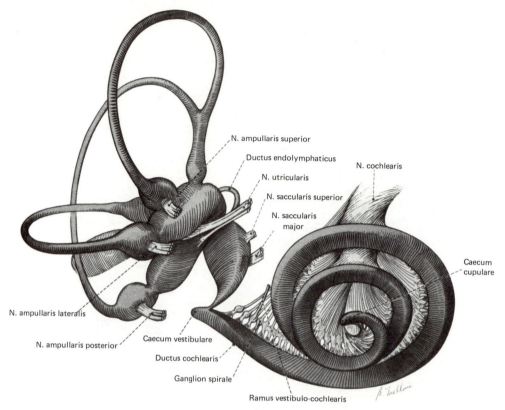

N. ampullaris superior

Ductus endolymphaticus

N. cochlearis

N. utricularis

N. saccularis superior

N. saccularis major

Caecum cupulare

N. ampullaris lateralis

N. ampullaris posterior

Caecum vestibulare

Ductus cochlearis

Ganglion spirale

Ramus vestibulo-cochlearis

FIGURE 2-20.   The membranous labyrinth showing the nerves arising from the end organs in the semicircular canals, the utricle, and the saccule, which combine to form the vestibular branch of the VIIIth nerve. The cochlear portion of the VIIIth nerve (N. cochlearis) consists of nerve fibers from the spiral ganglion of the cochlea. (Reproduced with permission from "The Internal Ear," *What's New,* North Chicago: Abbott Laboratories, Spring 1957.)

hair cells through the *reticular membrane* and then make contact with the *tectorial membrane,* which extends over them. Each inner hair cell sprouts from 30 to 60 cilia, and each outer hair cell sprouts from 75 to 100 cilia. On each outer hair cell, the cilia are arranged in a W-shaped pattern. In addition to the hair cells, the organ of Corti contains supporting cell structures. The hair cells themselves are supported by *phalangeal* (fingerlike) cells called *Deiters* cells. Between the outer hair cells and the spiral ligament are other supporting cells: the cells of *Hensen,* the cells of *Boettcher,* and the cells of *Claudius.* The interior of the organ of Corti apparently is isolated from the endolymph in the rest of the cochlear duct and contains a fluid called *cortilymph,* which is similar

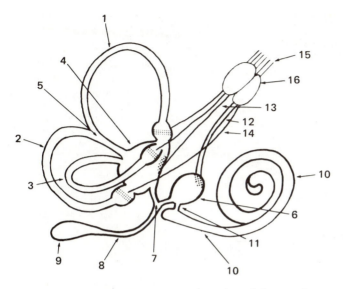

FIGURE 2-21. Diagramatic representation of the membranous labyrinth and the components of the vestibular portion of the VIIIth nerve. These components are (1) superior (anterior vertical) semicircular canal, (2) posterior (posterior vertical) semicircular canal, (3) lateral (horizontal) semicircular canal, (4) utricle, (5) common crus of superior and posterior canals, (6) saccule, (7) utriculo-saccular duct, (8) endolymphatic duct, (9) endolymphatic sac, (10) cochlear duct, (11) ductus reuniens, (12) nerve fibers from the macula of the saccule, (13) nerve fibers from the macula of the utricle and from the ampullae of the superior and lateral semicircular canals, (14) nerve fibers from the ampulla of the posterior semicircular canal, (15) vestibular portion of the VIIIth nerve in the internal auditory meatus, and (16) vestibular ganglion. (Reproduced with permission from George H. Paff, *Anatomy of the Head and Neck,* Philadelphia: W. B. Saunders Co., 1973.)

to perilymph.[8] The basilar membrane is 32 mm long from the base to the apex of the cochlea. It contains some 24,000 transverse fibers and varies in width from about 1/20 mm at the base to about 1/2 mm at the apex. The hair cells are connected in a complex fashion with some 20,000 to 30,000 nerve fibers that run into the central core of the cochlea to the *spiral ganglion,* where they synapse with second-order neurons that unite to form the *cochlear* branch of the VIIIth nerve. The cochlear branch then joins the vestibular branch, and the VIIIth nerve, called the *auditory* or *vestibulocochlear* nerve, in company with the VIIth (facial) nerve, proceeds through the *internal auditory meatus* to nuclei in the brain stem. From there, the auditory pathway extends through

[8]W. Lawrence Gulick, *Hearing: Physiology and Psychophysics* (New York: Oxford University Press, 1971), pp. 39–41.

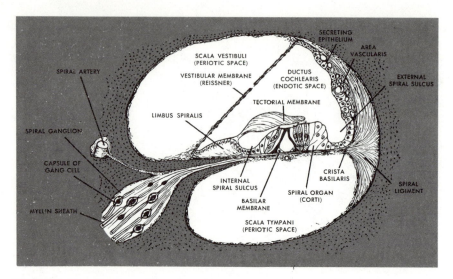

FIGURE 2-22. Cross section of cochlear canal. (From A. T. Rasmussen, *Outlines of Neuro-Anatomy,* 3rd ed., Dubuque, Ia.: Wm. C. Brown Co., 1943. Reproduced by permission of the publishers.)

FIGURE 2-23. Details of the organ of Corti. (From *Hearing: Physiology and Psychophysics* by W. Lawrence Gulick. Copyright © 1971 by Oxford University Press, Inc. Reprinted by permission.)

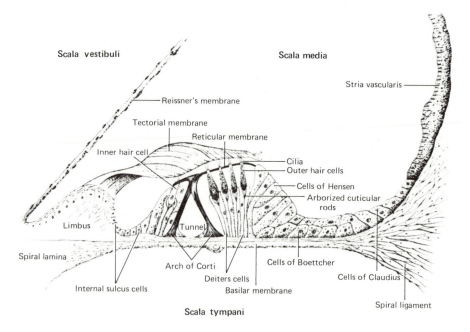

various nuclei to the cerebral cortex in the temporal lobes of the brain, as will be detailed in the next section of this chapter.

THE PHYSIOLOGY OF HEARING

For centuries, the problem of how the hearing mechanism functions has been in dispute, and many books and articles have been written on the subject. No attempt will be made here to explain how the cochlea functions as a sound analyzer, and only brief mention will be made of the various theories of hearing. Here we shall be concerned primarily with how sound reaches the cochlea, not with what occurs electrically, chemically, and/or mechanically within the cochlea.

Hearing by Air Conduction

Normally, we hear by the mechanism of air conduction, because most sounds to which we attend are airborne and because the mechanism of air conduction is much more sensitive than that of bone conduction. Sound waves in the air around us are directed by the pinna into the external acoustic meatus, where they impinge on the eardrum. The eardrum is thus set into vibration by the movements of the air particles adjacent to it.

Because the handle of the malleus is imbedded in the eardrum, the ossicular chain is set into vibration. These tiny bones vibrate as a unit and act as a lever, increasing the energy from the eardrum to the oval window by a factor of 1.31 to 1.[9] Further enhancement of sound energy is provided by the difference in area between the eardrum and the stapes footplate, computed as 21 to 1. Because only two-thirds of the eardrum is an effective vibrator, the effective areal difference between the eardrum and the stapes footplate is only 14 to 1. Multiplying the effective areal difference (14) by the lever action (1.31) gives an energy increase of 18.3 to 1, which translates into an amplification factor of 25.25 dB on the pressure scale.[10] This calculation agrees well with clinical experience that following a successful fenestration operation, the operated ear will have a residual loss of from 20 to 25 dB because of the elimination of the ossicular chain. By changing the energy collected by the eardrum into greater force and less excursion, the middle ear acts as a transformer, thus matching the impedance of sound waves in air to that in fluid.

When the sound stimulus striking the eardrum is sufficiently intense—a sensation level of from 65 to 105 dB in the normal ear, depending on the fre-

---

[9] Willard R. Zemlin, *Speech and Hearing Science* (Englewood Cliffs, N.J.: Prentice-Hall, 1981), p. 575.

[10] Ibid., p. 576.

quency of the stimulus—the acoustic reflex is elicited.[11] This reflex, which is due primarily to the contraction of the stapedius muscle, reduces the energy transmitted through the oval window to the perilymph in the vestibule. The greatest reduction in sound transmission as a function of the acoustic reflex—from 20 to 30 dB—occurs for low frequencies.[12] Little attenuation occurs for frequencies above 2000 Hz. The latency of the stapedial reflex —"dead" time between the onset of the stimulus and onset of muscle contraction—is reported to be between 25 and 160 msec,[13] although some investigators have reported latencies as short as 10 msec.[14] Latency of the muscle decreases as stimulus intensity increases. As stated earlier in this chapter, the reflex occurs in both ears, even though the evoking stimulus is presented to only one ear. Although various functions of the acoustic reflex have been proposed, certainly one important function is the protection of the end organ in the cochlea from overstimulation. As we shall see in a later chapter, measurement of the acoustic reflex has clinical utility in determining the site of lesion in cases of impaired hearing.

Because the fluid of the inner ear is virtually incompressible, there has to be some provision for the relief of the pressure produced by the inward movement of the footplate of the stapes. This relief is furnished by the round window, whose membrane reacts to the movements of the footplate of the stapes in the oval window. The interaction of the two windows is complex, but simply described, when the footplate is pushed into the vestibule, the membrane in the round window is bulged outward toward the middle-ear cavity. Without this reciprocal action of the two windows, the incompressibility of the perilymph would resist the action of the ossicular chain, which in turn would restrict the vibrations of the eardrum.

The fluid motion from the oval to the round window is transmitted through the cochlear duct. As the footplate of the stapes is pushed into the perilymph of the scala vestibuli, the vestibular membrane, or membrane of Reissner, is bulged into the cochlear duct, causing movement of the endolymph within the cochlear duct and movement of the basilar membrane. The cilia of the hair cells are imbedded in the gelatinous tectorial membrane, so that when the basilar membrane is displaced there is a "shearing" action on the cilia by the tectorial membrane (as illustrated diagramatically in Figure 2-24). This shearing action causes an alternating current to be generated by the hair cells, called the *cochlear microphonic* (CM), or *cochlear potential* (CP).

---

[11] Gisle Djupesland, "Advanced Reflex Considerations," in *Handbook of Clinical Impedance Audiometry*, ed. James Jerger (Dobbs Ferry, N.Y.: American Electromedics Corp., 1975), chap. 5, p. 93.

[12] Peter Dallos, *The Auditory Periphery* (New York: Academic Press, 1973), p. 481.

[13] Ibid., p. 487; Djupesland, "Advance Reflex Consideration," p. 100; and Aage R. Møller, "The Middle Ear," in *Foundations of Modern Auditory Theory*, vol. 2, ed. Jerry V. Tobias (New York: Academic Press, 1972), chap. 4, p. 179.

[14] Zemlin, *Speech and Hearing Science*, p. 568.

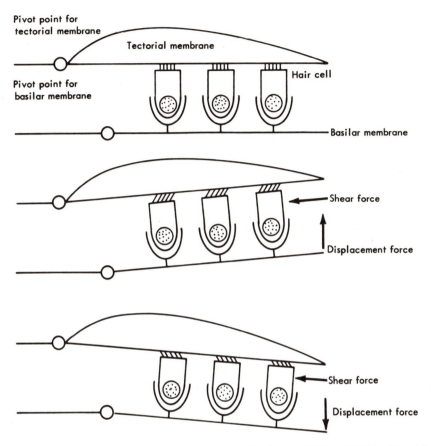

FIGURE 2-24.   How shearing action of the tectorial membrane and the cilia of the hair cells is produced. (From *Speech and Hearing Science,* 2nd ed., by Willard R. Zemlin, copyright © 1981. Reprinted by permission of Prentice-Hall, Inc.)

The CM can be recorded by an electrode on the round window or within the cochlea, or even in the vicinity of the cochlea.[15] The CM generally mirrors the waveform and within certain limits the amplitude of an auditory stimulus. The CM is also referred to as the Wever-Bray effect, because these two investigators discovered in 1930 that speech delivered to a cat's ear could be understood when the signal was picked up from the cochlear nerve and amplified.[16] The CM triggers responses in the neurons connected to the hair cells. Figure 2–25 illustrates the electrical activity in a neuron associated with its "firing." Impulses are carried by nerve fibers to the main trunk of the

[15] Dallos, *Auditory Periphery,* p. 25.
[16] Gulick, *Hearing: Physiology,* p. 54.

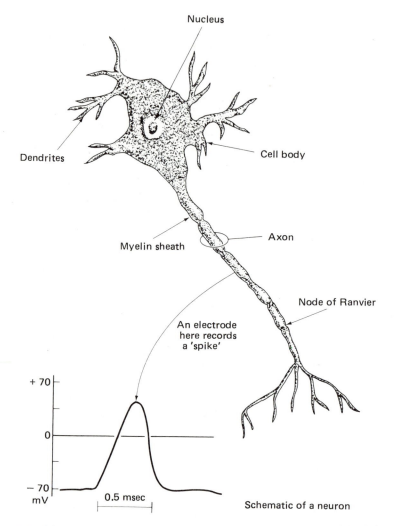

FIGURE 2-25. Electrical activity during discharge of a neuron. (From Theodore J. Glattke, "Elements of Auditory Physiology," Chapter 8 in Fred D. Minifie, Thomas J. Hixon, and Frederick Williams, eds., *Normal Aspects of Speech, Hearing, and Language,* copyright © 1973. Reprinted by permission of Prentice-Hall, Inc.)

cochlear portion of the VIIIth nerve, and thence to the brain. Thus, it is the cerebral cortex that eventually "hears" the vibrations impinged on the eardrum. The movement of the basilar membrane is transmitted to the perilymph in the scala tympani, and the bulge produced by the inward movement of the footplate of the stapes thus reaches the round window, the membrane of which is bulged into the middle-ear cavity.

Experimental studies have demonstrated that sounds of very high frequency cause movements of the basilar membrane and the hair cells of the organ of Corti at the basal end of the cochlea, or in other words, at the part of the cochlea nearest the middle ear; whereas sounds of very low frequency affect the cochlear duct at the apical end, near or at the helicotrema. Figure 2–26 schematically illustrates the frequency response of the organ of Corti at various distances along the basilar membrane from the base of the cochlea. Figure 2–27 illustrates the manner in which vibrations are transmitted from the eardrum to the cochlea, the transmission of energy through the cochlear duct, and the reciprocal action of the two windows that connect the middle ear with the inner ear. Figure 2–28 is an enlarged view of the transmission of energy through the cochlear duct.

The nerve fibers leading from the hair cells collect at the *spiral ganglion* and then emerge from the temporal bone through the *internal acoustic meatus*, in company with the fibers of the vestibular branch of the VIIIth nerve and the VIIth, or facial, nerve. The neurons of the cochlear portion of the VIIIth nerve proceed to the *ventral* and *dorsal cochlear nuclei* on the ipsilateral (same) side of the upper medulla and pons of the brain stem. Next, the neurons proceed to the *superior olivary complex* of the pons. Some neurons decussate (cross) through the *trapezoid body* to the contralateral (opposite) superior olivary complex. From the superior olivary complex on each side of the pons, the neurons proceed in tracts called the *lateral lemnisci* to nuclei called the *inferior colliculi* at the level of the midbrain. Some additional decussation occurs at this level. The neurons then proceed to the thalamic nuclei called the *medial geniculate bodies*. From these points, *auditory radiations* spread to the cortex of the cerebrum—specifically to *Heschl's gyrus* in

FIGURE 2–26.   Location along the basilar membrane of various frequency receptors. For purposes of illustration, the cochlea is shown uncoiled. (From *Speech and Hearing Science,* 2nd ed., by Willard R. Zemlin, copyright © 1981.) Reprinted by permission of Prentice-Hall, Inc.

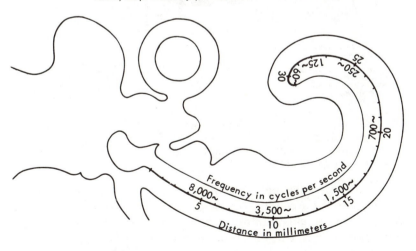

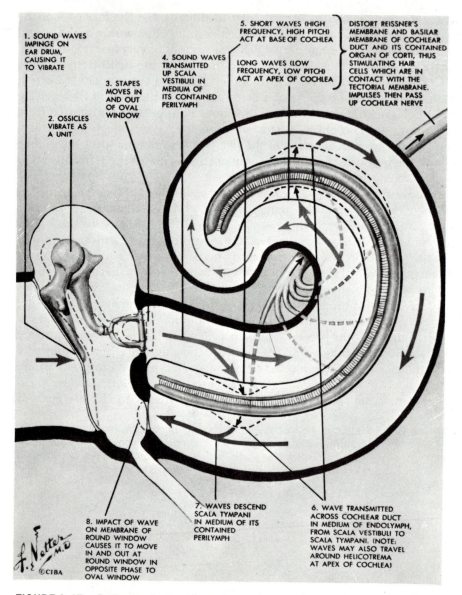

1. SOUND WAVES IMPINGE ON EAR DRUM, CAUSING IT TO VIBRATE

2. OSSICLES VIBRATE AS A UNIT

3. STAPES MOVES IN AND OUT OF OVAL WINDOW

4. SOUND WAVES TRANSMITTED UP SCALA VESTIBULI IN MEDIUM OF ITS CONTAINED PERILYMPH

5. SHORT WAVES (HIGH FREQUENCY, HIGH PITCH) ACT AT BASE OF COCHLEA

LONG WAVES (LOW FREQUENCY, LOW PITCH) ACT AT APEX OF COCHLEA

DISTORT REISSNER'S MEMBRANE AND BASILAR MEMBRANE OF COCHLEAR DUCT AND ITS CONTAINED ORGAN OF CORTI, THUS STIMULATING HAIR CELLS WHICH ARE IN CONTACT WITH THE TECTORIAL MEMBRANE. IMPULSES THEN PASS UP COCHLEAR NERVE

6. WAVE TRANSMITTED ACROSS COCHLEAR DUCT IN MEDIUM OF ENDOLYMPH, FROM SCALA VESTIBULI TO SCALA TYMPANI. (NOTE: WAVES MAY ALSO TRAVEL AROUND HELICOTREMA AT APEX OF COCHLEA)

7. WAVES DESCEND SCALA TYMPANI IN MEDIUM OF ITS CONTAINED PERILYMPH

8. IMPACT OF WAVE ON MEMBRANE OF ROUND WINDOW CAUSES IT TO MOVE IN AND OUT AT ROUND WINDOW IN OPPOSITE PHASE TO OVAL WINDOW

FIGURE 2-27.   Pathway of sound from the eardrum through the cochlea. (© Copyright 1970 CIBA Pharmaceutical Company, Division of CIBA-GEIGY Corporation. Reprinted with permission from *Clinical Symposia,* illustrated by Frank H. Netter, M.D.)

the temporal lobe. As we have seen, there is a crossing over of some neurons at two different levels in the ascending tracts, so that impulses originating in one cochlea eventually reach both auditory cortices. Because of this bilateral cortical representation of each ear, interruption of the ascending auditory tract on one side of the brain stem above the level of the cochlear nuclei, or the

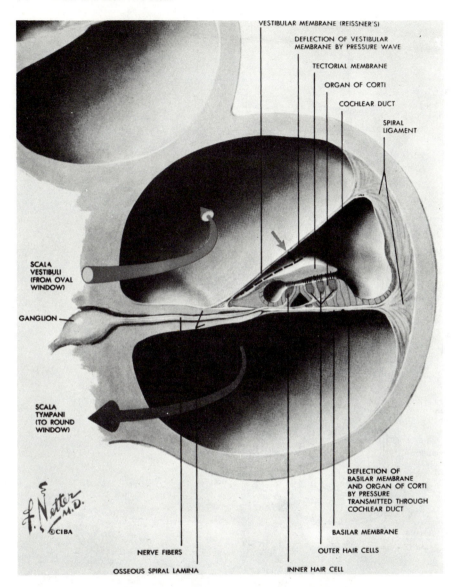

VESTIBULAR MEMBRANE (REISSNER'S)

DEFLECTION OF VESTIBULAR
MEMBRANE BY PRESSURE WAVE

TECTORIAL MEMBRANE

ORGAN OF CORTI

COCHLEAR DUCT

SPIRAL
LIGAMENT

SCALA
VESTIBULI
(FROM OVAL
WINDOW)

GANGLION

SCALA
TYMPANI
(TO ROUND
WINDOW)

DEFLECTION OF
BASILAR MEMBRANE
AND ORGAN OF CORTI
BY PRESSURE
TRANSMITTED THROUGH
COCHLEAR DUCT

BASILAR MEMBRANE

OUTER HAIR CELLS

NERVE FIBERS

OSSEOUS SPIRAL LAMINA

INNER HAIR CELL

FIGURE 2-28.   Transmission of sound energy through the cochlear duct. (© Copyright 1970 CIBA Pharmaceutical Company, Division of CIBA-GEIGY Corporation. Reproduced with permission from *Clinical Symposia,* illustrated by Frank H. Netter, M.D.)

removal of one temporal lobe, does not result in a loss of hearing sensitivity in either ear. Figure 2–29 diagrams the pathways of the cochlear branch of the VIIIth nerve.

Although the VIIIth nerve is primarily a sensory nerve—that is, it carries sensory information from the cochlea and the vestibular system to the brain—there are a limited number of efferent fibers—about 500—proceeding

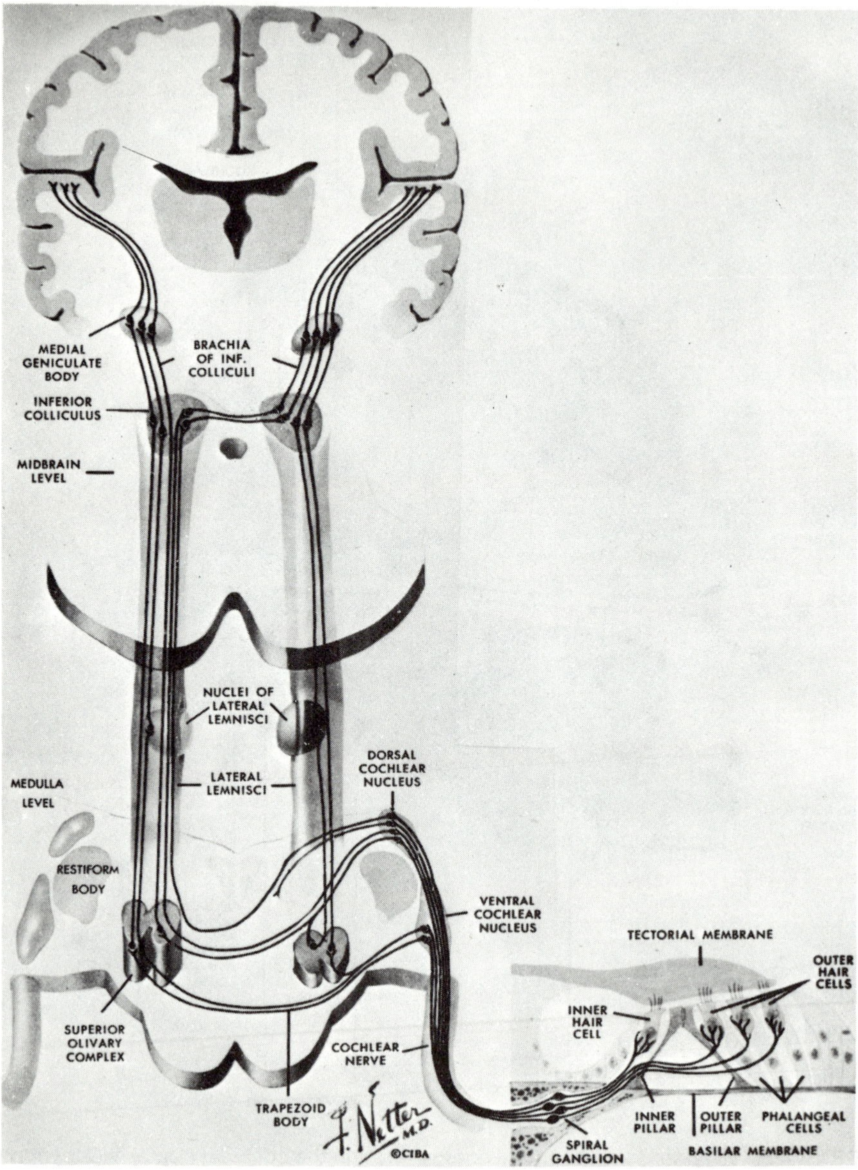

FIGURE 2–29. Ascending pathways of the cochlear branch of the VIIIth nerve. (© Copyright 1970 CIBA Pharmaceutical Company, Division of CIBA-GEIGY Corporation. Reproduced with permission from *Clinical Symposia*, illustrated by Frank H. Netter, M.D.)

from the superior olivary complex to the cochlea. Most are crossed fibers, connecting with the cochlea of the opposite side. This descending tract is called the *olivo-cochlear* tract (shown in Figure 2–30), or Rasmussen's bundle. Although its function is still not clear, the olivo-cochlear tract apparently ex-

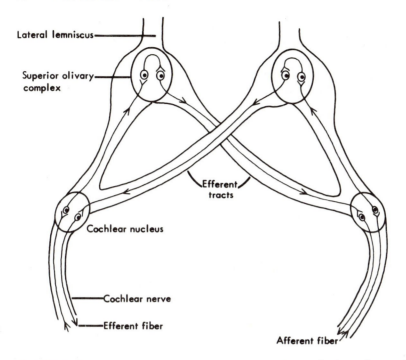

Lateral lemniscus

Superior olivary complex

Efferent tracts

Cochlear nucleus

Cochlear nerve

Efferent fiber

Afferent fiber

FIGURE 2-30. Simplified schematic representation of the olivo-cochlear tract (Rasmussen's bundle)—the fibers descending toward the cochlea (efferent). (From *Speech and Hearing Science,* 2nd ed., by Willard R. Zemlin, copyright © 1981. Reprinted by permission of Prentice-Hall, Inc.)

erts primarily an inhibitory effect on the hair cells, thus enabling us to listen selectively to certain sounds by "tuning out" competing stimuli.

Hearing by Bone Conduction

Because the inner ear is encased in bone (the *petrous* portion of the temporal bone), vibrations of this bone will cause movement of the fluid of the inner ear directly. Thus, the sensation of hearing can be produced without vibrations proceeding through the eardrum and the ossicular chain. The mechanism for transmission of sound by *bone conduction* is much less efficient than for air-conducted sound because vibrations must be sufficiently intense to set the bones of the skull into movement before they can be heard. Moreover, in going through skin, flesh, and bone, sound waves are not accurately transmitted because sounds of longer wavelength (lower frequency) are impeded less by these obstructions than are sounds of shorter wavelength (higher frequency). Thus, hearing by bone conduction tends to be somewhat distorted when compared with that by air conduction.

At least two modes of vibration are known to occur in bone conduction: *inertial,* or *translatory,* motion and *compressional* motion. Sounds of low frequency (roughly below 800 Hz) excite the hair cells because of the inertia of the ossicular chain. The skull apparently moves as a whole in response to low-frequency stimulation. If the ossicles lag behind the movement of the skull, vibrations are transmitted through the oval window in the same way as when airborne vibrations set the ossicular chain in motion. A different kind of vibratory motion of the skull results from high-frequency stimulation (roughly above 1500 Hz). Instead of moving as a whole, the skull vibrates so that opposite surfaces move in an out-of-phase relationship. As the front and back of the skull move outward, the sides of the skull move inward. The effect of this skull movement is to produce a compression of the cochlea. Because the round window is the point of least resistance within the cochlea, when compression of the cochlea occurs, the fluid within causes displacement of the round window. The fluid movement within the cochlea initiates nerve impulses. Both inertial and compressional motions result from bone-conduction stimulation by frequencies between 800 and 1500 Hz. Figure 2–31 illustrates the modes of vibration of the skull for various frequencies.

Ordinarily, we are not conscious of hearing by bone conduction because most sounds we are interested in are carried by air, and the air-conducting mechanism of hearing is so much more efficient than the bone-conduction mechanism. If our heads are in contact with a solid surface, however, such as the floor, the bones of the skull receive vibrations, such as footsteps, and the bone-conducting mechanism is thus activated. Moreover, we tend to hear our own voices partly through the mechanism of bone conduction. This occurs because the vibrations of our vocal folds in the larynx are transmitted to the air in cavities of the head and neck, and thus also to the bones of the skull. The fluid of the inner ear is then set into motion directly. Of course, we are also hearing our own voices through air conduction if we have normal outer and

FIGURE 2-31.   Vibrations of the skull in bone-conduction hearing according to Békésy. (From *Speech and Hearing Science,* 2nd ed., by Willard R. Zemlin, copyright © 1981. Reprinted by permission of Prentice-Hall, Inc.)

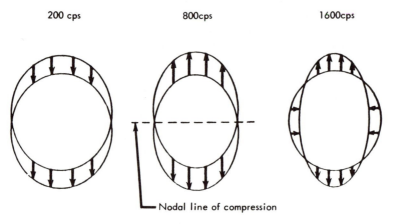

200 cps   800cps   1600cps

Nodal line of compression

middle ears. The shock that many of us receive when we first hear our recorded voices is due in part to the fact that this is the first time we have heard ourselves "as others hear us," through air conduction alone.

The mechanism of bone conduction provides an alternate pathway for sound that can be utilized by people who have suffered an impairment of the air-conduction system, that is, an impairment of the outer or middle ear. If the inner ear is functioning normally, they can "hear," provided that sound can reach the inner ear. Such individuals usually do quite well with the amplification that a wearable hearing aid furnishes. Sound can be made intense enough through amplification, delivered to either an air-conduction or to a bone-conduction type of receiver, to activate the bone-conducting mechanism.

Theories of Hearing

As was previously stated, this book is not concerned with the controversy of how the cochlea functions in analyzing sound. The serious student of audiology will, of course, want to pursue this subject in detail. Only the briefest mention will be made here of the principal theories of hearing.

The place theory. This theory, originally popularized by the famous German scientist Helmholtz, states that pitch perception is related to the place of maximum stimulation of the basilar membrane. Experimental evidence, as we have mentioned, indicates that the basal end of the cochlea is sensitive to high frequencies and the apical end of the cochlea is stimulated by low frequencies. The place theory holds that it is the *exact* place of stimulation of the organ of Corti along the basilar membrane that determines the pitch perceived. Helmholtz proposed that structures of the cochlear duct act as resonators, much as the strings of a piano vibrate in response to particular frequencies. Later exponents of the place theory do not believe that the tuning of the cochlea is as precise as Helmholtz thought. Nevertheless, the principle of the theory is the same—it is the particular region of stimulation of the basilar membrane that is responsible for the sensation of pitch.

The frequency theory. This theory explains pitch perception on the basis of the frequency of occurrence of impulses in the auditory nerve. Thus, a sound stimulus of a frequency of 500 Hz would cause fibers within the auditory nerve to discharge at the rate of 500 times per second. Rutherford and, more recently, Boring were exponents of this theory. The development of techniques for recording action potentials of nerve fibers disclosed that no fiber of the auditory nerve is capable of "firing" at a rate greater than about 1000 times per second. This experimental finding meant that discrimination of high pitches could therefore not be explained on the basis of a frequency theory. Even making allowance for the synchronized action of several nerve fibers discharging at slightly different times, the frequency theory could account for pitch perceptions only of frequencies below about 5000 Hz.

The volley theory.   This theory is a compromise between the place and frequency theories. It holds that perception of pitch for frequencies up to 5000 Hz can be explained primarily on the basis of the frequency of nerve impulses firing in "volleys," and that the primary explanation for perception of pitch for frequencies in excess of 5000 Hz is the place of greatest excitation along the basilar membrane. Figure 2–32 illustrates the principle of the volley theory. It is achieving popularity because it utilizes the experimental information available, which does indicate that place of stimulation within the cochlea is important and that pitch discriminations are correlated with frequency of nerve impulses, at least for the lower frequencies of sound vibration.

The traveling wave theory.   No discussion of theories of hearing can ignore the contributions of Békésy, who received the Nobel prize for his many years of detailed and meticulous research in regard to the functioning of the hearing mechanism. Békésy's experimentation with cochlear models led him to formulate a theory that sound is propagated in the cochlea in the form of a traveling wave in the basilar membrane. This wave travels from the base to the apex of the cochlea. The maximum amplitude of the wave occurs at a point along the basilar membrane that corresponds to the frequency of the stimulus; that is, the point of maximum amplitude is at the point that resonates to the stimulating frequency. See Figure 2–33 for a schematic representation of Békésy's traveling wave theory.

FIGURE 2-32.   The volley principle. (Reproduced with permission from Ernest Glen Wever, *Theory of Hearing,* New York: John Wiley & Sons, Inc., 1949.)

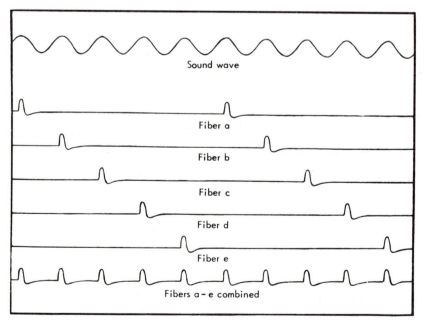

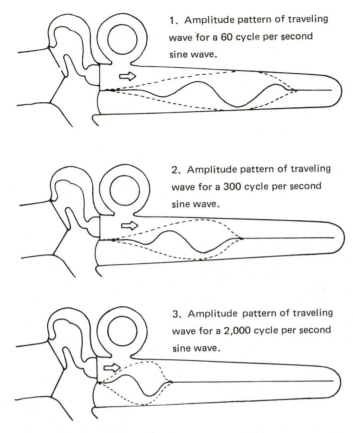

1. Amplitude pattern of traveling wave for a 60 cycle per second sine wave.

2. Amplitude pattern of traveling wave for a 300 cycle per second sine wave.

3. Amplitude pattern of traveling wave for a 2,000 cycle per second sine wave.

FIGURE 2-33.   Traveling waves along the basilar membrane. (From *Speech and Hearing Science,* 2nd ed., by Willard R. Zemlin, copyright © 1981. Reprinted by permission of Prentice-Hall, Inc.)

These theories of hearing are concerned primarily with the way in which the ear discriminates frequency. Intensity discrimination apparently is dependent on the number of nerve fibers activated by the stimulus, the total number of impulses per second in all fibers, and possibly the existence of certain fibers that respond only to stimuli of high intensity.

REFERENCES

Bast, Theodore H., and Anson, Barry J.   *The Temporal Bone and the Ear.* Springfield, Ill.: Charles C. Thomas, 1949.

Békésy, Georg von.   *Experiments in Hearing.* New York: McGraw-Hill, 1960.

Bradford, Larry J., ed.   *Physiological Measures of the Audio-Vestibular System.* New York: Academic Press, 1975.

Dallos, Peter.   *The Auditory Periphery.* New York: Academic Press, 1973.

DAVIS, HALLOWELL, and SILVERMAN, S. RICHARD, eds.   *Hearing and Deafness,* 4th ed. Chaps. 2 and 3. New York: Holt, Rinehart and Winston, 1978.

DENES, PETER B., and PINSON, ELLIOT N.   *The Speech Chain.* Chap. 3. Garden City, N.Y.: Doubleday, Anchor Press, 1973.

DeWEESE, DAVID D., and SAUNDERS, WILLIAM H.   *Textbook of Otolaryngology.* Chaps. 18, 19, and 21. Saint Louis: C. V. Mosby, 1973.

DURRANT, JOHN D., and LOVRINIC, JEAN H., eds.   *Bases of Hearing Science.* Baltimore, Md.: Williams & Wilkins, 1977.

EAGLES, ELDON L., ed.   *Human Communication and Its Disorders. The Nervous System* edited by Donald B. Tower, vol. 3. New York: Raven Press, 1975.

FLETCHER, HARVEY.   *Speech and Hearing in Communication.* New York: Van Nostrand, 1953.

GELFAND, STANLEY A.   *Hearing,* New York: Marcel Dekker, 1981.

GERBER, SANFORD E., ed.   *Introductory Hearing Science.* Philadelphia: W. B. Saunders, 1974.

GLORIG, ARAM, ed.   *Audiometry: Principles and Practices.* Chaps. 2 and 3. Baltimore: Williams & Wilkins, 1965.

GRAHAM, A. BRUCE, ed.   *Sensorineural Hearing Processes and Disorders.* Chaps. 1–6. Boston: Little, Brown and Company, 1967.

GULICK, W. LAWRENCE.   *Hearing: Physiology and Psychophysics.* Chap. 3. New York: Oxford University Press, 1971.

HARRIS, J. DONALD.   *Anatomy and Physiology of the Peripheral Hearing Mechanism.* New York: Bobbs-Merrill, 1974.

———.   *Psychoacoustics.* New York: Bobbs-Merrill, 1974.

———., ed.   *Forty Germinal Papers in Human Hearing.* Groton, Conn.: The Journal of Auditory Research, 1969.

HIRSH, IRA J.   *The Measurement of Hearing.* New York: McGraw-Hill, 1952.

McNALLY, W. J., and STUART, E. A.   *Physiology of the Labyrinth.* Rochester, Minn.: American Academy of Ophthalmology and Otolaryngology, 1967.

MARTIN, FREDERICK N.   *Introduction to Audiology,* 2nd ed. Englewood Cliffs, N.J.: Prentice-Hall, 1981.

———, ed.   *Medical Audiology: Disorders of Hearing.* Englewood Cliffs, N.J.: Prentice-Hall, 1981.

MINIFIE, FRED D.; HIXON, THOMAS J., and WILLIAMS, FREDERICK, eds.   *Normal Aspects of Speech, Hearing, and Language.* Chaps. 2, 8, and 9. Englewood Cliffs, N.J.: Prentice-Hall, 1973.

NORTHERN, JERRY L., ed.   *Hearing Disorders,* 2nd ed. Chaps. 21–22. Boston: Little, Brown and Company, 1984.

PAFF, GEORGE H.   *Anatomy of the Head and Neck.* Philadelphia: W. B. Saunders, 1973.

PETERSON, ARNOLD P. G., and GROSS, ERVIN E., JR.   *Handbook of Noise Measurement.* Concord, Mass.: General Radio, 1972.

PIERCE, JOHN R., and DAVID, EDWARD E., JR.   *Man's World of Sound.* Garden City, N.Y.: Doubleday, 1958.

POLYAK, STEPHEN L.; McHUGH, GLADYS; and JUDD, DELBERT K.   *The Human Ear in Anatomical Transparencies.* New York: Sonotone Corp., 1946.

RASMUSSEN, GRANT L., and WINDLE, WILLIAM F.   *Neural Mechanisms of the Auditory and Vestibular Systems.* Springfield, Ill.: Charles C. Thomas, 1960.

ROSE, DARRELL E., ed.   *Audiological Assessment,* 2nd ed. Chaps. 1 and 2. Englewood Cliffs, N.J.: Prentice-Hall, 1978.

ROSENBLITH, WALTER A., ed.   *Sensory Communication.* New York: Wiley and the M.I.T. Press, 1961.

SMALL, ARNOLD M.   *Elements of Hearing Science: A Programmed Text.* New York: Wiley, 1978.

STEVENS, S. S., ed.   *Handbook of Experimental Psychology.* Chaps. 25–28. New York: Wiley, 1951.

STEVENS, S. S., and DAVIS, HALLOWELL.   *Hearing.* New York: Wiley, 1938.

STEVENS, S. S.; WARSHOFSKY, FRED, and the Editors of *Life.   Sound and Hearing.* New York: Time, Inc., *Life* Science Library, 1967.

TOBIAS, JERRY V., ed.   *Foundations of Modern Auditory Theory,* vols. 1 and 2. New York: Academic Press, 1970 and 1972.

TOBIAS, JERRY V., and SCHUBERT, EARL D., eds.   *Hearing Research and Theory.* New York: Academic Press, 1981.

TRAVIS, LEE EDWARD, ed.   *Handbook of Speech Pathology and Audiology.* Chaps. 10–12. Englewood Cliffs, N.J.: Prentice-Hall, 1971.

VAN BERGEIJK, WILLEM A.; PIERCE, JOHN R.; and DAVID, EDWARD E., JR.   *Waves and the Ear.* Garden City, N.Y.: Doubleday, Anchor Books, 1960.

WEVER, ERNEST GLEN.   *Theory of Hearing.* New York: Wiley, 1949.

WEVER, E. G., and LAWRENCE, MERLE.   *Physiological Acoustics.* Princeton, N.J.: Princeton University Press, 1954.

YOST, WILLIAM, and NIELSEN, DONALD W., eds.   *Fundamentals of Hearing: An Introduction.* New York: Holt, Rinehart and Winston, 1977.

ZEMLIN, WILLARD R.   *Speech and Hearing Science,* 2nd ed. Chap. 6. Englewood Cliffs, N.J.: Prentice-Hall, 1981.

CHAPTER THREE
DISORDERS OF HEARING

So far we have been concerned with the functioning of the normal ear. In audiology, so much reference is made to the normal ear that some definition is in order. By "normal" ear, we mean the ear of a young adult (from eighteen to twenty-two years of age), which has had no known pathology—no history of infection nor any kind of disorder. Actually, the phrase *normal ear* refers not to any one ear but to a hypothetical average normal ear. As we shall see in subsequent chapters, the concept of average normal ear is frequently adopted in the calibration of equipment for testing the hearing function.

In this chapter, we shall be concerned with impairment of hearing. A *disorder of hearing* we shall define as any significant deviation from the behavior of the average normal ear. In later chapters, we shall see how hearing impairments are measured. Here, the principal types of hearing disorders and their symptoms, causes, and treatment are discussed.

There are three main categories of hearing disorders: peripheral impairments, central auditory disorders, and functional or nonorganic hearing problems. The terms *peripheral* and *central* cover the entire auditory system, from the external ear to the cerebrum. Lesions (injuries) that occur within the central nervous system, specifically the brain stem and the cerebrum, are termed *central* disorders. They are subdivided into brain-stem lesions and "higher-level," primarily temporal lobe, lesions. Lesions outside the central nervous system are called *peripheral.* A peripheral disorder may involve the outer ear (auricle or external canal), the middle ear, the cochlea, or the auditory portion of the VIIIth nerve up to the point where it first synapses within the brain stem. Functional or nonorganic problems are psychological rather than physiological disorders, although there may be a combination of an organic and a nonorganic problem, which is termed a *functional* or *nonorganic "overlay."* When we refer to actual organic hearing impairment—people with diminished auditory acuity or sensitivity who are hard of hearing or deaf, depending on the degree—we are talking about peripheral disorders. Peripheral disorders, which are subdivided into conductive, sensorineural, and mixed impairments, constitute almost 100 percent of the otologist's and the audiologist's caseloads; the bulk of this chapter will be concerned, therefore, with peripheral disorders.

CONDUCTIVE IMPAIRMENTS

Any dysfunction of the outer or middle ear in the presence of a normal inner ear is termed a *conductive* impairment of hearing. In other words, the difficulty is not with the perception of sound but with the conduction of sound to the analyzing system. Acquired hearing losses in children will most likely be of the conductive type.

Symptoms

Although it is not possible to specify with absolute accuracy the symptoms that indicate conductive impairment, some generalizations can be made. For example, it has sometimes been observed that persons with conductive loss tend to speak in a relatively quiet voice, so that it may be difficult for others to hear them. Because by definition persons with "pure" conductive loss have a normal inner ear, and because we tend to hear our own voices to some extent through the mechanism of bone conduction, such persons hear themselves with adequate loudness at all times and, because of the air-conduction loss, may be unaware of the presence of noise that makes it difficult for others to hear.

Another symptom of conductive impairment is that speech discrimination is relatively unimpaired. In other words, a patient with a conductive loss understands well what is heard provided that speech is made loud enough. It may be necessary, therefore, to shout at such a patient or at least to speak with more than ordinary loudness. Because loud speech is heard well, the conductively impaired patient can usually hear better in the presence of noise than can the person with normal hearing. The reason is that when it is noisy, as in a factory, for example, people with normal hearing have to speak loudly in order to hear each other above the noise, which serves as a masking device. The patient with the conductive loss is largely unaware of the noise and benefits from the increased loudness with which those nearby are speaking. The term for this phenomenon is *paracusis willisiana (Willisii).*

The ability of this patient to hear loud speech satisfactorily is related to another symptom of conductive impairment, namely, the ability to tolerate loud speech and other sounds of an intensity sufficient to reach the threshold of discomfort of the normal ear. The conductive impairment serves as a protection to the inner ear, giving the same effect as that of wearing an ear plug. A patient with a conductive loss of 40 dB hears a sound having an intensity of 60 dB above the normal threshold with the loudness that a person with normal hearing would perceive for a sound of 20 dB intensity. The protective feature of a conductive loss does not extend to very high sound-pressure levels, however. In other words, the conductively impaired patient and a person with normal hearing would both find sounds to be painful at extreme intensities.

The patient with a conductive loss tends to have about the same loss of sensitivity for sounds of any frequency. Sometimes hearing is better for the higher frequencies than it is for the lower ones, and occasionally the reverse may be true, but by and large the loss pattern is "flat."

Frequently, the conductively impaired individual complains of subjective head noises that may be localized in one ear or in both ears or unlocalized in the head. The otologist refers to head noises as *tinnitus.* We all have experienced tinnitus at some time. After the shooting of a gun, our ears may "ring" for several hours. In a very quiet room, we may be conscious of hearing our pulse beat or of other physiologic noises in our head. With most of us, however, tinnitus has been of a transient nature. Many hard-of-hearing people experience tinnitus every hour of the day. It is one of the most annoying features of impaired hearing. In the case of a conductive impairment, the tinnitus tends to be of relatively low frequency. An experimental study of tinnitus revealed that subjects with conductive hearing impairments matched their tinnitus to pure tones in the range from 120 to 1400 Hz.[1]

Etiology (Causes)

Conditions of the outer ear.   The commonest cause of an impairment of hearing due to the improper functioning of the outer ear is a blocking or plugging of the external meatus or canal by an excess accumulation of cerumen (wax). Of course it is possible for the canal to be blocked by other substances also. Sometimes, children will stuff objects such as beans or even wads of paper in the canal. The blockage will cause a conductive impairment that will persist until the object is removed. Some people produce much more cerumen than they need for the ordinary protection of the eardrum, with the result that

---

[1] James T. Graham and Hayes A. Newby, "Acoustical Characteristics of Tinnitus," A.M.A. *Archives of Otolaryngology* 75 (February 1962):165.

the cerumen builds up into a plug, which effectively prevents sound waves from reaching the eardrum. The remedy is simple: Remove the cerumen, and the hearing is restored to normal. Yet patients have been known to purchase hearing aids to compensate for a loss that later turns out to be caused only by a blocking of the external canal. The importance of seeing a physician when a hearing loss is noticed cannot be overemphasized. Also, the importance of having a physician remove excess cerumen or other objects in the canal should be stressed. The skin lining the external canal is very sensitive and easily scratched. Probing the canal with a hairpin or any other object can result in painful lacerations of the skin, with the ensuing danger of infection, to say nothing of the danger of injuring the eardrum by probing too deeply. It is not uncommon for mothers to try to remove cerumen from children's ears, using large cotton-tipped swabs. Instead of removing the cerumen, the applicator pushes it deeper into the canal, perhaps impacting it against the eardrum and making the eventual task of removal more difficult. An old saying that has a lot of sense is "Don't stick anything in your ear smaller than your elbow!"

Occasionally, babies are born with missing or occluded canals. The occlusion may be soft tissue or it may be bone. One or both ears may be affected. This condition, which is an embryonic defect, is referred to as *congenital atresia*. The auricle may be deformed or absent (*agenesis* of the auricle), or it may be normal. Naturally, a complete bony atresia of the canal produces a complete conductive loss, and if the condition is bilateral the infant will definitely be handicapped in language development. The remedy depends on the extent of functioning of the cochlea and on whether or not the middle-ear mechanism is intact. If middle and inner ears are normal, it is necessary for the surgeon only to open up the occluded canals for hearing to be made functional. More often than not, however, congenital atresia is accompanied by an anomaly of the middle ear as well. Frequently, the eardrum and ossicles are missing entirely, which would call for rather extensive surgery to construct a tympanic membrane and a substitute ossicular chain. Such surgery would, of course, presuppose a normally functioning inner ear, and fortunately the cochlea usually is normal because its embryology follows a different course from that of the outer and middle ears.[2]

A special instance of congenital atresia with accompanying deformation of the auricles and ossicles is Treacher-Collins syndrome, a genetic defect, characterized in addition by "facial bone abnormalities of structures formed from the first branchial arch including downward sloping palpebral fissures, depressed cheek bones . . . receding chin, and large fish-like mouth with frequent dental abnormalities."[3] Perhaps the most distinctive facial feature of

[2] Joseph Sataloff, *Hearing Loss* (Philadelphia: J. B. Lippincott Co., 1966), pp. 32–33.

[3] Jerry L. Northern and Marion P. Downs, *Hearing in Children* (Baltimore: Williams & Wilkins, 1974), p. 306.

these patients is the downward slant of the outer corners of the eyes in what Sataloff terms the "antimongoloid fashion."[4] Although children with Treacher-Collins syndrome have a grotesque appearance, which, together with the complete conductive impairment affecting their language development suggests mental retardation, actually 95 percent of them are not mentally retarded. Usually, their sensori-neural mechanisms are normal, so their hearing can be improved by surgery.

Conditions of the middle ear.   1. *Otitis media.*   The most common cause of conductive impairment is an inflammation or infection of the middle ear known as *otitis media.* Almost everyone at sometime has had otitis media in some form. Frequently, it accompanies an upper respiratory infection, particularly in children. The connection between the middle ear and the nasopharynx, the Eustachian tube, provides an easy pathway for infection or inflammation to reach the ear. The common "earache" in children is usually a manifestation of otitis media.

Various terms are employed by otologists to categorize otitis media. Broadly, there are two main types: suppurative (or purulent) and nonsuppurative (or nonpurulent). *Suppurative* and *purulent* are synonymous terms that refer to the presence of pus. So, if pus is present in the middle ear, there is a suppurative otitis media. Any middle-ear inflammation that is not characterized by the presence of pus is, therefore, a nonsuppurative otitis media, although there may or may not be fluid in the middle ear.

The terms *acute* and *chronic* are frequently applied to otitis media, "An acute otitis media is an ear infection of comparatively short duration. If the acute otitis media does not respond satisfactorily to therapy and the infection persists for many months, it then becomes a chronic otitis media."[5] There may be repeated attacks of acute otitis media interspersed with periods of normal middle-ear conditions. Some people mistakenly refer to a lengthy period of alternating infections and normal middle ears as *chronic* otitis media, when the proper descriptive term is *recurrent* acute otitis media.[6]

Two types of middle-ear conditions are nonsuppurative: *secretory* and *serous* otitis media. In secretory otitis media, the mucosa of the middle ear is edematous (swollen) and thickened, and the fluid in the middle ear is mucus, secreted by the glands of the mucous membrane.[7] The mucoid fluid is straw colored, it may be thick and gel-like, and it may continue to accumulate despite treatment. In serous otitis media, the fluid in the middle ear is a tran-

[4] Sataloff, *Hearing Loss*, p. 35.

[5] Ibid., p. 70.

[6] Ibid.

[7] Elizabeth E. Payne and Michael M. Paparella, "Otitis Media," in *Hearing Disorders*, ed. Jerry L. Northern (Boston: Little, Brown and Company, 1976), chap. 10, p. 121.

sudate through the mucous membrane that closely resembles serum bio-chemically. The mucosa may be edematous but not thickened as it is in secretory otitis media.[8] Some authorities make no distinction between secretory and serous otitis media,[9] and some of those who differentiate the two conditions admit that it is hard to tell them apart.[10]

Acute suppurative otitis media is commonly seen in children. It is generally an extension of an upper respiratory infection that reaches the middle ear by way of the Eustachian tube. In rare cases, the infection may enter the middle ear through a perforation in the eardrum. The main symptom of the condition is a throbbing earache—*otalgia*—and a fever that may rise as high as 104 to 105 degrees Fahrenheit in children.[11] Some hearing loss will result from decreased mobility of the drum and ossicles and from the increased vibratory mass in the middle ear. The eardrum is red, thickened, and distended—that is, bulged outward—from the pressure built up within the middle ear, and if the pressure is not relieved, the eardrum may rupture spontaneously. The rupture releases the pressure, producing a discharge of purulent matter (*otorrhea*) in the canal and alleviating the pain. In most cases, the perforation resulting from a rupture of the eardrum will heal spontaneously, but a rupture may destroy a sizable portion of the drum or create a perforation too large to heal. That is why in the case of a threatened rupture the otologist prefers to incise the eardrum surgically to relieve pressure and produce drainage, as will be discussed in a later section on treatment.

Improper noseblowing may contribute to the secondary involvement of the ear during an upper respiratory infection. When the nostrils are pressed tightly together in blowing the nose, pressure is built up in the nasal passage, which forces mucous into the orifice of the Eustachian tube. The proper way to blow the nose is to press lightly on each nostril with the fingers without pinching the nostrils together.

If not controlled by antibiotics, the infection in the middle ear may spread into the air cells of the mastoid portion of the temporal bone by way of the aditus and antrum and produce acute *mastoiditis*, which has the potential for involving the meninges and the brain in life-threatening situations. Before the days of antibiotics, acute mastoiditis was one of the most common causes of death in young children.

The treatment of acute suppurative otitis media with antibiotics without also providing for complete drainage of the middle ear can result in what

[8] Ibid.

[9] D. Thane R. Cody, "Otologic Assessment and Treatment," in *Audiological Assessment*, ed. Darrell E. Rose (Englewood Cliffs, N.J.: Prentice-Hall, 1978), chap. 3, p. 79; David D. DeWeese and William H. Saunders, *Textbook of Otolaryngology* (St. Louis: C. V. Mosby, 1973), pp. 353–54.

[10] Sataloff, *Hearing Loss*, p. 67.

[11] DeWeese and Saunders, *Textbook of Otolaryngology*, p. 351.

Goodhill and Guggenheim have termed "unresolved" otitis media. This is a situation characterized by hearing loss associated with the retention of fluid in the middle ear. Goodhill and Guggenheim state,

> Acute otitis media with secretion deserves prompt surgical drainage . . . along with proper and adequate antibiotic therapy. Even though the acute inflammatory process may subside with antibiotic therapy alone, the persistence of even sterile fluid as a sequel of otitis media not only is a temporary threat to hearing, but may also produce permanent deafness by long-range damage to tympanic structures (fibrosis, necrosis of incudal long process, etc.).[12]

When the infection in the middle ear persists for long periods despite antibiotic treatment, the condition becomes a chronic suppurative otitis media. "There is invariably a perforation in the eardrum."[13] The most common symptoms of the condition are hearing loss and discharge of foul-smelling matter.[14] Chronic suppurative otitis media may produce pathological changes in the mucosa of the middle ear and erosion of the ossicles. Not uncommonly, the erosion may produce a disarticulation of the incus and the stapes. Central perforations of the eardrum are not as serious as perforations that involve the margin of the drum. The danger with a marginal perforation is that a pseudotumor called *cholesteatoma* will develop and invade the middle ear. According to DeWeese and Saunders,

> It (cholesteatoma) occurs most often when there is a marginal perforation of the eardrum that allows squamous epithelium from the external auditory canal to grow into the middle ear. The epitympanum (attic) of the middle ear may then become lined by squamous epithelium. As squamous epithelium grows, it desquamates, and keratin and cellular debris collect inside the middle ear. Slow enlargement of the cholesteatoma leads to expansion into the mastoid antrum.[15]

Goodhill and Guggenheim say that cholesteatoma is really a misnomer because the growth contains little cholesterol. They use the term *keratoma* synonymously with cholesteatoma because the growths consist of concentric layers of squamous epithelium that are predominantly keratin.[16] They also point out that keratomas may occur spontaneously behind an intact eardrum and in the absence of any infection in the middle ear. Cholesteatomas represent a threat to life because they can invade the cranial cavity, and so they must be removed. The potential of cholesteatoma occurring is a compelling

---

[12] Victor Goodhill and Paul Guggenheim, "Pathology, Diagnosis, and Therapy of Deafness," in *Handbook of Speech Pathology and Audiology,* ed. Lee Edward Travis (Englewood Cliffs, N.J.: Prentice-Hall, 1971), chap. 12, pp. 302–303.

[13] Sataloff, *Hearing Loss,* p. 71.

[14] Payne and Paparella, "Otitis Media," p. 125.

[15] DeWeese and Saunders, *Textbook of Otolaryngology,* p. 359.

[16] Goodhill and Guggenheim, "Pathology of Deafness," p. 307.

reason for the surgical repair of any perforation in the eardrum. According to Goodhill and Guggenheim, cholesteatomas occur in about 50 percent of cases of chronic suppurative otitis media.[17]

As we said earlier, in secretory otitis media the middle ear contains a straw-colored fluid that may be thick. According to Sataloff, the Eustachian tube may be *patent* (functional), and the fluid in the ear may continue to form and distend the eardrum until it ruptures. Thus, there is a situation akin to suppurative otitis media except that the discharge is virtually sterile.[18] In serous otitis media, the fluid is a transudate associated with a nonfunctioning Eustachian tube and resulting retracted eardrum. The middle ear receives its ventilation and oxygen through the Eustachian tube. The tube is the pressure-regulating device for the middle ear, enabling us to undergo changes in atmospheric pressure without suffering discomfort in the ears or loss of any hearing function. Blockage of the Eustachian tube will lower the air pressure within the middle ear as the oxygen is absorbed by tissue, and the eardrum will be forced inward (retracted) owing to the greater pressure on the outside surface of the drum. Retraction of the drum interferes with its mobility and thus with its ability to vibrate in response to sound waves. A hearing loss is the result. If the condition producing the drum retraction persists, the middle ear will gradually fill with a serous fluid. If the middle ear contains both air and fluid, the otologist can see through the drum membrane a fluid line or *meniscus*; but if the middle-ear cavity is completely filled with fluid there is no meniscus, and it is difficult to tell by inspection alone whether or not the middle ear contains fluid. If the eardrum does not move when the otologist applies pressure to it, the presence of fluid in the ear is suspected.

The Eustachian tube blockage responsible for serous otitis media may be due to edema of the lining of the tube, resulting from allergy or infection, or it may be caused by adenoid tissue around the orifice of the tube, or sometimes—following adenoidectomy—by scar tissue. The child who is an habitual mouth-breather is evidencing blockage of the nasopharynx owing to enlarged adenoids and/or allergy and may very well have some hearing loss if the adenoid growth or swollen tissue prevents normal functioning of the Eustachian tube.

Serous otitis media does not cause pain, and often the hearing loss is slight. Sataloff says, "The diagnosis of serous otitis as a cause of hearing loss in children often is overlooked, because the hearing loss rarely exceeds 30 dB, and children generally are addressed in a loud voice. Thus their hearing difficulty is not detected until the school audiogram is performed, or until the symptom has persisted for a long time."[19] The longer fluid is allowed to remain in the middle-ear cavity, the greater the danger of permanent damage to the

[17] Ibid.
[18] Sataloff, *Hearing Loss*, p. 65.
[19] Ibid., p. 68.

mucosa and to the ossicles, and also the more difficult it is to remove. In time, the fluid thickens and becomes gluelike in consistency, and adhesions may form on the ossicles, damaging or destroying them. Such a condition is referred to as *adhesive* otitis media. Whenever a child has an upper respiratory infection, parents should be alert to any indications that the ears are becoming involved. At the first sign of such involvement, they should seek the assistance of an otolaryngologist. Likewise, after the acute phase of an upper respiratory infection has passed, parents should be aware of the possibility of "unresolved" otitis media, that is, the continuation of fluid in the ear, and carefully observe the child for any indication that hearing may be impaired.

When the Eustachian tube is not functioning normally, changes in outside air pressure can cause middle-ear problems and hearing loss. It is for this reason that it is inadvisable to fly when one has a cold. If the tube cannot enable the ear to accommodate to changes in outside pressure, the eardrum will be forced outward as the plane gains altitude and inward as the plane descends. So many flyers in World War II suffered from Eustachian tube malfunctioning that the name *aerotitis* was attached to the condition. Divers, who must work under conditions of increased atmospheric pressure, will also be subject to considerable pain and distress if their Eustachian tubes are not functioning properly. Sometimes the term *barotrauma* is used to refer to middle-ear difficulties resulting from exposure to abnormal atmospheric pressure. If one's Eustachian tubes do not open spontaneously when descending in an airplane, and the eardrums retract with resulting hearing loss and discomfort—*and if one is not suffering from an upper respiratory infection*—it is possible to "clear the ears" (return the eardrums to their normal positions and restore hearing to normal) by means of what is called the *Valsalva* technique. This is performed by pinching the nostrils together and gently forcing air into the blocked-off nasal passage. The increased air pressure forces the Eustachian tube to open and sends air to the middle ear, balancing the pressures on both sides of the eardrum. It may be necessary to repeat this maneuver two or three times in the course of the descent. Each time the eardrums return to their normal positions, the restoration of hearing to normal levels is dramatic. Suddenly, the noises of the aircraft and conversations of one's fellow passengers increase in loudness. Then as the eardrums begin to retract again, there is a gradual fading away of environmental noises until the Valsalva technique is applied again. The reason for cautioning against utilizing this method of clearing the ears when one has an upper respiratory infection should be obvious. Forcing the Eustachian tubes to open could result in extending the infection to the middle ears. Of course, anyone with an upper respiratory infection should not be flying in the first place.

2. *Otosclerosis.* This is a disease process that affects the bony capsule of the inner ear, turning the normally hard bone into vascularized, spongy bone. It produces a progressive hearing loss through the fixation, or *ankylosis,* of the stapes in the oval window, owing to the invasion of the spongy bone. Ac-

tually, otosclerosis is a misnomer for this condition because "sclerosis" means "hardening." Some authorities have proposed the term *otospongiosis* as being more descriptive of the disease process. In any event, the disease apparently is hereditary; for some unknown reason it affects the Caucasian race primarily, and women are more susceptible than men. So far, no one has been able to discover what causes it. Apparently, many people are otosclerotics without being aware of it because, although the disease is limited to the otic capsule, it does not necessarily occur at or around the oval window. According to Walsh, otosclerosis is responsible for about one million cases of hearing loss in the United States.[20]

A diagnosis of clinical otosclerosis is made when a hearing loss of a conductive type occurs in a relatively young person (late teens or early twenties, usually), and there is no other apparent explanation for the loss. In other words, the eardrum is normal in appearance, and there is no history of a middle-ear type of disorder. Occasionally, there may be a pinkness or redness visible through the eardrum, called *Schwartze's sign*, which apparently is caused by vascularization of the bony promontory. Frequently, there is a history of progressive hearing loss in the family, although not necessarily so, because several generations of the family may have had otosclerosis without an effect on their hearing. Occasionally, otosclerosis will be diagnosed in a child, but generally it is a disease of early adulthood. The hearing loss may progress quite rapidly, so that noticeable changes in the degree of loss occur from year to year. Often a pregnancy is blamed for a marked, sudden drop in hearing acuity in an otosclerotic woman. Although usually otosclerosis produces a conductive loss because the problem is one of transmitting vibrations to the fluid of the inner ear, occasionally the disease may invade the inner ear and cause a pure sensori-neural impairment that has been designated by some as *labyrinthine* or *cochlear otosclerosis*.[21] Even though in its initial stages the loss produced may be a purely conductive one, it is quite common for the inner ear to become involved in later stages of the disease.

Otosclerosis is almost always accompanied by an annoying tinnitus. Frequently, the tinnitus will be much more disturbing to the patient than the hearing loss.

3. *Other conditions.*   Other middle-ear conditions that may produce conductive impairments include tumors, tympanosclerosis, myringitis bullosa, Paget's disease, and Van der Hoeve's syndrome. Although tumors in the middle ear are rare, they do occur. Carcinoma in the middle ear has a high mortality rate. It may occur after a long-standing chronic suppurative otitis media, or it may occur spontaneously. A *glomus jugulare* tumor is a vascular growth that

---

[20]T. E. Walsh, "The Surgical Treatment of Hearing Loss," in *Hearing and Deafness*, 1st ed., ed. Hallowell Davis (New York: Rinehart, 1947), chap. 5, p. 104.

[21]Eugene L. Derlacki, "Otosclerosis," in *Hearing Disorders*, ed. Jerry L. Northern, chap. 11, p. 131.

originates from the glomus bodies—small vascular structures around the dome of the jugular bulb, located just beneath the floor of the middle ear. The bulb is a dilation of the internal jugular vein. The tumor may expand into the middle ear, where it causes hearing loss because of pressure on the ossicles and a pulsating tinnitus synchronous with the heart beat;[22] it may even cause a rupture of the eardrum and protrude into the canal. The tumor must be surgically removed, and controlling the bleeding during surgery can be a serious problem.

Following a chronic suppurative otitis media, there may be a deposit of layers of bone over the promontory and around the oval window. According to Sataloff, the incus and stapes may be "enveloped by stratified bone that can be peeled off in layers."[23] The name for this condition is *tympanosclerosis*. It may resemble otosclerosis audiologically because of fixation of the ossicular chain, but it is an entirely different disease process. Usually, the eardrum is thickened and scarred and only one ear is affected.

Myringitis bullosa is a viral infection of the outer layer of the eardrum in which blisters appear on the drum. The mobility of the drum is impaired, and a slight hearing loss results. Usually, the condition is unilateral. When the blisters are punctured or spontaneously rupture, they discharge a thin fluid that may be tinged with blood. This is one instance in which a discharge into the canal does not represent a perforated eardrum.

Paget's disease and *Van der Hoeve's syndrome* are both conditions that pathologically are similar to otosclerosis. Paget's disease is a systemic disease "manifested by an uncontrolled growth of a dystrophic type of bone strongly resembling the spongiose stage of otosclerosis."[24] The disease primarily affects the skull, spine, and shins. It can produce either a conductive impairment through fixation of the stapes or a sensori-neural impairment because of a serous exudate into the labyrinth or pressure on the VIIIth nerve in the internal acoustic meatus.[25] Van der Hoeve's syndrome is a combination of *osteogenesis imperfecta, blue sclera,* and hearing loss. In osteogenesis imperfecta, the bones are extremely brittle and easily fractured. Blue sclera refers to a distinctive bluish cast to the white of the eye. Each of these conditions may occur in isolation or in combination. Osteogenesis imperfecta and blue sclera appear to be genetically related to otosclerosis.

Treatment

Fortunately, patients with conductive hearing losses have available to them medical and surgical treatment, which usually can improve the hearing and frequently restore it completely. The simplest type of hearing loss to

[22] Goodhill and Guggenheim, "Pathology of Deafness," p. 308.
[23] Sataloff, *Hearing Loss,* p. 73.
[24] Goodhill and Guggenheim, "Pathology of Deafness, p. 316.
[25] Sataloff, *Hearing Loss,* p. 100.

remedy is, of course, that occasioned by obstruction caused by cerumen or a foreign object in the external meatus. The wax or foreign matter is removed by means of instruments and/or irrigation. If no other causative factor is operating, the removal of the obstruction will restore the hearing. Mention has already been made that in the case of congenital atresia the surgeon opens up the occluded canals. If the middle and inner ears are normal, no additional surgery is required.

The treatment for acute suppurative otitis media is usually the administration of one or more of the antibiotic drugs, in order to control the infection in the ear as well as to remove the original source of infection. If there is any danger that the drum might spontaneously rupture, the physician will make an incision in the drum to allow the middle ear to drain. This operation is called a *myringotomy*. The advantage of a myringotomy is that the surgical incision is made in the best place in the drum for drainage and for quick healing to occur—usually the posterior-inferior quadrant—whereas a spontaneous rupture may occur anywhere on the drum and may be slow to heal, with the formation of scar tissue that can impede the vibration of the drum. Also, of course, a spontaneous rupture may destroy so much of the drum that a permanent perforation results.

In chronic otitis media, with drainage through a perforation and possibly with the presence of cholesteatoma, there is always the danger that the infection or the growth will reach the covering of the brain and cause meningitis or other complications. Where this danger exists, it may be necessary as a preventive measure for the otologist to perform an operation on the middle ear. The operation of choice is a *modified radical mastoidectomy*, in which an attempt is made to clear up the disease process without sacrificing any of the middle-ear structures. A successful modified radical mastoidectomy does not produce additional hearing loss and may even succeed in restoring some hearing function that has been lost as a result of the disease process. Occasionally, it is not possible to clear up the disease process except by removing the eardrum, the malleus, and the incus—a procedure called a *radical mastoidectomy*. Naturally, a radical mastoidectomy produces a marked hearing loss by destroying the sound-conducting mechanism. The operation is not designed to improve the hearing but to remove a threat to life. If the inner-ear apparatus is normal, even a patient who has had a bilateral radical mastoidectomy can receive considerable benefit from a hearing aid.

Spontaneous rupture of the eardrum may result in a perforation that will not heal. As mentioned previously in this chapter, such perforations produce some hearing impairment, the degree depending on the size and location of the perforation. Perforated drums pose a constant potential hazard to the middle ear. Fortunately, techniques have evolved that are successful in many instances in eliminating the perforation and restoring the normal vibratory function of the drum. One of these procedures induces healing of the drum by irritating the edges of the perforation with acid. Sometimes, a thin paper patch placed over the perforation will assist in the healing, especially when the patch is used in conjunction with acid treatment of the edges of the perforation. With a patch in place, the patient's hearing is improved, although the patch, of course, is only to assist the healing process and is not intended as a prosthesis. If healing will not occur as a result of repeated acid treatments, with or without the assistance of a patch, surgical repair of the eardrum, called *myringoplasty,* may be performed.

Until relatively recently, the preferred material for grafting on the eardrum was vein wall, *perichondreum* (the fibrous membrane covering cartilage) obtained from the tragus of the auricle, or *fascia* (the fibrous material covering muscle), usually taken from the temporalis muscle that closes the jaw. Since the mid-1960s, transplants of human eardrums, referred to as *homografts,* have been used successfully to repair perforated eardrums. Homografts are obtained from temporal bones removed from cadavers at the time of autopsy and stored in temporal bone banks. In reporting on five years of experience with almost 400 cases of homograft transplants in myringoplasty, Wehrs stated that the primary advantage of the homograft was its natural cone shape. He reported a graft survival rate of 94 percent of his patients and a good hearing result in 87 percent.[26] In an audiological study comparing the postmyringoplasty results of patients with homografts and patients with temporalis fascia grafts, Gladstone found that the former achieved more normal tympanic membrane function than did the latter.[27]

Today, a great deal of otological surgery is devoted to the preservation or improvement of function, in contrast to the preantibiotic times when most surgery was of the life-saving variety. Naturally, where a life was at stake, little attention was paid by surgeon or patient to the preservation of hearing. The myringoplasty is one of a class of reconstructive operations called *tympanoplasty.* All the tympanoplasty procedures have as their objective the restoration of hearing through repair or reconstruction of damaged parts of the middle ear. The principle followed in tympanoplasty is that there must be reciprocal action of the oval and round windows in order for maximum movement of the cochlear fluids to occur. In the normal ear, the eardrum and ossicular chain provide a magnification of sound pressure at the oval window that is greatly in excess of any pressure exerted through the middle-ear cavity on the round window. Moreover, energy that reaches the round window from the eardrum is transmitted through the air in the middle-ear cavity and is in opposite phase to the vibrations reaching the oval window through the ossicular chain. If the mechanical advantage of the oval window is reduced or

[26] R. Wehrs, "The Homograft Tympanic Membrane: A Five-Year Study," *Transactions of the American Academy of Ophthalmology and Otolaryngology* 82 (1976): 39–43.

[27] Vic S. Gladstone, "A Comparison of the Effects of Middle Ear Grafting Material on Acoustic Impedance Measurements and Audiometry," Unpublished Ph.D. Dissertation, University of Maryland, 1977.

eliminated through an interruption in the ossicular chain, or if the phase difference between the two windows is altered because of a large perforation in the eardrum, a hearing loss results. The tympanoplasty seeks to restore the mechanical advantage of the oval window and the reciprocal action of the two windows to permit maximum fluid motion in the cochlea. According to Shambaugh, "The ideal tympanoplasty restores sound protection for the round window by constructing a closed, air-containing middle ear against the round window membrane, and restores sound pressure transformation for the oval window by connecting a large tympanic membrane or substitute membrane with the stapes footplate either via an intact ossicular chain, or the stapes alone or a substitute stapes."[28]

There are five basic types of tympanoplasty as described originally by Wullstein.[29] Type I is the repair of a perforated eardrum—a myringoplasty. Type II is performed when there is a perforated drum with an eroded malleus, and the perforation is closed with a graft attached to the incus. In Type III, both malleus and incus are missing, but the stapes is present and mobile. The graft is attached directly to the head of the stapes. Type IV is performed when only the footplate of the stapes is present; but it is mobile. The eardrum graft is attached directly to the footplate. In Type V, the stapes is fixed in the oval window so a fenestration of the horizontal semicircular canal is performed (as described later in this section under surgery for otosclerosis). Figure 3–1 illustrates the types of tympanoplasty, except for Type I. In theory, Types I, II, and III should provide normal or close to normal hearing. Because with Types IV and V there is no transformer action of the middle ear, the best hearing that can result is a loss of around 25 dB. Just as homografts may be used to repair perforations in the tympanic membrane, so transplants of cadaver eardrums plus one or two attached ossicles can be used to repair the middle ear in lieu of one of the original types of tympanoplasty just described.

Treatment of otitis media of the drum-retracted type is directed toward restoring the patency of the Eustachian tubes. If the tubes have been blocked because of edematous tissue in the nasopharynx, treatment will be directed toward controlling the condition that has produced the swelling of the nasal tissue. Even after the swelling in the nasal passages has been controlled, the tube will not regain patency immediately. Frequently, it will require from a week to ten days before the tube regains its normal function and the drum returns to its normal position. In the meantime, of course, any hearing loss that has been caused by the retraction of the drum will persist. The otolaryngologist may help the tube regain its function by a technique called *inflation*. Usually, in inflation the physician inserts a catheter through the nostril

[28] George E. Shambaugh, Jr., *Surgery of the Ear* (Philadelphia: W. B. Saunders, 1967), p. 451.

[29] H. Wullstein, "Theory and Practice of Tympanoplasty," *Laryngoscope* 66 (July 1956):1076–93.

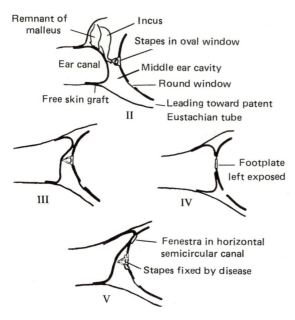

FIGURE 3-1.   Types II, III, IV, and V tympanoplasty. (From David D. DeWeese and
William H. Saunders, *Textbook of Otolaryngology,* 4th ed., St. Louis: C.
V. Mosby Co., 1973. Reproduced by permission.)

until its tip makes contact with the orifice of the Eustachian tube; the physician then forces a small amount of air through the tube into the middle ear. The air forced into the middle ear restores normal air pressure in the middle ear, which permits the drum to move from its position of retraction to its normal position. An immediate improvement in hearing is noted by the patient. Unless the Eustachian tube retains patency, however, the oxygen will soon be absorbed from the air in the middle ear, and the drum will retract again. The process of inflation may speed up the recovery of the proper functioning of the tube, however. This is a technique that should be applied sparingly, as resorting to inflation too frequently may cause the eardrum to become "floppy" and lose its normal resilience. Inflation should not be used when there is a danger of spreading infection from the nasopharynx to the middle ear.

When the drum retraction is due to the presence of excess lymphoid tissue around the orifice of the Eustachian tube in the nasopharynx, the only remedy is to remove the tissue through adenoidectomy. Formerly, irradiation, usually by x-ray but sometimes by direct application of a radium capsule, was used to remove any adenoid tags around the orifice of the Eustachian tube remaining after an adenoidectomy. Because of the remote danger of thyroid cancer occurring twenty to thirty years following irradiation in the nasopharynx, however, this practice has been discontinued.

The treatment for serous otitis media is aimed at removing the fluid in the middle ear. Usually, a myringotomy will suffice, but on occasion it may be necessary to employ suction, particularly if the fluid in the middle ear has thickened, or to insert tubing through the myringotomy incision to provide continual drainage. Figure 3–2 shows two polyethylene (PE) tubes placed in myringotomy incisions in the eardrum to promote drainage and aeration of the middle ear. Without the tubes, the myringotomy incisions would heal, probably before the middle ear was completely drained. The PE tubes may be left in place for weeks or months. Sometimes, a myringotomy combined with inflation will serve to evacuate the fluid from the middle ear.

Surgery for otosclerosis has posed a challenge of great interest to otologists since the latter part of the nineteenth century. The first attempts at improving hearing in cases of otosclerosis were directed at mobilizing the fixated stapes. In 1890, Miot reported on a series of 200 stapes mobilization procedures performed in a manner similar to the technique described by Rosen in the 1950s.[30] Stapes mobilization consists of laying back the eardrum and manipulating the ossicular chain with an instrument, usually at the point of

FIGURE 3–2.   Drainage tubes placed through anterior and posterior myringotomy incisions in a right tympanic membrane. (From Victor Goodhill and Paul Guggenheim, "Pathology, Diagnosis, and Therapy of Deafness," chap. 12 in Lee Edward Travis, ed., *Handbook of Speech Pathology and Audiology,* copyright © 1971. Reprinted by permission of Prentice-Hall, Inc.)

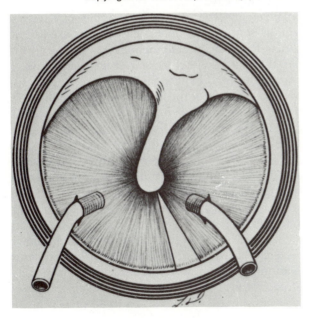

[30] Shambaugh, *Surgery of the Ear*, p. 502.

the incudo-stapedial joint, until the stapes is broken free of the otosclerotic growth that surrounds it. For reasons that are not clear, the stapes mobilization operation was abandoned around the turn of the twentieth century. Shambaugh speculates that it may have resulted in some serious infections of the middle ear and the labyrinth, which discouraged otologists from attempting operations on the ear.[31]

Also late in the nineteenth century, there were some attempts to correct hearing impairment due to otosclerosis by bypassing the fixated stapes and creating a new window (*fenestra*) in the wall of the labyrinth. Early in the twentieth century, the first *fenestration* operation on the horizontal semicircular canal was performed. Holmgren in Sweden pioneered in fenestration surgery and was the first to employ the operating microscope in ear surgery. He had difficulty in keeping the labyrinthine window free from bony closure, but he inspired others, notably Sourdille of France, to experiment with techniques of fenestration that finally succeeded in maintaining a mobile window. Sourdille, in the 1920s and 1930s, performed many successful fenestration operations through a procedure involving two or more stages. In this country, Lempert, in the late 1930s and 1940s, perfected a one-stage fenestration operation that became very popular. Otologists from all over the world flocked to New York to receive instruction on the revolutionary new technique that was to restore the hearing of thousands of otosclerotics to useful levels.

Briefly, the operation consists of making an endaural approach (through the external canal) to the middle-ear cavity, laying aside the eardrum, and removing the head of the malleus and the incus. The middle-ear cavity is enlarged so that the horizontal semicircular canal can be exposed. The surgeon then creates a fenestra in the horizontal semicircular canal and covers this window with the skin flap that has been cut loose in laying aside the eardrum. The purpose of the operation is to bypass the oval window that has been made inoperative through the fixation of the stapes and to provide a new window through which sound vibrations can reach the inner ear. Because the perilymph of the semicircular canals is continuous with the perilymph of the cochlea, movement of the fluid in the horizontal canal will be transmitted to the end organ of hearing. For the operation to be successful, it is necessary that the round window membrane be mobile, as two windows are essential for the transmission of sound through the incompressible fluid of the inner ear.

The fenestration operation cannot restore a patient's hearing to normal, because in the course of the operation the ossicular chain, an important part of the sound-conducting mechanism, has been broken by the elimination of the malleus and incus. Experience has shown that the maximum result obtainable through the fenestration operation is restoration of the hearing to within 20 to 30 dB of normal. This is not to say that the operation is undesirable, however, because a residual loss of only 20 to 30 dB will seem

[31] Ibid., p. 503.

almost like normal hearing to a patient whose preoperative loss may have been as great as 70 dB.

In 1952, while testing the mobility of the ossicular chain in a patient whom he was considering as a candidate for fenestration, Rosen, a New York otologist, "accidentally" performed a stapes mobilization that resulted in a sudden, dramatic improvement in the patient's hearing. The following year, Rosen reported on the results of a number of operations in which he was successful at purposely mobilizing the stapes. His experience of "rediscovering" the principle of improving the hearing in otosclerotics by restoring the mobility of the ossicular chain resulted in a swing away from the fenestration operation by most otologists. The stapes mobilization was a simpler operation from the standpoint of the patient, and when successful it could restore hearing to normal or close to normal levels, whereas the fenestration operation, even at its best, left the patient with a residual hearing deficit of about 20 dB. The chances for a "successful" operative result from the fenestration procedure, however, were about eight in ten as compared with about five in ten for the stapes mobilization.

In 1956, a new technique of surgery for otosclerosis was reported by Shea of Memphis, Tennessee. This technique, called *stapedectomy*, consisted of completely removing the stapes. A vein graft was used to close the oval window, and a polyethylene "strut" was inserted between the lenticular process of the incus and the vein graft. Other otologists followed Shea's lead in removing the stapes and creating a prosthetic link between the incus and the oval window, and at the present writing the stapedectomy procedure is the operation of choice for restoring hearing in cases of otosclerosis. Otologists differ in their preferences for materials to close the oval window (vein; fatty tissue from the ear lobe; gelfoam; fascia, for example, from the temporalis muscle; periosteum; perichondreum; or other connective tissue)[32] and to connect the incus with the oval window (polyethylene, teflon, stainless steel, tantalum, or platinum).[33] Regardless of the materials used, the principle of the operation is the same: the stapes in its entirety is removed and a substitute "ossicle" is inserted in its place, connecting the incus with the oval window, which has been closed by means of gelfoam or transplanted tissue. Figure 3–3 illustrates steps in a stapedectomy in which a stainless steel wire attached to fatty tissue is used as the prosthesis. An alternative to complete removal of the stapes is a procedure in which the footplate of the stapes is left in the oval window and the remainder of the bone is removed. A hole is drilled through the footplate (fenestration of the footplate) and a piston of teflon or steel is fitted in the hole and attached to the long process of the incus, usually with a stainless steel wire. This procedure may be employed when the extent of otosclerotic growth obliterates the footplate and makes its removal difficult or inadvisable. Most

[32] Derlacki, "Otosclerosis," p. 133.
[33] Goodhill and Guggenheim, "Pathology of Deafness," p. 315.

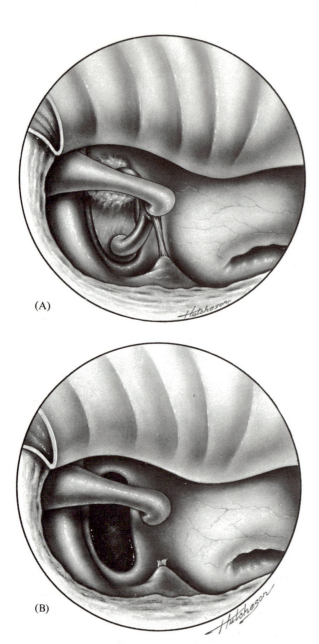

FIGURE 3–3. Three steps in a stapedectomy. (A) The eardrum has been laid back exposing the incus and stapes. Otosclerotic growth can be seen on the anterior of the stapes footplate. (B) The tendon of the stapedius muscle has been cut and the entire stapes has been removed. (C) The oval window has been closed with fatty tissue attached to a stainless steel wire crimped around the long process of the incus. (From D. Thane R. Cody, "Otologic Assessment and Treatment," chap. 3 in Darrell E. Rose, ed., *Audiological Assessment,* copyright © 1978. Reprinted by permission of Prentice-Hall, Inc.)

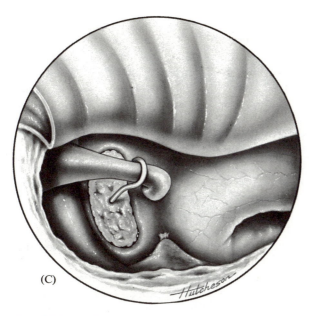

(C)

FIGURE 3-3. *Continued.*

surgeons perform the stapedectomy operation under local anesthesia. A binocular microscope provides excellent visualization of the middle ear through the ear canal, once the eardrum has been incised and elevated. It may be necessary to remove some bone from around the ear canal in order to bring the stapes into view. The stapes is removed with appropriate instruments, and the prosthesis is put in place, after which the eardrum is replaced and held in position by packing. The patient frequently will experience a dramatic improvement in hearing while on the operating table. Later, there may be a decline in hearing until healing has taken place, a process that requires from one to two weeks. A month following the operation, the hearing should be at its maximum, although there may be some slight additional gain noticed through the next six months.

As in the case of stapes mobilization, the stapedectomy procedure is, for the patient, a minor operation compared with the fenestration. The patient usually leaves the hospital the day after the operation, and rarely is there any complication such as a persistent dizziness. In contrast, the patient who has a fenestration operation must spend up to two weeks in the hospital, the operation must be performed under general anesthesia, and frequently the patient will have severe dizziness for weeks or months following the operation. Moreover, the fenestration operation permanently alters the anatomy of the ear and imposes limitations on the patient, such as inability to go swimming, whereas stapedectomy provides a minimum of modification of the ear's anatomy, and the patient is not limited in activities following the operation.

As is true also with stapes mobilization, the potential improvement in hearing is much greater with the stapedectomy than with fenestration. If the operation is completely successful, the entire conductive block can be eliminated. The operation is considered to be successful if air-conduction hearing can be restored to within 10 dB of bone-conduction hearing. According to Schuknecht, excellent results are obtained in over 90 percent of "carefully done" stapedectomy operations, which exceeds the percentage of success achieved with fenestration. Many patients, having had greatly improved hearing in the operated ear, will want the other ear operated on also. If the hearing in the operated ear remains good for from six months to a year, there is no reason for not operating on the other ear. To date, there have been very few complications resulting from reactions to the plastic strut or steel wire. The operation has a low rate of failure; in only 2 percent of stapedectomies is there a greater loss following the operation. Ninety-five percent of the patients who have been periodically checked have maintained their improved hearing over a three- to five-year period.[34]

Two other operative procedures for improvement of hearing in cases of otosclerosis should be mentioned. One of these is called "partial" stapedectomy. The usual site of origin of otosclerotic bone is just anterior to the oval window, and the first part of the stapes to be involved is the anterior portion of the footplate.[35] Hough suggested a way to separate the fixated part of the footplate from the rest of the stapes by cutting the anterior crus and bisecting the footplate. The posterior crus then transmits motion from the incus to the freed posterior half of the footplate.[36] The other procedure is called *stapedoplasty* and was described by Goodhill and Guggenheim. It involves removing the anterior crus and the footplate of the stapes and closing the oval window with a perichondrium graft or with gelfoam. The connection between the incus and the oval window is maintained by the posterior crus.[37] The advantages of partial stapedectomy and stapedoplasty are that the stapedial reflex is maintained, and it is not necessary to utilize a foreign substance in connecting the incus with the oval window. Figure 3–4 illustrates partial and complete stapedectomy procedures.

None of these operations can succeed in restoring hearing that has been lost as a result of inner-ear pathology; they are successful only in removing the block in the sound-conducting system. It is important, therefore, to evaluate as precisely as possible the function of the inner ear in selecting candidates for these operations. The audiologist can be of great assistance to the otologist in

---

[34] Harold F. Schuknecht, "Stapedectomy Operation for Hearing Loss from Otosclerosis," *Sound* 1 (July–August 1962):21.

[35] DeWeese and Saunders, *Textbook of Otolaryngology*, p. 377.

[36] J. V. D. Hough, "Partial Stapedectomy: A Physiological Approach to Stapedial Ankylosis," *Journal of the American Medical Association* 187 (March 7, 1964):697–702.

[37] Goodhill and Guggenheim, "Pathology of Deafness," pp. 315–16.

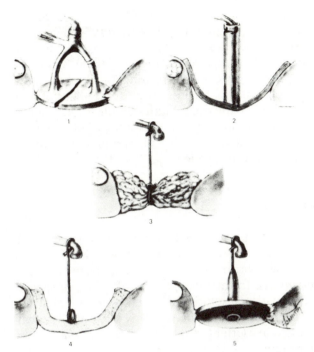

FIGURE 3-4. A partial stapedectomy is illustrated in 1; 2, 3, and 4 show complete stapedectomies. In 2, a polyethylene strut connects the incus with a vein graft in the oval window. In 3, a wire attached to fatty tissue replaces the stapes. In 4, the oval window is closed with gelfoam and a wire makes the connection. In 5, the footplate of the stapes remains in the oval window. A teflon piston attached to a wire crimped on the incus fits in a hole bored through the footplate. (From David D. DeWeese and William H. Saunders, *Textbook of Otolaryngology,* 5th ed., Saint Louis: C. V. Mosby Co., 1977. Reproduced by permission.)

the selection of patients who may be expected to receive reasonable benefit from one of these operations, as we shall see in a subsequent chapter.

Before leaving the subject of surgery for otosclerosis, mention should be made of a treatment suggested by Shambaugh, one of the pioneers in this type of surgery. The treatment consists of administering tablets of sodium fluoride to patients discovered to have progressive hearing loss because of otosclerosis. This produces recalcification of the spongy bone in the ear and arrests the progression of the hearing loss in most patients. Shambaugh was inspired to try this treatment by the finding that osteoporosis, a disease of bone characterized by increased porosity and decalcification, was much more prevalent in areas low in fluorides than in areas in which the fluoride count in water was high. A similar finding was reported in a study of the prevalence of otosclerosis. In 1964, he began prescribing sodium fluoride to otosclerotic patients and in ten years treated 2000 patients. Dr. Causse of Beziers, France, treated 2000 patients with sodium fluoride between 1969 and 1974. Shambaugh and Causse reported their findings jointly at the spring 1974 meeting of the American Otologic Society. They reported that some improvement in hearing was noted in 3 percent of the patients. Eighty percent achieved stabilization of what had been a progressive loss of hearing. In 17 percent, the treatment failed to arrest the progression of the loss. None of the 4000 patients received any permanent harm from taking the sodium fluoride.[38] Early detection of hearing loss and the prompt administration of sodium fluoride to those individuals diagnosed as otosclerotic may arrest the disease process before a handicapping hearing loss occurs, at least in the majority of those treated.

SENSORI-NEURAL IMPAIRMENTS

When the loss of hearing function is due to pathology in the inner ear or along the nerve pathway from the inner ear to the brain stem, the loss is referred to as a sensori-neural impairment (also written *sensorineural* or *sensory-neural*, or sometimes reversed, *neuro-sensory*). In this book, the word has been spelled "sensori-neural" in accordance with a resolution adopted by the Committee on the Conservation of Hearing of the American Academy of Ophthalmology and Otolaryngology and reported in a letter to the editor of the *Transactions of the Academy*. The resolution states,

> Since the end organ precedes the nerve functionally, this should be stressed by placing sensori before neural when speaking of hearing loss. The first part of the word should be written "sensori" instead of "sensory" because sensory is a complete word whereas sensori is not. Therefore, employment of the latter spelling tends to imply more positively that while some lesions are purely sensory and others are purely neural, a substantial fraction are probably composite. This is an important possibility to keep in mind pending the day when we can positively separate cochlear lesions from neural lesions, and these from true sensory-neural composites.
>
> The second part of the word should be written "neural" with a hyphen separating sensori from neural. The inclusion of the hyphen helps remind us that the term is really a wastebasket term, covering some cases with pure sense organ lesions, some with pure nerve fiber lesions, and some which are composites of the two. Omission of the hyphen would tend to imply that most lesions are composite.[39]

Formerly, the terms *perceptive impairment* and *nerve loss* were used in place of what we now call sensori-neural impairment. A "pure" sensori-neural

---

[38] George E. Shambaugh, Jr., "Research Completed: Analysis of Results of Fluoride Treatment for Otospongiosis," *Newsletter of the Mid America Hearing Research Foundation* 5 (Autumn 1974):4–5.

[39] Henry L. Williams, Letter to the Editor, *Transactions of the American Academy of Ophthalmology and Otolaryngology* 67 (March–April 1963):225.

impairment exists when the sound-conducting mechanism, that is, the outer and middle ear, is normal in every respect. In other words, sound is conducted properly to the fluid of the inner ear, but it cannot be analyzed or perceived normally.

Symptoms

Just as certain generalizations could be made about patients with conductive losses, so we can generalize to some extent about the symptoms exhibited by patients with sensori-neural losses. The patient may speak with excessive loudness of voice in many situations where a loud voice is inappropriate. The reason is that, as we have seen, we hear our own voices to some degree through the mechanism of bone conduction. A person with a sensori-neural loss does not have normal hearing by bone conduction because the source of the difficulty is in the inner ear or nerve. Hence, the patient's own voice or others' voices are not heard normally. In order to achieve what appears to be adequate loudness, the patient's voice may be raised more loudly than is necessary for others to hear in comfort. The "shouting" type of hard-of-hearing person, therefore, is exhibiting one symptom of a sensori-neural loss. Although we may make generalizations concerning the relationship of a patient's voice level and the type of impairment, it should be realized, of course, that individuals with sensori-neural problems do not always speak in a loud voice, nor are people with conductive losses always difficult to hear. Many patients learn to regulate their voice levels appropriately, probably because of their sensitivity to the reactions of their listeners, acquired over a long period of time.

Generally, although not always, a sensori-neural impairment causes some difficulty in speech discrimination, even for speech at levels well above threshold. Although a sensori-neural loss may be severe or profound at all frequencies, the typical loss is characterized by better hearing for the lower frequencies than for the high frequencies. In fact, many people with sensori-neural losses may have normal or close-to-normal hearing sensitivity through 500 or even 1000 Hz and then drop off rapidly on the audiogram at higher frequencies. Such people have no difficulty in hearing voices at normal intensities because their low-frequency hearing sensitivity is unimpaired. Many consonants of the English language are characterized by high frequencies and weak intensities (such as *f, k,* and *s*). Thus, a sensori-neural impairment that affects chiefly the high frequencies would result in the inability of the patient to differentiate among many words that sound similar but contain different high-frequency consonants. For example, this patient might confuse the words *fake, cake,* and *sake* on the basis of hearing alone, because the initial or final consonant sound in any of the words is not heard. A patient with sensori-neural impairment might hear all these words as *a* because only the vowel sound would be heard. Because such a patient hears low frequencies well and high frequencies poorly, confusion may occur. There is no difficulty in hearing voices because low-frequency hearing is good, but there is difficulty in understanding what is said because of the inability to hear many consonants. It is useless to shout because speech can be heard easily and the patient would react to shouting as would a person with normal hearing. The difficulty is in understanding, and shouting may not help; in fact, it may hinder understanding. In speaking to a person with sensori-neural impairment, it is important to enunciate clearly and not to speak too rapidly. One should not exaggerate the sounds of speech but simply speak carefully and clearly. Many older patients with high-frequency-type sensori-neural losses complain that the present generation does not speak as carefully and precisely as people did when they were young. Although this may be true, it is probable that the difference is not in how people speak now and how they spoke then, but rather in how well the patient's hearing functioned in the past compared with its present functioning.

The negative reaction of patients with sensori-neural impairment to shouting is related to another characteristic of sensori-neural loss, at least of loss due to malfunctioning of the inner ear. This is the rapid increase of the sensation of loudness once the patient's threshold of hearing has been crossed. As we have seen previously, a conductive impairment acts to reduce the intensity of all sounds reaching the inner ear by the same amount, regardless of the strength of the sound wave (that is, up to the point of its reaching the patient's threshold of discomfort). The situation with some patients who have sensori-neural impairment is different; once a sound is intense enough to be perceived, an increase in intensity causes a disproportionate increase in the sensation of loudness. Thus, such a patient, with a sensori-neural loss of 40 dB, can just barely detect the presence of a sound with an intensity of 40 dB above the normal threshold. However, a sound with an intensity of 5 dB above threshold may be perceived by the patient with a loudness greater than that heard by a normal-hearing person at 5 dB above threshold. Further increases in the intensity of the stimulus would result in more rapid increases in the patient's sensation of loudness, so that a sound of 60 dB intensity above the normal threshold might be perceived with the same loudness as a normal ear would perceive a sound of that intensity. Thus, over a range of 20 dB in intensity of the stimulus, in this example, the patient's loudness perception has increased as much as the normal ear's over a range of 60 dB. This rapid increase in the sensation of loudness once threshold has been reached is referred to as *loudness recruitment,* or the *recruitment factor,* sometimes abbreviated as *RF.* Recruitment of loudness is characteristic of sensori-neural impairment because of cochlear involvement; it does not exist in cases of sensori-neural impairment resulting from lesions of the VIIIth nerve. Because of recruitment, and because of the speech-sound discrimination difficulty associated with this type of sensori-neural impairment, these patients do not hear well in noisy surroundings, in contrast to patients with conductive impairment.

Figure 3-5 illustrates the growth of loudness with increasing intensity in

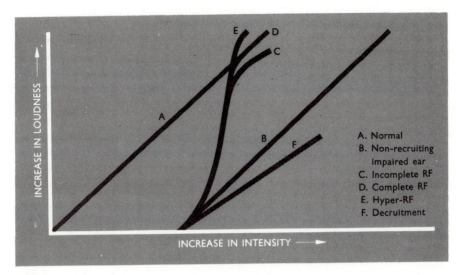

INCREASE IN LOUDNESS

A. Normal
B. Non-recruiting
   impaired ear
C. Incomplete RF
D. Complete RF
E. Hyper-RF
F. Decruitment

INCREASE IN INTENSITY ——▶

FIGURE 3-5. Three degrees of loudness recruitment compared with the growth of loudness in the normal ear and in the nonrecruiting impaired ear.

the normal ear, in the nonrecruiting impaired ear, in recruiting ears, and in an ear that exhibits the opposite of recruitment—*decruitment.* In both the normal and the nonrecruiting impaired ears, the growth of loudness is proportional to the increase of intensity. In the recruiting ears, the sensation of loudness increases out of proportion with increases in intensity. Three degrees of recruitment are illustrated in Figure 3-5. In complete recruitment the impaired ear catches up with the normal ear's sensation of loudness at some intensity above the impaired ear's threshold. In incomplete recruitment, the impaired ear's sensation of loudness increases disproportionately but never reaches the level of the normal ear's sensation of loudness. Hyper-recruitment occurs when a given intensity evokes a sensation of loudness that exceeds a normal ear's sensation of loudness for that intensity of the stimulus. Decruitment refers to a disproportionately slow increase in loudness with increasing intensity. It has been reported in association with a neural or *retrocochlear* impairment, in contrast with recruitment, which is associated with a cochlear type of sensori-neural impairment. Tests for determining the presence and degree of recruitment will be described in Chapter 7.

Sensori-neural impairment may be accompanied by a distortion in the sensation of pitch called *diplacusis.* In binaural diplacusis, the two ears respond to a given frequency in different ways. There may be simply a noticeable pitch difference between the ears, or one ear may perceive a pure tone normally, whereas the other perceives it as noise or something other than a pure tone. If a single stimulus produces two different sensations in the same ear, we call it *monaural diplacusis.*

The patient with sensori-neural impairment is usually subject to tinnitus

of a somewhat different sort from that associated with conductive impairment. Generally, the patient reports a constant "ringing" or "buzzing" noise,
which may be localized in either ear or may not be localized. In the experimental study of tinnitus referred to previously, it was found that patients with
sensori-neural impairment matched their tinnitus to pure tones covering a
wide frequency range, from 155 to 7800 Hz.[40] In general, the pitch of tinnitus
tends to be higher in sensori-neural impairment than in conductive impairment. Patients have reported getting up in the night to answer the telephone
or the doorbell, only to find that the noise was "in their heads."

Etiology

Most babies born with impaired hearing have sensori-neural impairments, with the principal exception of congenital atresia and its associated
middle-ear anomalies, referred to previously in the section on conductive impairments. Sensori-neural impairments may also be acquired at any time during life.

Congenital causes.   *Congenital* means existing at the time of birth.
Congenital defects may be hereditary (genetic) or nonhereditary (nongenetic).
In a study of 427 patients who had been hearing impaired at a very young age,
it was found that the etiology could be ascribed to heredity in 40.5 percent and
to nonhereditary factors in 31.5 percent. The etiology was unknown in 28 percent of the cases.[41] Inherited traits may be *dominant, recessive,* or *X-linked*
(sex-linked). In dominant inheritance, a trait can be transmitted if one parent
has an abnormal gene, and the trait generally appears in each generation of an
affected family. In recessive inheritance, each parent must have an abnormal
gene, and a child must inherit an abnormal gene from each parent in order to
display the trait. There is only one chance in four that this will happen. In
X-linked inheritance, a trait can be transmitted only from a mother to a son.
Females serve only as carriers and do not display the abnormal trait themselves. Hereditary hearing impairments can be either dominant or recessive
but rarely X-linked. Although hearing impairment can be inherited without
any other abnormality being present, in many cases it is only one of several inherited traits that constitute a *syndrome.* In the section on conductive impairments, mention was made of Treacher-Collins syndrome, a dominantly inherited condition including among its manifestations hearing loss because of
atresia. An example of a dominantly inherited syndrome including sensori-
neural hearing impairment is Waardenberg's syndrome. According to
Bergstrom,

---

[40] Graham and Newby, "Acoustical Characteristics of Tinnitus."
    [41] LaVonne Bergstrom, "Congenital Deafness," in *Hearing Disorders,* ed. Jerry L.
Northern, chap. 15, p. 173.

. . . A patient with all the manifestations has outward or lateral displacement (dystopia) of the medial canthi (slits between the eyelids) of the eyes; heterochromia of the irides (one iris may be pale blue, the other brown or a blue iris may have a brown quadrant); median white forelock of the hair; area of depigmentation of the skin; confluence of the eyebrows over the bridge of the nose; premature greying; obstruction of the nasolacrimal duct; a rather pinched-together appearance of the nostril area of the nose; a small, downturned mouth; and sensorineural CHL (congenital hearing loss).[42]

Not every patient may have every trait. For example, hearing impairment is present in only 20 percent of the cases, and it may be unilateral or bilateral, and mild to profound. Waardenburg's article describing the syndrome that now bears his name included in the title the primary traits that characterize the syndrome.[43] An example of a recessive disorder is Usher's syndrome, which combines a serious eye problem—retinitis pigmentosa, progressive loss of visual acuity and developing night blindness—with a profound degree of late-developing sensori-neural hearing impairment and ataxia.

Many times, congenital deafness can be explained in terms of damage to the embryo *in utero*. It is known, for example, that when the mother incurs certain diseases in pregnancy, usually but not always during the first three months, the embryo is subject to injury of various sorts, including impairments of hearing. German measles (rubella) is one of the most insidious diseases in its effects on the embryo. It may produce such anomalies, singly or in combination, as deafness or some lesser degree of hearing impairment, blindness, heart defects, cerebral palsy, and mental deficiency. Other diseases incurred by the mother during pregnancy may have harmful effects on the embryo or fetus—influenza, for example—but more is known about the effect of rubella than is known about the effect of any other disease.

Acquired causes.   Sensori-neural impairments may be acquired at any time during life. The causative agent may be disease, injury, toxic effect of drugs, or simply the inexorable process of growing older. By far, the most common cause of sensori-neural hearing impairment is the aging process. As the human organism grows older, sensory processes tend to deteriorate. In hearing, sensitivity for higher frequencies gradually diminishes with increasing years. The study of large samples of the population demonstrates that the process starts at about the age of twenty and becomes increasingly noticeable with each succeeding decade. This progressive loss of hearing because of increasing age is called *presbycusis* (also spelled *presbyacusis*). With medical science extending the life span more and more, problems of hearing loss due

[42] Ibid., p. 175.

[43] P. J. Waardenburg, "A New Syndrome Combining Developmental Anomalies of the Eyelids, Eyebrows and Nose Root with Pigmentary Defects of the Iris and Head Hair and with Congenital Deafness," *American Journal of Human Genetics* 3 (September 1951):195–253.

to presbycusis are increasing. Not all old people are hard of hearing, but the curves based on surveys of thousands of people show the mean hearing loss increasing and extending into the lower frequencies with each succeeding decade of life after age twenty. Surveys differ in the mean or median hearing-level values reported for various ages because of differences in sampling, differences in the age groupings reported, and perhaps also differences in testing environment and techniques. Table 3–1 presents information from one study of hearing levels (audiometric levels) of a select sample of males and females of various ages. Females tend to have better hearing than males except at frequencies below 1000 Hz in the older age groups. Recently, as we shall see in Chapter 9, evidence has been presented that in populations protected from the noises and other stresses of modern civilization, the effects on hearing that can be attributed to aging per se may be rather negligible. It is difficult if not impossible to separate the long-term effects on hearing of our exposure to modern civilization from the effects of the aging process. However, the hearing levels reported in Table 3–1 should represent reasonably good estimates of the effects of aging on males and females in our culture, because individuals with known otological problems or history of exposure to noise were excluded from the sample. Although presbycusis is listed here as a sensori-neural impairment, there is evidence that aging also affects the structures in the middle ear. The very elderly may have a substantial conductive component of their presbycusis.[44]

The diseases that may cause sensori-neural hearing impairment include measles, mumps, scarlet fever, diphtheria, whooping cough, influenza, and any of the unnamed virus infections. Such diseases may also cause conductive impairments through otitis media originating in an infection of the nasal passages. When these diseases produce a sensori-neural impairment, it is due to the toxic effect of the disease process on the sensitive nerve endings in the cochlea. Infections of the cerebrospinal fluid, such as meningitis, also cause sensori-neural impairments from cochlear damage. Tumorous growths in the region of the pathway of the VIIIth nerve between the cochlea and the brain stem may cause sensori-neural loss through pressure exerted on the nerve trunk. The most common tumor is an *acoustic neurinoma*, also known as an *acoustic neuroma* and an *acoustic nerve tumor*.[45] This benign (noncancerous) tumor apparently originates in the cells of the sheath of Schwann covering the vestibular portion of the VIIIth nerve and, according to Weaver and Northern, might more accurately be called a *vestibular neurilemmoma* or *schwannoma*.[46]

[44] Hallowell Davis, "Abnormal Hearing and Deafness," in *Hearing and Deafness,* 4th ed., eds. Hallowell Davis and S. Richard Silverman (New York: Holt, Rinehart and Winston, 1978), chap. 4, p. 115.

[45] J. Lawrence Pool and Arthur A. Pava, *The Early Diagnosis and Treatment of Acoustic Nerve Tumors* (Springfield, Ill.: Charles C. Thomas, 1957), p. 9.

[46] Marlin Weaver and Jerry L. Northern, "The Acoustic Nerve Tumor," in *Hearing Disorders,* ed. Jerry L. Northern, chap. 17, p. 185.

TABLE 3–1.   Median hearing levels by age groups and sex of both ears of selected subjects (N = 1247) "who passed the rigid screening criteria related to otological disorders and extent of noise exposure."

Age	Sex	Frequencies in Hz								
		250	500	1000	1500	2000	3000	4000	6000	8000
18–24	M	1.3	0.2	−0.5	0.1	−1.8	3.8	2.0	20.8	13.5
	F	−0.3	−1.0	−0.2	−0.8	−3.7	−0.2	0.7	13.0	8.3
26–32	M	0.5	0.9	0.2	−0.5	−1.5	4.2	4.1	26.0	20.5
	F	0.2	0.9	−0.3	0.4	−1.2	−0.8	−0.6	13.7	12.1
34–40	M	−1.3	0.1	0.4	0.5	−0.1	5.8	10.4	27.4	24.8
	F	0.0	0.0	−0.3	0.9	−0.2	0.7	2.6	17.5	16.5
43–49	M	−0.7	3.4	−1.0	8.0	5.5	17.6	23.0	37.5	26.5
	F	−0.3	2.1	−0.6	4.8	2.9	3.8	6.8	25.4	16.3
51–57	M	2.0	3.9	4.4	5.1	6.1	16.9	17.8	33.7	32.5
	F	4.5	5.8	6.2	6.0	9.0	10.8	12.7	27.2	24.5
59–65	M	8.1	5.9	7.1	10.3	14.4	28.6	39.8	52.3	47.7
	F	10.4	8.0	5.3	8.1	9.2	13.2	16.9	34.5	32.3

These hearing levels in dB re ANSI-1969 audiometric zero were computed from sound pressure levels presented by John F. Corso, "Age and Sex Differences in Pure-Tone Thresholds," *A.M.A. Archives of Otolaryngology* 77 (April 1963): 398–99.

Typically, the tumor grows within the internal auditory meatus, causing compression of both the VIIth (facial) and VIIIth nerves and sometimes erosion of the bony canal, which may be seen in x-rays. Sometimes the tumor originates in the angle formed by the cerebellum and the pons, and the internal auditory meatus is unaffected. Although these are still acoustic neurinomas, they may be called *cerebellopontine angle* tumors because of their location. As the tumor expands, other cranial nerves may be affected. Although cases of bilateral acoustic nerve tumors have been reported, typically only one side is affected, and the hearing impairment and tinnitus that usually are the first symptoms of the tumor are unilateral.

Special mention should be made of *Ménière's disease* or *syndrome* as a cause of sensori-neural impairment, as this is a condition confined to the inner ear. The symptoms of Ménière's disease constitute a triad—tinnitus, vertigo (whirling dizziness), and hearing loss. In addition, patients may report a feeling of pressure or fullness in the ear. The immediate cause of these symptoms is apparently increased fluid pressure within the membranous labyrinth, causing distention throughout its length, so that Ménière's disease is also referred to as *endolymphatic* or *labyrinthine hydrops*. Authorities disagree as to whether it is proper to call the condition Ménière's disease if one of the three symptoms is missing. Although apparently the endolymphatic hydrops that is characteristic of the disease may be caused by various identifiable conditions, in almost half the cases of Ménière's disease it is not possible to determine the etiology. According to Pulec, the single most important cause of Ménière's is allergy, particularly for foods. Other causes he identifies are inadequate functioning of the pituitary and adrenal glands, congenital or acquired syphilis, hypothyroidism, lack of adequate blood supply to the ear, and estrogen insufficiency.[47] Singly and in combination, these conditions accounted for 46 percent of the 55 percent of a group of patients for which a cause or causes for the Ménière's disease could be identified. Stenosis (narrowing) of the internal auditory meatus, physical trauma, acoustic trauma, and viral infections accounted for the remaining 9 percent. Pulec believes that many of the 45 percent classified as *idiopathic* (cause unknown) are related to viral infections, but so far he has been able to demonstrate a viral cause in no more than 1 percent of the patients he studied.[48]

Ménière's disease usually consists of "attacks" of vertigo with nausea and accompanying tinnitus and hearing impairment. The acute episodes may last from a few minutes to several hours, followed by periods of remission. Weeks or months may intervene between acute episodes, or they may increase in severity and frequency so that a patient is effectively incapacitated by the repeated episodes of vertigo and nausea. The hearing loss fluctuates with the other symptoms, although a certain amount of permanent damage apparently occurs with repeated episodes. In an acute episode, the low frequencies may show a greater loss than the high frequencies. In later stages of the disease when there is a minimum of fluctuation, the loss is usually greater for the higher frequencies. The patient with Ménière's is typically affected in only one ear. Pulec states that both ears are affected in 24 percent of the cases,[49] but most authorities would feel this is much too high an incidence. The hearing loss in Ménière's is characterized by severe loudness recruitment. In fact, the affected ear generally builds up loudness so rapidly once threshold is reached that the sensation of loudness in that ear exceeds the sensation of loudness in the better ear for a stimulus of fixed intensity, or in other words, the affected ear exhibits hyper-recruitment. The serious student of audiology will want to pursue the study of Ménière's disease in detail, as this is a condition affecting hearing in which the audiologist plays a particularly important role in assisting the otologist in a diagnosis. The various otological journals contain a wealth of information about research and clinical experience, and entire books have been devoted to a discussion of the disease.

Related to Ménière's disease in its symptomatology is sudden, severe hearing loss in which the patient overnight may lose almost all the hearing in one ear or sometimes both ears. Tinnitus is almost always present and there may or may not be an accompanying vertigo. Although there may be many possible causes for sudden sensori-neural losses (Jaffe refers to over 200 possible etiologies[50]), they are in many cases thought to be caused by an interrup-

[47] Jack L. Pulec, "Ménière's Disease," in *Hearing Disorders,* ed. Jerry L. Northern, chap. 13, pp. 154–56.

[48] Ibid., p. 156.

[49] Ibid., p. 154.

[50] Burton F. Jaffe, "Sudden Sensori-neural Deafness," *Maico Audiological Library Series* 11, report 2 (1972).

tion of the blood supply to the cochlea, probably a blockage or spasm of the cochlear artery. If the condition persists more than a few hours, the cochlea may suffer irreparable damage and the hearing loss could become permanent.

Other cases of sudden hearing loss may be associated with *perilymphatic fistulas.* "A perilymphatic fistula is a slow microscopic leak of perilymphatic fluid through the oval or round window membrane, causing gradual and chronic decompression of the perilymphatic space."[51] Frequently, a patient will have a sudden unilateral hearing loss following a period of physical exertion or perhaps during an upper respiratory infection, and a *tympanotomy,* a surgical exploration of the middle ear, will reveal a perilymphatic fistula. It is presumed that the oval or round window membranes rupture as a result of increased intracranial pressure, which produces an increase in perilymphatic pressure through the cochlear aqueduct and an "explosive" force against the oval or round window membranes, or from excessive pressure within the middle ear, which creates an "implosive" force against the oval or round window.[52] Fistulas have been found, however, in patients with an absence of a history of exertion or of upper respiratory infection. In any event, the prompt surgical repair of a fistula, using a vein graft of perichondreum or like material, can frequently result in a dramatic improvement of what may have been a profound or extreme sensori-neural impairment.

Although it is rare in occurrence, sensori-neural loss due to mechanical injury of the inner ear is possible. Thus, in the case of a fracture of the temporal bone, the inner ear may be damaged, producing a sensori-neural hearing impairment on that side. Automobile accidents and wartime injuries contribute to sensori-neural impairments of this character.

Trauma of a different sort is responsible for the occurrence of many cases of sensori-neural impairment. Exposure to intense noise can cause permanent damage to the hair cells in the cochlea. Actually, the term *acoustic trauma* is reserved for cases of damage to cochlear structures—and frequently also to middle-ear structures—resulting from a single exposure to a very intense noise, such as a blast or explosion. Much more common is the gradual, progressive loss of sensitivity resulting from years of exposure to noxious levels of sound, called *noise-induced hearing impairment.* People differ considerably in their ability to withstand intense noise. Our modern industrial civilization is a noisy one. In many vocations, noise-induced hearing loss is an accepted occupational hazard. "Boilermaker's ear" is a time-honored syndrome among otologists. Because of the intense noise in a boiler factory, it was taken for granted that sooner or later all the workers in such a vocation would develop some sensori-neural loss. In modern times, there are many occupations in

[51] Grace S. Sung, Donald B. Kamerer, and Richard J. Sung, "Perilymphatic Fistula and Its Interest to Audiologists," *Journal of Speech and Hearing Disorders* 41 (November 1976) :540–46.

[52] Victor Goodhill, "Sudden Deafness and Round Window Rupture," *Laryngoscope* 81 (September 1971) :1462–74.

which the worker is subject to an extremely noisy environment, and the whole question of industrial compensation for hearing loss is receiving concentrated attention from employers, labor organizations, and the legal and medical professions.

Military service, with its attendant exposure to noises of great intensity, is responsible for producing many cases of sensori-neural hearing impairment. People with delicate ears, that is, ears easily susceptible to damage from noise, may incur permanent damage to their hearing from even brief exposures to gunfire or to aircraft-engine noise. The entire matter of the effect of noise on hearing is justifiably receiving the attention of various experts, so that (1) methods of reducing or controlling the noise may be discovered, (2) ways to protect the worker's ears effectively from the noise may be found, and (3) techniques of discovering which individuals are most susceptible to loss of hearing from noise exposure may be devised and utilized in order to govern the proper placement of workers in industry or in the military service. Chapter 9 covers in detail the problems of industrial noise control and noise-induced hearing impairment.

Typically, noise exposure causes reduction in sensitivity for the higher frequencies first, presumably because the basal end of the basilar membrane is stimulated by traveling waves of all frequencies and thus receives more "wear and tear" than the more apical parts of the cochlea. The region of the basilar membrane corresponding to frequencies of 3000 to 6000 Hz seems to be the most susceptible to injury from noise exposure. In fact, it is so common to see audiograms showing the greatest amount of impairment in this area that a "4000-Hz dip" is taken to be an indication of damage through exposure to noise (see Figure 5–10, Chapter 5). Although the point of greatest impairment may be localized at or around the 4000-Hz level, loss due to noise exposure will extend below and above this point, if the person with noise-susceptible ears incurs exposures to noise over a period of years. Most noise-induced hearing impairment results from continued exposure to wide-band noise of high intensity. When the noxious stimulus is a pure tone, or a narrow-band noise approaching a pure tone, the greatest loss will usually be found for frequencies that are from a half-octave to an octave higher than the frequency of the stimulus. Ward explains the susceptibility of the ear to impairment in the region of 4000 Hz on the basis that the ear is most sensitive to the frequencies from 1000 to 4000 Hz. The aural reflex (stapedius reflex) reduces the intensity of stimuli below 2000 Hz but not of stimuli above 2000 Hz. Therefore, stimuli between 2000 and 4000 Hz reach the cochlea at full strength, and the maximum loss of sensitivity occurs from a half-octave to an octave higher than the frequency of the stimulus.[53]

[53] W. Dixon Ward, "Adaptation and Fatigue," in *Sensorineural Hearing Processes and Disorders*, ed. A. Bruce Graham (Boston: Little, Brown and Company, 1967), p. 117; "Effects of Noise on Hearing Thresholds," in *Noise as a Public Health Hazard*, eds. W. Dixon Ward and James E. Fricke (Washington, D.C.: The American Speech and Hearing Association, 1969), p. 44.

Brief exposures to intense noise can produce a temporary hearing loss or threshold shift, and after a period of rest the ear will regain its former sensitivity. We have all experienced temporary threshold shift. A good example is the decrease of auditory sensitivity for several hours after completing a flight in a noisy airplane. The effect of exposure to noise is cumulative, however. If we were to fly in this noisy plane every day, we would find that our hearing would not recover completely after each flight, or in other words, that we were acquiring a permanent hearing loss. It is not uncommon to find veteran commercial pilots whose hearing is markedly diminished as the result of the accumulation of their many years of exposure to the noise of aircraft engines. The ground crew around jet aircraft are more likely to incur noise-induced hearing impairment.

Just as ears differ in their susceptibility to damage through exposure to noise, so also do they differ in their reaction to drugs that may have a toxic effect on the inner ear. In the past, quinine was responsible for producing sensori-neural impairment, as it was a popular agent in the treatment of malaria and even of the common cold. With the control of malaria, and the development of other drugs for treating it, quinine is no longer extensively used. Acetylsalicylic acid (aspirin) can have an ototoxic effect if taken in high daily doses, as for the treatment of arthritis, for example. Generally, the hearing loss is reversible if the dosage is lowered or discontinued. Today, the drugs that are chiefly responsible for causing sensori-neural hearing loss are in the family of *aminoglycoside antibiotics,* which "are an essential part of the therapeutic regimen of many life-threatening infectious diseases and in many instances are the only drugs of choice."[54] The best known of these drugs are *streptomycin, dihydrostreptomycin, neomycin,* and *kanamycin.* Incidentally, not all drugs whose names end in *mycin* are ototoxic. Streptomycin, developed to treat tuberculous infections, is much more likely to cause vestibular damage than hearing impairment. Dihydrostreptomycin, also an antitubercular drug, proved to be more ototoxic than streptomycin and affected primarily the hearing. It is no longer in use. Neomycin is effective against a wide range of infections. It is highly ototoxic when administered by injection, primarily affecting the auditory system. The effect may not be evident until weeks or months after the drug has been discontinued. Kanamycin is used for treating various bacterial infections and also affects the cochlea primarily, but its effect is not delayed. Other aminoglycosides that are ototoxic but appear to be less so than the ones just discussed are *gentamicin, vancomycin,* and *tobramycin.*[55] The effect of ototoxic drugs on hearing may range from mild to extreme, depending on the dosage, interaction with other drugs, kidney function, and other factors peculiar to the individual. Because physicians are well aware of the danger to the hearing from these drugs, large doses are prescribed only when urgent as a

[54]LaVonne Bergstrom and Patricia Thompson, "Ototoxicity," in *Hearing Disorders,* ed. Jerry L. Northern, chap. 12, p. 138.

[55] Ibid., p. 143.

life-saving measure. Mention should be made that ototoxicity may be a cause of congenital as well as acquired hearing loss if ototoxic drugs are administered to pregnant women.

Treatment

In contrast to conductive impairments, which are frequently responsive to medical or surgical treatment, sensori-neural hearing loss generally cannot be helped through treatment, with the exception of the loss due to Ménieère's disease and sudden, severe deafness due to an interruption of the blood supply to the cochlea or to a perilymphatic fistula. In the special case of Ménieère's, the hearing loss, as well as the other symptoms, is subject to remissions. In the case of sudden, severe hearing loss, the prompt administration of a vasodilator, perhaps in combination with an anticoagulant, will sometimes result in a dramatic restoration of hearing. Should the sudden loss be caused by a perilymphatic fistula of the oval or round window membrane, prompt surgical closure of the fistula will frequently result in the complete or nearly complete return of hearing. From time to time, there have been reports in the literature concerning the beneficial effects of vitamin therapy in improving the hearing, but the medical consensus is that sensori-neural impairment is irreversible. Once the nerve fibers in the cochlea or in the VIIIth nerve are destroyed, there is no regeneration, and because the cochlear portion of the VIIIth nerve is specific to the sensation of hearing, no other pathway for sound is possible. Of course, if the cochlear structures are only fatigued and not destroyed, as in the case of temporary threshold shift from noise exposure, hearing will return to normal in time after the noise exposure has ceased.

Thus, medical care of patients with sensori-neural impairment (with the exception of Ménieère's disease and vascular disturbances, of course) is limited to the prevention of further loss. If the causative factor of the loss is noise exposure, the physician can only advise the patient to try in the future to avoid exposure to noise or to use ear protectors (plugs or muffs). About the only other tack that the physician can take with patients who have sensori-neural impairments is to advise proper nutrition, rest, and personal hygiene, so that the patient's general resistance will be at an optimum level.

In the case of sensori-neural loss due to Ménieère's disease, the treatment would be directed toward correcting the condition responsible for the Ménieère's, if that can be determined. If a specific etiology cannot be identified, administration of a vasodilator, such as nicotinic acid, is frequently successful in controlling symptoms.[56] DeWeese and Saunders believe that a salt-free diet will provide relief of vertigo to more than 75 percent of Ménieère's patients. They also favor the use of a vasodilator in addition to the salt-free diet.[57]

---

[56] Pulec, "Ménieère's Disease," p. 158.
[57] DeWeese and Saunders, *Textbook of Otolaryngology*, pp. 429–30.

For patients not helped by medical treatment, Pulec recommends an operation called the *endolymphatic subarachnoid shunt,* which connects the blind endolymphatic sac, which lies between the arachnoid and the dura mater, with the subarachnoid space so that excess endolymph can be disposed of, thus relieving the hydropic condition in the endolymphatic system.[58] If medical treatment is ineffective in eliminating the vertigo and if the hearing in the affected ear is essentially nonfunctional, surgical destruction of the labyrinth (*labyrinthectomy*) may be recommended. This may be accomplished by an endaural approach, removal of the stapes, and removal of the membranous labyrinth with a hook, or by a postauricular approach to the lateral semicircular canal and removal of the membranous labyrinth through a hole bored in the canal, as in a fenestration operation. Alternate procedures employ electrocoagulation through the fenestra or destruction of the contents of the labyrinth by application of an ultrasonic generator on the horizontal canal.[59] Cryosurgery—applying intense cold to the horizontal (lateral) semicircular canal—has been reported to yield "excellent" results in 80 of 100 patients in whom vertigo was eliminated without further impairment to the hearing.[60] On occasion, the VIIIth nerve may be sectioned in cases where a labyrinthectomy has not succeeded in alleviating symptoms, or as the operation of choice in the most severe cases.

When the sensori-neural loss is due to the presence of an acoustic neurinoma, whenever possible the tumor must be removed, unless it is felt that the tumor does not pose a threat to the patient's life. The tumor grows slowly, so a patient may "outlive" it. Radiation is not effective against acoustic neurinomas. If the tumor is to be removed, the procedure may be to perform a craniotomy and gain access to the tumor without affecting the inner ear, or to make a *translabyrinthine* approach, going through the middle ear and the vestibular portion of the inner ear to reach the internal auditory meatus. The craniotomy approach presents the danger of damage to the brain or other cranial nerves. The translabyrinthine approach is less dangerous to the patient but does sacrifice the inner ear. It can be used only for comparatively small tumors, however.[61]

Since the early 1960s, there has been active experimental work in trying to restore hearing by direct electrical stimulation of the VIIIth nerve in individuals who have complete sensori-neural loss because of cochlear pathology. Because the stimulation usually takes place within the cochlea—in the modiolus or within the scala tympani—the technique is frequently termed a

[58] Pulec, "Ménière's Disease, p. 159.

[59] DeWeese and Saunders, *Textbook of Otolaryngology,* pp. 431–32.

[60] David Myers, Woodrow D. Schlosser, Robert J. Wolfson, Richard A. Winchester, and Norman H. Carmel, "Otologic Diagnosis and the Treatment of Deafness," *Clinical Symposia* 22, no. 2, CIBA Pharmaceutical Company (1970):64.

[61] Weaver and Northern, "Acoustic Nerve Tumor," pp. 189–90.

cochlear implant.[62] What is implanted is an electrode or multiple electrodes connected to an external transducer or, in some cases, to an induction coil implanted in the mastoid portion of the temporal bone. An external device is then used to activate the electrodes. To date, very few patients have had cochlear implants, the large majority being adults with acquired deafness although a few children have been implanted. No experimental subject has been able to achieve more than a primitive awareness of sound upon stimulation that, insofar as hearing speech is concerned, conveys at most a sense of the rhythm of speech. The cochlear implant is experimental and not generally available as a clinical procedure. Many basic questions remain to be answered, especially those related to the long-term viability of the devices, the long-term viability of the tissue, and the relative benefits between a cochlear implant and other strategies such as those involving devices external to the cochlea that activate the VIII nerve or devices that activate the tactile system. The hope is that a multichannel stimulator can be constructed that will function somewhat like the actual cochlea and provide sufficient information to the auditory nerve to make comprehension of speech possible. Brackmann and House conclude their discussion of the state of the art by saying ". . . the engineering aspects of direct eighth nerve stimulation are within the scope of current technology. The problem that remains is to outline the specifications necessary for the unit, which is not an easy task."[63]

The resumption of relations between the United States and China has resulted in a renewal of interest in this country in the use of acupuncture as a means of treating a variety of disorders. Some practitioners have claimed to "cure" sensori-neural hearing impairment through a series of acupuncture treatments. Unfortunately, otological and audiological studies of patients who have received these treatments fail to substantiate the practitioners' claims. Simmons says,

> . . . there is no evidence that acupuncture can help hearing loss as measured by standard audiometric criteria administered by trained professionals. This unfortunate, unexciting conclusion to the latest "miracle" in hearing cures will probably not drown out the claims for acupuncture from patient testimonials, if we pay attention to the history of medicine in other therapeutic arenas where cures by any means are equally few and far between. A vacuum exists in the treatment of deafness; the popularity of acupuncture is a symptom of this void.[64]

[62] Derald E. Brackmann and William F. House, "Direct Stimulation of the Auditory Nerve," in *Hearing Disorders*, ed. Jerry L. Northern, 2nd ed., 1984, chap. 24, pp. 279–89.

[63] Ibid., p. 288.

[64] F. Blair Simmons, "Acupuncture and Hearing Loss," in *Hearing Disorders*, ed. Jerry L. Northern, chap. 22, pp. 246–47.

OTHER HEARING DISORDERS

So far in this chapter, we have been concerned with the symptoms, etiology, and treatment of the two principal types of organic hearing disorders: conductive and sensori-neural losses. Now, brief mention will be made of other kinds of auditory disturbances.

Mixed Impairments

In the preceding sections of this chapter, conductive and sensori-neural losses were discussed as separate entities. In other words, only "pure" conductive and "pure" sensori-neural losses were considered. Actually, there are many instances of patients exhibiting symptoms of both types of loss. An elderly patient with presbycusis may also have some conductive loss because of otitis media, for example, or an otosclerotic may have some secondary nerve involvement. Such cases, demonstrating some degree of both types of hearing loss, are referred to as "mixed" impairments.

Central Auditory Disorders

Sensori-neural impairments refer to losses that occur because of improper functioning of the inner ear or damage to the VIIIth nerve between the inner ear and the brain stem. Once the nerve fibers enter the brain stem, they proceed by various pathways to the temporal lobes of the cerebral cortex. Any interference with these pathways from the brain stem to and including the cortex produces a *central* auditory disorder. The cause of the disorder may be a brain tumor or abscess, vascular changes in the brain (arteriosclerosis or a cerebral vascular accident), infections such as encephalitis or meningitis, degenerative diseases such as Parkinson's disease or multiple sclerosis, and brain damage resulting from trauma or asphyxia or from *kernicterus* associated with *erythroblastosis fetalis*.

Erythroblastosis fetalis is a congenital hemolytic disease that results from blood-group incompatibilities of the mother and fetus. One such incompatibility is that concerned with the *Rh factor*. In the 1940s, scientists discovered that human blood could be subclassified from the major blood groups (A, B, AB, and O) as either positive or negative in regard to the presence or absence of a substance referred to as the Rh factor. This factor is present in the blood in about 85 percent of the white population, who would therefore be classified as Rh positive. The remainder of the population would be classified as Rh negative. When Rh positive blood is mixed with Rh negative blood, antibodies are formed that attack the red blood cells of the Rh positive blood. Thus, Rh positive and Rh negative blood are said to be incompatible. Antibodies are created when a person with Rh negative blood is transfused with blood that is Rh positive, or when the Rh positive blood of a fetus crosses the placenta in the course of the pregnancy of a woman whose blood is Rh negative. When a child is conceived by an Rh negative mother and an Rh positive father, the fetus may be Rh positive. If so, antibodies are created in the mother's bloodstream that destroy the Rh positive cells in the blood of the fetus (erythroblastosis). Generally, the first child born of Rh-incompatible parents will not be harmed, as the antibodies in the mother's blood are not created in sufficient number to affect the child's blood. After the first pregnancy, however, the antibodies may be present in sufficient number to cause trouble to any child with Rh positive blood.

If extensive fetal damage occurs, the result may be a miscarriage or a stillbirth. If the physician is alerted to the existence of the Rh incompatibility, however, it is possible to save the lives of many of these babies and even to prevent serious brain damage from occurring by completely transfusing the baby's blood within a few hours of birth. Repeated complete exchange transfusions may be necessary to prevent *kernicterus*, which is the pathologic process that results in the jaundicing of nuclei in the brain. This process begins at birth as a result of the destruction of the infant's red blood cells and subsequent deposition of blood pigments in the brain stem. Without exchange transfusions, the kernicterus may cause cerebral palsy (usually of the athetoid type), mental deficiency, and/or an auditory disturbance. Children with auditory disorders due to erythroblastosis and kernicterus may give the appearance of being deaf, and audiologic testing may demonstrate various degrees of what would seem to be sensori-neural impairment. The evidence is contradictory, however, as to whether or not such children have peripheral or central impairments of hearing.[65]

The evidence from postmortem studies of kernicteric athetoids is also contradictory. The preponderance of such evidence, however, seems to point to normal cochleas but to abnormalities within the ventral and dorsal cochlear nuclei in the brain stem, which as early as 1949 led Goodhill to suggest the term "nuclear deafness" as appropriate with erythroblastotic children.[66] Carhart theorized that lesions in the cochlear nuclei could produce audiometric results suggestive of peripheral sensori-neural involvement of cochlear

[65] Victor Goodhill, Peter Cohen, Helen Hannigan, Jack Rosen, and Helmer Myklebust, "The Rh Child: Deaf or 'Aphasic'?" *Journal of Speech and Hearing Disorders* 21 (December 1956):407–25; Robert W. Blakely, "Erythroblastosis and Perceptive Hearing Loss: Responses of Athetoids to Tests of Cochlear Function," *Journal of Speech and Hearing Research* 2 (March 1959):5–15; Richard M. Flower, Richard Viehweg, and William F. Ruzicka, "The Communicative Disorders of Children with Kernicteric Athetosis: 1. Auditory Disorders," *Journal of Speech and Hearing Disorders* 31 (February 1966) :41–59.

[66] Victor Goodhill, "Auditory Pathway Lesions Resulting from Rh Incompatibility," in *Deafness in Childhood*, eds. Freeman McConnell and Paul H. Ward (Nashville, Tenn.: Vanderbilt University Press, 1967), chap. 14, pp. 215–28.

origin and thus lead to misdiagnoses.[67] To confound the diagnostic problem further, the possibility exists that a particular kernicteric child may in fact have a peripheral hearing impairment from causes unrelated to erythroblastosis.

Central auditory disorders can result from lesions that occur anywhere along the pathway of the auditory nerve, from the ventral and dorsal cochlear nuclei to Heschl's gyrus in the temporal lobe, or lesions in pathways to intra- and interhemispheric auditory association areas. Lesions can produce breakdown in monaural or binaural transmission of auditory information at various levels from the brain stem to the cortex.[68] Because fibers of the auditory nerve travel up both ipsilateral and contralateral pathways—with a majority crossing over to the contralateral side—a central lesion on one side will not result in loss of sensitivity in one ear. As a matter of fact, central auditory lesions acquired after language has been established cannot be identified through routine audiometric procedures because the ears will respond normally to the demands placed on them in routine tests. Only when the auditory system is subjected to special stresses will there be obvious breakdown in the transmission of information (see Chapter 7), and patients with central auditory disorders will demonstrate difficulty in the comprehension of what is heard. The term *auditory imperception* is used to refer to this lack of understanding.[69]

Another term sometimes used to describe the auditory behavior of aphasic patients is *auditory agnosia,* which refers to the inability to recognize sound, or more specifically, *auditory verbal agnosia,* meaning the inability to recognize speech sounds. In other words, the patient can "hear" but does not understand what is heard. *Aphasia,* which is a broad term referring to language disorders associated with injury to the "dominant" cerebral hemisphere resulting from trauma or from cerebrovascular accidents (strokes), is frequently described as being expressive, receptive, or a combination of the two types. In expressive aphasia, patients are unable to express themselves adequately in either the spoken or written form of language. In the receptive type, the difficulty is in comprehending language as it is heard or read. Agnosia, therefore, is a receptive disorder. Children of normal intelligence and normal hearing sensitivity who do not develop language abilities at the usual time are frequently designated aphasic. The assumption is that they incurred some brain injury *in utero* or at the time of birth that affected their ability to process auditory verbal stimuli—a situation analogous to an adult aphasic's problem.

[67] Raymond Carhart, "Audiologic Tests: Questions and Speculations," ibid., chap. 15.

[68] George E. Lynn and John Gilroy, "Central Aspects of Audition," in *Hearing Disorders,* ed. Jerry L. Northern, chap. 9, p. 104.

[69] Davis, "Abnormal Hearing and Deafness," p. 136.

Children with so-called congenital aphasia may exhibit visual imperception, auditory imperception, or both.

Central auditory disorders are thus not hearing-loss problems in the sense in which we have been applying the term in this chapter. Because it is a neurological disorder, a central problem falls within the domain of the neurologist, the neurosurgeon, and the psychiatrist rather than that of the otologist. The audiologist, however, is interested in central auditory disorders because part of the audiologist's responsibility is to differentiate peripheral from central impairments.

Functional or Nonorganic Hearing Loss

Another condition of auditory disturbance not caused by an impairment of the peripheral hearing mechanism is *functional* or *nonorganic* hearing loss, sometimes referred to as *psychogenic* hearing loss. In other words, the cause of the auditory disorder is psychological rather than organic. Occasionally, under emotional stress an individual unconsciously develops a "hearing loss" as a protective device or an escape from an intolerable situation. The terms *hysterical deafness* and *conversion deafness* serve to describe such a condition. Patients with hysterical deafness are not trying to "fool" anybody. They are convinced that a genuine hearing loss exists. Sometimes the patient may have a mild-to-moderate degree of actual organic impairment but behaves as if a profound hearing loss exists. This patient would be described as having a *functional overlay* on a true hearing loss.

Both the otologist and the audiologist are concerned with the job of differentiating true organic loss from functional loss. In children who have never developed language, differential diagnosis presents special problems. The treatment of functional hearing loss of the hysterical or conversion type is in the province of psychiatry, however, because the assumed loss is a symptom of an underlying psychological disturbance. Demonstration to these patients that they actually can hear destroys their defenses without solving their problems, and it can be expected that other psychogenic disturbances will develop in place of the hearing loss. These disturbances may take the form of blindness, inability to vocalize (aphonia), or paralysis of one or more limbs. It must be emphasized that all such psychogenic manifestations are on an unconscious level. The patient is convinced that the disorder is genuine.

An entirely different sort of assumed hearing loss occurs in the case of the *malingerer,* who adopts the role of deafness or hearing impairment consciously and deliberately for various purposes. Usually these purposes are concerned with financial reimbursement for "injury." The motive, then, is purely pecuniary, and the "patient" is well aware of the true state of hearing. Sometimes, a hearing loss will be assumed by an individual in order to be relieved of an onerous duty. This form of "goldbricking" has been employed by servicepeople in order to avoid unpleasant duty or perhaps to obtain a medical discharge.

In Chapter 7, the problems of differential diagnosis of genuine hearing loss and functional or nonorganic hearing loss will be discussed in detail.

REFERENCES

BESS, FRED H., ed.   *Childhood Deafness: Causation, Assessment, and Management.* Chaps. 1–6, 16–17. New York: Grune & Stratton, 1977.

BRADFORD, LARRY J., and HARDY, WILLIAM G., eds.   *Hearing and Hearing Impairment.* New York: Grune & Stratton, 1979.

DAVIS, HALLOWELL, and SILVERMAN, S. RICHARD, eds.   *Hearing and Deafness,* 4th ed. Chaps. 4, 5, and 6. New York: Holt, Rinehart and Winston, 1978.

DeWEESE, DAVID D., and SAUNDERS, WILLIAM H.   *Textbook of Otolaryngology.* Saint Louis: C. V. Mosby, 1973.

GRAHAM, A. BRUCE, ed.   *Sensorineural Hearing Processes and Disorders.* Boston: Little, Brown and Company, 1967.

HENDERSON, DONALD; HAMERNIK, ROGER P.; DOSANJH, DARSHAN S.; and MILLS, JOHN H., eds.   *Effects of Noise on Hearing.* New York: Raven Press, 1976.

JAFFE, BURTON F., ed.   *Hearing Loss in Children.* Chaps. 9–41. Baltimore: University Park Press, 1977.

NORTHERN, JERRY L., ed.   *Hearing Disorders,* 2nd ed.   Boston: Little, Brown and Company, 1984.

POOL, J. LAWRENCE, and PAVA, ARTHUR A.   *Acoustic Nerve Tumors.* Springfield, Ill.: Charles C. Thomas, 1957.

SATALOFF, JOSEPH.   *Hearing Loss.* Philadelphia: J. B. Lippincott Company, 1966.

SCHUKNECHT, HAROLD F.   *Pathology of the Ear.* Cambridge, Mass.: Harvard University Press, 1974.

SHAMBAUGH, GEORGE E., JR.   *Surgery of the Ear.* Philadelphia: W. B. Saunders Co., 1967.

TRAVIS, LEE EDWARD, ed.   *Handbook of Speech Pathology and Audiology.* Chap. 12. Englewood Cliffs, N.J.: Prentice-Hall, 1971.

CHAPTER FOUR
THE DEVELOPMENT
OF HEARING TESTS

Hearing impairment is a matter of *degree* and also of *pattern*. When a patient complains to the otologist that hearing is defective, the physician needs to know certain things about the patient's hearing loss—information that together with the patient's medical history and the results of the physical examination, will enable the otologist to make a diagnosis of the type of hearing impairment that the patient has and to provide some basis for estimating the possible effect of medical or surgical treatment. To perform these functions of diagnosis and prognosis, the otologist needs to know: (1) How much hearing loss is there in the low-, middle-, and high-frequency ranges of the ear? (2) How does the patient's air-conduction hearing compare with the bone-conduction hearing? (3) How seriously is this patient handicapped by the hearing loss?

To provide the answers to these questions, otologists have devised various tests of patients' hearing, ranging from the crude watch-tick and coin-click tests to the extensive quantitative measurements made possible by the development of pure-tone and speech audiometers. Between these extremes fall such time-honored tests (among otologists) as the spoken- and whispered-voice test and the various tuning-fork tests. Even with today's modern audiometric instrumentation, many otologists prefer to diagnose and "measure" hearing loss by voice and tuning-fork tests. Perhaps the reason for this preference is that measurement of the hearing function with modern equipment requires technical skill on the part of the tester and more time than most otologists can spend with their patients, whereas the voice and tuning-fork tests are administered easily by the otologist in a brief space of time.

Because the audiologist frequently will receive reports from otologists referring to the results of nonaudiometric hearing tests, and also because our modern audiometric tests are merely refinements of some of these earlier tests, we shall now briefly examine the so-called noninstrumental tests of hearing, except for the watch-tick and coin-click tests, which are not really useful in evaluating hearing loss and are seldom used today.

CONVERSATIONAL VOICE TEST

When it is employed by an experienced examiner aware of its limitations, the conversational voice test is useful in detecting gross deviations from normal hearing. Unfortunately, this test has been applied extensively as a way to quantify hearing sensitivity for speech, particularly by the armed forces. In World War II, the conversational voice test was given as part of the routine physical examination at induction and separation centers, just as the Snellen chart was used to measure visual acuity. If, at a distance of 20 feet, we can identify letters on the Snellen chart that "normal" eyes can identify at that distance, we are said to have 20/20 vision. In the same manner, it was assumed that if we were able to identify spoken words at a prescribed distance our hearing was normal. The conversational voice test was administered at a distance of either 20 or 15 feet. "Normal" hearing was represented by a test score of 20/20 or 15/15. Whereas every induction or separation center used a standard visual chart, there was no attempt to control the intensity of speech stimuli or the specific words used for hearing tests. In visual testing, it is necessary only to light the chart properly and measure off distances on the floor; it does not matter in what kind of room the test is administered. In hearing testing, the size, shape, and acoustic characteristics of a room influence how the voice is heard at some distance from the speaker. Naturally, it was not feasible for the armed forces to construct "standard" rooms for testing in every center, so the conversational voice test was not given under the same physical conditions in various places. Although the manner of scoring the test suggests that hearing might be measured with the same degree of precision as vision, actually there is no comparison in the control of testing conditions between the two tests.

In administering the test, the patient is placed at the prescribed distance from the examiner so that first one ear and then the other is directed toward the examiner. The patient plugs the ear not being tested with the index finger and is instructed to repeat the words the examiner speaks. Then, in a "normal" level of voice, the examiner says some numbers, simple words, and simple phrases. If the patient is unable to repeat these, the examiner moves forward until the patient is able to repeat what the examiner is saying. A score of 10/20 means that the examiner had to move to a distance of 10 feet before the patient was able to repeat what the "normal" ear is supposed to hear at 20 feet.

In the armed forces, the responsibility for administering the conversational voice test was usually vested in a medical corpsman who may have had only a vague conception of how the test should be administered. Different examiners made their own interpretation of what was meant by a "normal" level of conversational voice. As a result of this slipshod method of "measuring," many men with impaired hearing were inducted into the service during World War II with a clean bill of health. If, at the time of their discharge, these men requested a careful audiometric examination that disclosed a hearing loss, the armed services had no evidence that the loss had not occurred during the claimant's period of service. The Veterans Administration today is paying hundreds of thousands of dollars annually in compensation to veterans whose hearing loss antedates their entrance into the service because, by the crude methods of hearing testing at the time of their induction, their hearing was considered to be normal. Fortunately, the situation has changed, so that today most recruits are given audiometric tests. In many cases, their hearing is checked with "automatic" audiometers (discussed in Chapter 9).

TUNING-FORK TESTS

In otology, the classic method of measuring, or more properly, describing, hearing loss is by noting the patient's responses to vibrating tuning forks. Forks of various frequencies are selected for administering the standard tests. These frequencies are octaves of C on the scientific scale, from 128 Hz through 8192 Hz. The most common fork tests are the Rinne, Weber, Bing, and Schwabach, named after their nineteenth-century German originators.

The Rinne Test[1]

The purpose of this test is to differentiate between conductive and sensori-neural hearing loss and thus assist the otologist in a diagnosis of the type of hearing impairment that a particular patient exhibits. To perform the test, the otologist sets a tuning fork into vibration (by pinching and then releasing the tines with the fingers, or by striking the fork with a soft mallet) and holds it close to the patient's external ear. When the patient reports that the sound produced by the fork can no longer be heard, the otologist quickly

[1] In passing, it is interesting to note that although the originator of this test was of German nationality, many authors in the past have written his name as if it were French, *Rinné*. As a matter of fact, it appeared this way in the first edition of this book. The authors are grateful to the late Dr. Walter Heck ["Dr. A. Rinne," *Laryngoscope* 72 (May 1962):647–52] for correcting this error.

places the handle of the vibrating fork against the patient's mastoid process and asks if the patient can again hear the fork. If the patient replies affirmatively, the result of the test is said to be a *Rinne negative,* which indicates a conductive-type lesion. If the patient hears the fork longer by air conduction than by bone conduction, the result is labeled a *Rinne positive* and indicates a sensori-neural loss. A Rinne test on a normal ear will yield a positive result also, since normally our hearing is more sensitive by air conduction than by bone conduction.

The method of administering the Rinne test may be just the reverse of that described. That is, the examiner may begin by pressing the handle of the fork against the patient's mastoid and then shift the fork to the external ear. Or the test may be performed first by one method and then the other in order to validate the result obtained. Standard procedure calls for the use of three forks: forks with frequencies of 128, 256, and 512 Hz. Most otologists will want to test at 1024 and 2048 Hz as well, because hearing speech depends to a considerable extent on hearing frequencies higher than 512 Hz. Instead of expressing the results in terms of positive or negative, some otologists prefer to say that air conduction is greater than bone conduction (in the case of a positive Rinne), or that bone conduction is greater than air conduction (in the case of a negative Rinne).

There are limitations to the use of the Rinne, of which the otologist must be aware. In the first place, before a negative Rinne can be obtained, the patient must have more than a slight conductive loss. Because normally the ear is much more sensitive to airborne sounds, a slight conductive impairment will not overcome the normal differential between air and bone conduction, and the test result will be a positive Rinne, even though the patient's impairment is actually of the conductive type. Another limitation involves the testing of a patient who has a severe sensori-neural impairment in one ear, the other ear having normal, or close to normal, bone conduction sensitivity. Then the Rinne test result will be negative (bone conduction better than air conduction) on the severely impaired ear that actually has a sensori-neural loss. The result might lead the otologist to diagnose a conductive loss, which, of course, would be grossly wrong. What produces this misleading test result is the participation of the ear with normal bone conduction when the handle of the fork is pressed against the mastoid of the poorer ear. When the fork is placed on the mastoid, the bones of the skull are set into vibration, and the fluid in both inner ears is agitated. If the nerve endings in only one cochlea are insensitive to the vibrations in the fluid, the sound will be heard by the other, normal cochlea. The patient with a unilateral loss who states that the sound is heard longer by bone conduction than by air conduction, therefore, might actually be responding to the bone-conducted vibrations in the better ear. To safeguard against making a false diagnosis in this situation, the otologist must prevent the participation of the better ear by introducing a masking noise of sufficient intensity to make it impossible for the better ear to hear the bone-conducted sound. With a unilateral hearing loss, however, the otologist can check the results of the Rinne against the results of the next test to be described, the Weber.

The Weber Test

This test also has as its purpose the differentiation between conductive and sensori-neural hearing impairment. The Weber, however, is used only in cases of unilateral loss or in losses characterized by better hearing in one ear. It is a test of lateralization, that is, a test to see to which of the ears the tone is referred, or lateralized, when the handle of the fork is placed on the midline of the skull. If when the fork is placed on the midline, the patient reports that the tone is heard in the *poorer* ear, a conductive impairment is indicated. If the tone is heard in the *better* ear, the impairment is sensori-neural. If there is no difference in sensitivity between the ears, the tone will be heard equally in the two ears. The tone refers to the poorer ear in cases of conductive impairment because of a phenomenon analogous to the *occlusion effect*. This can be demonstrated with a normal-hearing individual by closing each external canal alternately with finger pressure on the tragus while the vibrating fork is held on the midline of the skull. The tone will "shift" back and forth, always lateralizing to the ear that is occluded. A conductive impairment acts in the same way to occlude the passage of air-conducted sound, and thus the tone appears to be heard only in the ear having the greater occlusion, that is, the greater conductive impairment. In the case of unequally functioning inner ears, as would be true in unilateral sensori-neural impairment, the fork tone is referred to the side having the better cochlea. Caution must be exercised in evaluating the patient's responses to the Weber test. Unless informed that the tone may be heard in the poorer ear, the patient is likely to respond consistently that the tone is heard in the better ear, simply because it is not logical that the patient could ever hear better in the poorer ear.

The Bing Test

The Weber test is useful in cases of unilateral impairment, or where there is more than a slight difference in sensitivity between the ears. The Bing test, which is based on the occlusion effect, can be used in cases of bilateral impairment to distinguish between conductive and sensori-neural loss. The vibrating fork is placed on the mastoid as it is in the Rinne test. When the patient reports that the tone has become inaudible, the examiner immediately closes the external canal by light finger pressure on the tragus while the still vibrating fork is left in place. If the patient reports that the tone again becomes audible, it is evident that occluding the ear was responsible for enhancing the ear's sensitivity to the bone-conducted sound. Thus it can be presumed that there is no conductive impairment, or at least that there is some sensori-neural involvement. If the tone is not heard again when the canal is closed, the ear has a conductive impairment that is already effectively occluding the passage of air-conducted sound. When "secondary perception" occurs, the result is termed a *Bing positive* and is indicative of a sensori-neural impairment. Of course, a normal ear will also yield a Bing positive result, just as a normal ear yields a Rinne positive. If there is no secondary perception of the tone when the ear canal is closed, the result is a *Bing negative* and indicates a conductive impairment.

The Bing test provides valuable information to the audiologist in pure-tone audiometry when performed with the bone-conduction vibrator of the audiometer instead of a tuning fork. When a patient shifts from a negative to a positive Bing test result over a period of time, it is an indication that the middle-ear problem has improved—as a result of treatment or through a natural healing process.

The Schwabach Test

The Rinne, Weber, and Bing tests are qualitative tests of hearing; that is, they give information about what type of impairment the patient has. The Schwabach is a quantitative test; it attempts to tell how much impairment a patient has. Like the Weber and the Bing, the Schwabach involves bone conduction. In performing the test, the examiner places the handle of a vibrating tuning fork on the mastoid of the patient and tells the patient to indicate when the tone becomes inaudible. The handle of the fork is then placed on the examiner's mastoid, who then counts the number of seconds until the tone becomes inaudible. Of course this method of testing presumes that the examiner has normal hearing. The results of the test are expressed in terms of the time that the patient's hearing is diminished in comparison to the examiner's for each fork. Thus, if the examiner can hear the tone for ten seconds longer than the patient, the test result is expressed as "diminished ten." Because this is a test of bone-conduction sensitivity, it can be seen that the Schwabach test measures the amount of sensori-neural loss. Even with such "quantification" as the Schwabach provides, however, the test result is difficult to interpret in such terms because units of time rather than intensity serve to express the loss. Nevertheless, an experienced clinician can make effective use of this test to judge the severity of sensori-neural impairment.

PURE-TONE AUDIOMETRY

Tuning-fork tests provide information concerning a patient's hearing at discrete frequencies, but as we have seen, these tests are useful primarily for providing a qualitative description of a patient's loss. The next logical development in hearing tests was an instrument that would yield quantitative as well as qualitative information about a patient's hearing. Such an instrument is the pure-tone audiometer. Although some experimentation was conducted in the late nineteenth century with "electrical" hearing-testing devices, the prototype of the modern audiometer was not developed until the 1920s.

The audiometer is an instrument for electronically generating tones of essential "purity," such as those produced by the tuning fork. The intensity of these tones is accurately controlled by an *attenuator,* which is usually calibrated in 5-dB steps, although some audiometers are calibrated in steps of 1 or 2 dB. Zero-dB hearing level at each frequency is theoretically the lowest intensity at which the average normal ear can detect the presence of the test tone 50 percent of the time. Hearing "loss" is thus expressed as the number of dB in excess of this zero point that the intensity of the tone must be increased in order for the impaired ear just barely to detect its presence. The test tones produced by the audiometer are delivered to the patient's ear through an earphone for air-conduction tests and through a bone-conduction vibrator for tests of inner-ear functioning. Comparison of a patient's hearing sensitivity by air and by bone conduction yields information of diagnostic significance, as does the Rinne tuning-fork test, with the added advantage of measuring the amount of loss in dB by each method of testing. The audiometer provides a more accurate type of Schwabach test because it measures loss by bone conduction in dB rather than in units of time. Therefore, the audiometer performs both the Rinne and Schwabach tests, but in an improved manner. The Weber and Bing tests can also be administered with the audiometer, using the bone-conduction vibrator instead of a tuning fork, although there would be little point in performing an audiometric Weber test for routine diagnostic purposes, as the hearing loss in each ear can be accurately measured with the audiometer both by air and by bone. The audiometric Weber test for determining the need for masking will be discussed in the next chapter.

For many years, audiometers were designed to generate the same frequencies as those of tuning forks: octaves and mid-octaves of C on the scientific scale. Upon the recommendation of various scientific associations, audiometer manufacturers have standardized their instruments on a Hertz scale in the hundreds or thousands range. Thus, the modern audiometer may contain all the following test frequencies: 125, 250, 500, 750, 1000, 1500, 2000, 3000, 4000, 6000, and 8000 Hz.

So far in our discussion of intensity, we have been referring to sound-pressure levels, that is, the intensity in relation to a specified physical reference level, a pressure of 0.0002 dyne/cm^2 (20 μN/m^2 or 20 μPa). Another way to speak of intensity is by referring to the threshold of the "average normal ear" as a reference. The sound-pressure level required to make any frequency barely audible to the average normal ear is called *zero hearing level* or the *standard audiometric threshold.*[2] Audiometers are calibrated to national and international standards, based on studies of normal-hearing subjects, that specify the sound-pressure levels for zero hearing level—or audiometric zero—at each frequency. The intensity of any frequency can thus be specified in terms of its hearing level in dB, which means, of course, how much greater

---

[2] "Psychoacoustical Terminology," *American National Standard,* ANSI S3.20–1973 (New York: American National Standards Institute, 1973), p. 52.

its sound-pressure level is than the sound-pressure level for audiometric zero. The hearing level required to reach the threshold of any ear is the *hearing threshold level* (HTL) for that ear.[3] In discussing an impaired ear, the amount of hearing loss can be specified in terms of hearing threshold level.

As was seen in Figure 2–3 (Chapter 2), the sound-pressure level for audiometric zero is not the same for all frequencies. The human ear is more sensitive in the frequency region from 1000 to 1500 Hz than it is to lower and higher frequencies. The audiometer is compensated for this uneven response curve of the ear, so that the same zero-dB setting on the hearing-level control applies to every frequency. Because of the uneven response of the ear, higher sound-pressure levels are required to reach audiometric zero for the frequencies below 500 and above 6000 Hz. Because only so much amplification is available in the audiometer, there is less intensity available above audiometric zero at the extreme low and high frequencies than there is at the middle frequencies. The maximum hearing level available in most pure-tone audiometers is 110 dB. At the frequencies below 500 Hz and above 6000 Hz, the maximum hearing level available is less, for the reasons just discussed. Because zero hearing level represents a statistical average of threshold levels of normal ears, and some ears would have better than average normal hearing sensitivity, the hearing-level dial on some audiometers provides for the measurement of up to 10 db better than average normal hearing levels at all frequencies. A minus sign precedes the designation of a level that is lower than zero dB hearing level.

In addition to the frequency and intensity controls, an audiometer includes an interrupter switch, which enables the operator to turn the test tone on or off immediately and noiselessly; a masking circuit, so that the ear not under test can be prevented from participating; and a selector switch for directing the test signal to the right earphone, the left earphone, or the bone-conduction vibrator. In addition, some audiometers include a speech circuit, which enables the operator to amplify speech for the patient, making communication possible in cases of extreme loss and also providing for the administration of certain speech audiometric tests; and a patient-signaling device, usually a cord and push button connected with a small lamp on the face of the audiometer, so that the patient can indicate responses silently. The operation of the pure-tone audiometer will be explained in detail in the next chapter.

SPEECH AUDIOMETRY

Just as the pure-tone audiometer represents an extension and quantification of tuning-fork tests, so also the modern speech audiometer has developed from the early crude conversational voice test. Speech audiometry, as it is

[3] Ibid., p. 19.

practiced today, had its inception during World War II in the military aural rehabilitation centers. It is interesting to note that the test materials for speech audiometry were developed originally under government contract by the Harvard Psycho-Acoustic Laboratory for the purpose of comparing the efficiency of various communications systems in transmitting speech.[4] For this purpose, subjects with normal hearing were tested. Differences among communications systems in efficiency of speech transmission were represented by differences in test scores made by the same subject as listening was shifted from one system to another. Someone with clinical orientation soon saw that if the test materials were valuable in differentiating among communications systems used with normal ears, they should also be useful in differentiating normal from impaired hearing by means of a single communications system.

Speech audiometry should be performed in a two-room facility, with the patient in a room that is reasonably sound-isolated and the examiner in a separate control room. A two-way communications system provides for introducing the test materials to the patient and conveying responses to the tester. Ideally, the speech audiometer should provide inputs from a microphone, for live-voice testing; from a turn-table or tape recorder, for recorded speech tests; and from a white-noise generator, for masking purposes. The level of the test materials going into the amplifier is monitored by volume controls and one or more volume indicator meters. The output of the amplifier is directed through an attenuation system to one or both of a pair of earphones, or to one or two loudspeakers. The attenuation system controls the output in 1- or 2-dB steps over a range of hearing levels from zero or — 10 dB (that is, 10 dB better than the average normal threshold) to 100 or 110 dB. With such equipment, the following measures can be obtained monaurally and binaurally: (1) speech-reception threshold; (2) most comfortable listening level; (3) tolerance for loud speech; and (4) articulation, or word discrimination, ability. These measures, and procedures for obtaining them, will be explained in Chapter 6.

ACOUSTIC IMMITTANCE MEASUREMENTS

In addition to traditional pure-tone and speech audiometry, a standard audiological evaluation today includes some physical and physiological measures of the ear. These usually consist of *tympanometry* and measures of the intra-aural muscle reflex, collectively referred to as *acoustic immittance measures*. Such measures can be used to detect certain abnormal conditions of the physical structures of the ear as well as to assess the functional integrity of the ear. The usefulness of the measures falls into three categories. First, cer-

[4]J. P. Egan, *Articulation Testing Methods*, OSRD Rept. #3802 (Harvard University Psycho-Acoustic Laboratory, 1944).

tain abnormal conditions may be present which do not necessarily manifest themselves as changes in auditory function. Some of these conditions can be detected with physical measures so that proper medical intervention can occur. Second, certain conditions which affect the functional integrity of the ear may be difficult to detect with traditional behavioral measures. A physiologic measure can help solve this problem. Finally, physical and physiologic measures do not require behavioral responses from the patient, and they contribute important information about patients who are unwilling or unable to provide correct behavioral responses. This group of patients includes very young children, persons with limited mental abilities, and persons who demonstrate functional hearing loss.

The strategy is based on measurements of acoustic characteristics within the external meatus which are determined by the canal volume and the physical state of the structures forming the external canal cavity, primarily the tympanic membrane and certain middle-ear structures. By comparing measured values for an ear to values for normal ears, statements can be made concerning the physical condition of the ear. By measuring changes in the acoustic characteristics of the ear associated with manipulations, such as varying the air pressure in the external canal or causing a contraction of the middle-ear muscles, statements can be made about both the physical condition of the ear and certain auditory functions.

Acoustic characteristics are expressed in a wide variety of quantities collectively called *acoustic immittance quantities.* Immittance quantities fall into two categories, expressed either in terms of how much acoustic energy can enter the auditory system (the *admittance* analogy) or in terms of how much acoustic energy cannot enter the system (the *impedance* analogy). Thus, one category of quantities is simply complementary to the other. The impedance analogy uses *ohm* as the unit. Impedance is comprised of two components, *resistance* and *reactance.* The reactance component is further divided into *compliant* reactance and *inductive* reactance. The admittance analogy uses *mho* (the reverse spelling of *ohm*) as the unit. Its two components are called *conductance* and *susceptance,* and the susceptance component is further divided into *compliant* susceptance and *inductive* susceptance. There is a precise mathematical relation between the two analogies. Admittance is the reciprocal of impedance, conductance is associated with resistance, and susceptance is associated with reactance. The range of immittance values for the ear is generally in the thousands of ohms for the impedance analogy and, conversely, thousandths of a mho (millimhos) for the admittance analogy.

In practical terms, not all these quantities are used. All the devices are calibrated with a hard-walled cylinder whose physical acoustic characteristics can be specified precisely, based on the volume of the cylinder and the characteristics of the air it contains. Such a cylinder is an acoustic compliance by definition and produces a known compliant reactance. Some devices are calibrated to express the measured acoustic immittance quantity as equivalent to that resulting from the compliance of a volume of air. Thus, the units are in "equivalent" volume units, usually cubic centimeters (cc) or milliliters (ml). At 220 Hz the acoustic admittance of a 1 ml volume of air is ~ 1.0 millimho, and the acoustic compliance in equivalent volume units is 1.0 ml. The most common immittance units used are "compliance" (in cc or ml of equivalent volume), admittance (in millimhos), or the admittance components of conductance and susceptance (in millimhos).

The device used to obtain measures of immittance is called either an *electroacoustic bridge* or an *electroacoustic meter*. There are also mechanical impedance bridges, but these are seldom used clinically today. In electroacoustic bridges or meters, a so-called probe tone is introduced into the external ear canal by a miniature loudspeaker. The resulting sound is picked up by a miniature microphone. The more acoustic energy that enters the middle-ear, the less that will be reflected; and, conversely, the more energy that is reflected, the less that will be transmitted through the middle ear. The miniature speaker and microphone are mounted in a probe unit that is secured in the ear canal by a removable earpiece called a *probe tip*, which must be the proper size to provide a complete air-pressure seal between the probe and the canal wall. A third part of the probe unit is a tube through which air can be introduced to create positive or negative air pressure in the canal in relation to the ambient air pressure. The air pressure is controlled by a pump that either forces air into the external meatus or withdraws it from the meatus. The air pressure, specified in units of millimeters of water (mm H_2O), or its equivalent in dekaPascals (daPa), can be adjusted so that the measured immittance is at a maximum. This figure provides an estimate of the air pressure in the middle ear. The air pressure in the canal can be increased or decreased to put the eardrum under tension, which acoustically isolates its effect and results in a measurement of the immittance of the canal alone. The probe tone used in all immittance equipment is a low-frequency tone, generally 220 Hz. Some instruments employ a second probe tone, usually 660 Hz. For most measures the probe tone is kept at a constant sound-pressure level, typically 85 dB. An electroacoustic meter automatically keeps the sound-pressure level constant by means of an automatic volume-control circuit, whereas with an electroacoustic bridge, the operator must manually adjust an attenuator to keep the sound-pressure level constant.[5]

In tympanometry, the immittance of the eardrum is checked over a range of pressures in the external canal, from + 200 to − 200 mm of water. On occasion, this range may be extended from + 400 to − 400 mm of water. The immittance unit is plotted automatically on an X-Y plotter on the Y or vertical dimension, and air pressure in the ear canal is plotted on the X dimen-

[5]Alan S. Feldman, "Tympanometry—Procedures, Interpretations and Variables," in *Acoustic Impedance & Admittance—The Measurement of Middle Ear Function*, eds. Alan S. Feldman and Laura Ann Wilber (Baltimore: Williams & Wilkins, 1976), chap. 6, pp. 108–109.

sion. The plot is termed a *tympanogram*. The shape and configuration of the tympanogram convey information about the state of the middle ear, which helps the audiologist and otologist determine the causes of particular conductive impairments. Tympanometry can also be used to evaluate Eustachian tube functioning.

Immittance devices are used to study the acoustic intra-aural muscle reflex, which provides valuable diagnostic information. The presence or absence of the reflex has diagnostic significance, and if the reflex is present it is important to know at what sensation level it is activated and how much it decays over a ten-second period. The reflex is observed by introducing a tone at a high sensation level through a standard earphone connected with an audiometer and noting whether the audiometer tone causes a change in the immittance of the opposite ear. Testing is performed at the air-pressure level in the external canal that was determined in tympanometry to result in maximum immittance of the system. If a muscle contraction occurs, the drum immittance will change. The threshold of the acoustic reflex is determined by finding the lowest hearing level at which a definite immittance change can be detected. The threshold of the reflex is measured at several frequencies. As we learned in Chapter 2, the intra-aural muscles in both ears contract in response to an activating stimulus delivered to only one ear. Thus, in studying the reflex, changes in immittance can be observed with the probe in one ear while the contralateral ear receives the audiometer tone. Using a specially designed probe unit that contains a miniature loudspeaker connected to an audiometer, one can also observe whether a change in immittance occurs when the ipsilateral ear is stimulated with the audiometer tone. Evaluation of the results of acoustic reflex testing provides important diagnostic information regarding sensori-neural impairments as well as conductive losses, the function of the VIIIth nerve and low brain stem, and also the function of the VIIth nerve, which innervates the stapedius muscle. The response of the intra-aural muscles to nonacoustic stimuli can also be observed by noting changes in the immittance of the ear. The most commonly used nonacoustic stimuli are tactile or electrical stimulation in the ear canal or around the auricle, blowing air at the eyes, or lifting the upper eyelids.[6]

INSTRUMENTATION AND COMPUTERS

All the electronic equipment described so far was initially developed with analog instrumentation. Thus, within the instrument there is an electrical signal which is a direct analog of the acoustic signal of interest; that is, the

[6] Gisle Djupesland, "Nonacoustic Reflex Measurement—Procedures, Interpretations and Variables," in *Acoustic Impedance & Admittance*, eds. Feldman and Wilber, chap. 10, p. 218.

waveform of the electrical signal is directly analogous to the waveform of the acoustic signal. Technology has advanced greatly in recent years to allow the implementation of many functions with computers, which use digital techniques. The use of digital computers has several advantages over analog techniques. First, digital techniques are not as prone to calibration errors. For example, a pure tone generated with analog instrumentation will have a frequency that will vary from day to day, depending on the condition of the electronic components, the temperature of the components, and other factors. A pure tone generated by a digital computer and controlled by an inexpensive quartz clock will remain at a constant frequency even though the temperature and condition of the electronic components vary.

The second advantage of computer-based instruments is that they have the capability of accurately repeating specified tasks through the use of a program. For example, if a desired test sequence for a pure-tone audiogram is to start with a center frequency, proceed to the lower frequencies, and then conclude with the higher frequencies, a computer-based audiometer can be made to implement the precise sequence exactly, time after time.

A third advantage is that a computer can perform arithmetic tasks more easily than a human. As anyone who has used a small hand-held calculator can attest, it is much easier to perform arithmetic with the use of a computer than with a pencil and paper.

Finally, computers have the capacity to store, manipulate, and retrieve data. They are equally facile at these tasks whether the data are numbers or letters. Thus, computers can be used for digital data, such as threshold values, or textual data, such as a clinic report.

Fortunately for the clinician, there is a trend to incorporate computers into standard instrumentation rather than to develop totally new concepts in instruments. At the present time many standard instruments used in audiological practice are computer-based, although to the person using them they appear to be similar to older instruments. Throughout this book, standard instrumentation will be described in a conceptual manner, and it will make no difference if the inside of the device has a computer or not. The clinician need only be aware of what the device can do.

There is also a trend to incorporate computers into devices that allow totally new concepts to be implemented. At the present time these new approaches have not yet gained wide clinical usage so they will not be discussed in great detail. In the near future, however, computers may be used to perform a variety of new tasks, such as the reduction of noise and the processing of a speech signal in a hearing aid to make speech more intelligible to the hearing impaired, the presentation of synthetic speechreading stimuli for speechreading therapy, and the performance of a complete audiological evaluation under computer control so that the collection of data and the preparation of the final report can occur more efficiently than at present.

REFERENCES

FELDMAN, ALAN S., and WILBER, LAURA ANN, eds.   *Acoustic Impedance & Admittance—The Measurement of Middle Ear Function.* Baltimore: Williams & Wilkins, 1976.

JERGER, JAMES, ed.   *Handbook of Clinical Impedance Audiometry.* Dobbs Ferry, N.Y.: American Electromedics Corporation, 1975.

KATZ, JACK, ed.   *Handbook of Clinical Audiology,* 2nd ed. Baltimore: Williams & Wilkins, 1978.

MARTIN, FREDERICK N.   *Introduction to Audiology,* 2nd ed. Englewood Cliffs, N.J.: Prentice-Hall, 1981.

NORTHERN, JERRY L., ed.   *Hearing Disorders,* 2nd ed. Boston: Little, Brown, 1984.

RINTELMANN, WILLIAM F., ed.   *Hearing Assessment.* Baltimore: University Park Press, 1979.

ROSE, DARRELL E., ed.   *Audiological Assessment,* 2nd ed. Englewood Cliffs, N.J.: Prentice-Hall, 1978.

CHAPTER FIVE
TESTING
THE HEARING FUNCTION:
PURE-TONE AUDIOMETRY

EQUIPMENT REQUIRED

Several pure-tone audiometers are available commercially. These vary from simple portable models designed for school testing to elaborate "research"-type audiometers, with which it is possible to administer all kinds of special, advanced tests, in addition to the standard measures. To conduct the routine tests of pure-tone audiometry, it is necessary only to have an instrument that provides for air-conduction and bone-conduction testing and for introducing masking. Of course, any instrument must be properly calibrated. Methods of checking on the calibration of an audiometer will be given later.

Pure-tone audiometers are of two main types: discrete frequency and sweep frequency. The former provides tones only at octave and mid-octave steps as the frequency dial is turned; the latter provides a tone that is continuously variable in frequency. Most audiometers in use today are of the discrete-frequency type. The hearing-level dial is graduated in steps of 5 dB, and in most audiometers intensity changes of 5 dB only are possible. There is a trend today for audiometer manufacturers to provide intensity controls in 1-or 2-dB steps, although it is doubtful that the results of routine hearing tests will ever be presented in steps of less than 5 dB.

Regardless of the make and type of pure-tone audiometer, certain necessary controls will be common to all instruments, and the audiometrist must learn to operate them in order to give hearing tests. These basic controls are:

1. Power switch
2. Frequency selector
3. Hearing-level control (attenuator)
4. Output selector (bone, right, left)
5. Interrupter switch
6. Switch and attenuator for masking noise

As stated in the preceding chapter, audiometers do not produce the same maximum hearing level for all frequencies. Each audiometer indicates the maximum hearing level that is available for the specific frequency. For example, the figure 90 that appears beneath the frequency 250 means that 90 dB is the maximum hearing level that the audiometer will produce at the frequency of 250 Hz. With most audiometers, the maximum hearing level of 100 dB is available for the frequencies of 500 through 6000 Hz.

On most audiometers, the interrupter switch is able to work in either of two ways: (1) When depressed it turns the tone on, or (2) when depressed it turns the tone off. Some audiometrists prefer to have the interrupter function in one way, and some in the other. The interrupter switch is either spring-loaded or nonmechanical, so it returns to its on or off position, whichever the case may be, whenever the examiner releases it.

The design and arrangements of an audiometer's basic controls will differ from instrument to instrument. Figure 5–1 shows a typical arrangement.

To obtain valid testing results, there must be some control over the conditions under which the testing is performed. Ideally, all testing should be performed in a sound-isolated room in which ambient noise is at a minimum. Good sound-isolated rooms are expensive to construct. Some portable sound-treated rooms are on the market at less than it would cost to construct comparable facilities. Actually, however, unless it is intended for research studies involving precise measurement of normal ears, it is not necessary to have an expensive, highly isolated room. For purposes of ordinary testing to differentiate between normal and impaired ears, a room that provides a reduction in outside noise of about 40 dB will be adequate, provided, of course, that the room is not situated in a particularly noisy location. As a matter of fact, most of the testing done in the public schools must perforce be performed in rooms that are not specially treated, and unless the surroundings are unusually noisy, sufficiently accurate results can be obtained to differentiate those children who have hearing losses from those whose hearing is essentially normal. Of course, any follow-up testing of those discovered to have losses should be performed under better testing conditions than is found in the average school in order to obtain accurate threshold measurements. Refer to Chapter 9 for sug-

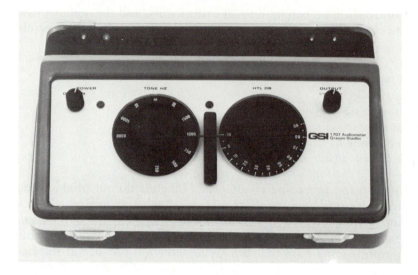

FIGURE 5-1.   A portable pure-tone audiometer (Reproduced by permission of Grason-
Stadler Inc., Littleton, Mass.)

gested maximum octave-band levels of ambient noise within test rooms where
hearing levels as low as zero dB are to be measured.

AIR-CONDUCTION TESTING

Before detailing the step-by-step procedure in administering a hearing test, it
is well to point out that the audiometer is not a magical instrument that can be
connected to a patient and yield automatically the exact amount of hearing
loss the patient has at each frequency. In the hands of an experienced clinician, the audiometer is a useful tool for obtaining measures of the extent and
type of hearing loss. The point is that the audiometer is a *tool,* and as such it
can be operated skillfully by the craftsperson or clumsily and ineffectively by
the amateur. The results of a hearing test must always be evaluated in terms of
the individual who performed the test. There is an unfortunate tendency for
some physicians and educators to accept audiograms at face value, without
regard for the conditions under which the tests were administered or by
whom. The audiogram is not a photograph of an individual's hearing loss; it is
the best estimate by the audiometrist of the state of the patient's hearing,
based on observation of the patient's behavior in the testing situation.
Because patients differ considerably in their reactions, it is not possible to
prescribe in detail the steps that should be followed invariably in obtaining an
audiogram. In hearing testing, as in almost every human activity, there is no
substitute for experience. The experienced clinician will adapt the testing
techniques to suit the situation instead of following a set procedure that

makes no allowance for individual differences from patient to patient. The beginner, however, must follow a rather rigid procedure if the results are to be at all reliable. It is urged, therefore, that those who are just beginning their hearing-testing experience follow the steps set forth in every case until they develop sufficient skill through experience to introduce their own modifications and improvisations. With this word of caution, then, let us proceed to the step-by-step procedure to be applied in administering a pure-tone audiometric test by air conduction. These steps assume that the examiner is using a portable audiometer, such as that shown in Figure 5–1, located in the same room with the patient, and that the test is the first one of the day. If the testing is performed in a two-room suite with a large multipurpose audiometer, some modification of these steps may be required; and if the test is not the first of the day, the first five steps can be dispensed with.

1. Plug in the audiometer, if it is the type that operates on "house current." Most audiometers are designed to operate on 60-cycle alternating current of 110 volts, although some may be operated on 220 volts as well. Just be sure that for the instrument being operated, the electric supply is proper.

2. Turn on the audiometer's power switch, ensuring that the instrument actually does receive power by seeing the indicator light up. Allow the audiometer to "warm up" for at least ten minutes to permit the electronic components to stabilize before starting the test.

3. If the earphones and the patient's signal cord are not already plugged into the audiometer, plug them in, seeing to it that they go in the proper jacks and are in the jacks all the way, making good contact.

4. Set the frequency control at 1000 Hz and the hearing-level control at 40 dB. Put on the earphones and listen to the tone as you switch from one ear to the other. When you are satisfied that the tone is present in equal strength in each earphone, listen to the tone as you gradually turn the hearing-level control toward zero-dB hearing level. If you have normal hearing, you should be able to hear the tone at near zero-dB hearing level. The purpose of this check is to verify that the audiometer and earphones are performing properly, and that the levels of sound in the phones are approximately as indicated on the hearing-level dial. This procedure is called a "biological check" on the calibration of the audiometer.

5. If you plan to have the patient use the signal cord and light in the course of the test, give them a trial to make sure they are working.

6. You are now ready to test with the audiometer, and it is time to instruct the patient, who should be sitting and facing you in such a position that the controls of the audiometer cannot be seen. Some examiners prefer to have the patient seated facing away from them. The disadvantage of this arrangement is that you cannot observe the facial expressions of the patient, which frequently are helpful in evaluating the patient's responses, and the patient cannot benefit from lipreading when given instructions.

In these instructions, and subsequently in this chapter, we shall assume that the patient is an adult or an older child. Special problems of testing young children will be dealt with in Chapter 7. The following instructions should be considered only as a guide. The words, and the manner of giving the instructions, may, of course, be varied to fit the situation.

> We are now going to test your hearing. I am going to place an earphone over each ear, but we shall test only one ear at a time. The object of the test is to find the point where you can just barely detect the presence of the tone. We shall start each time with the tone off. Then I shall gradually introduce the tone until you can just hear it. As soon as you first hear the tone, signal me. Then I'll make the tone louder so you can hear it well. I shall next make the tone softer until you signal me that you can no longer hear it. Then I'll make it louder and softer and turn it on and off while you tell me whether or not you can hear the tone each time, until I am satisfied that we have the point where you can just detect the presence of the tone. Then we'll shift to a different tone and start the process all over. You can signal that you hear the tone by pressing the button on the end of this cord, which will cause a light on the audiometer to turn on. Keep the button depressed as long as you hear the tone at all. When you no longer hear the tone, do not push the button. Do you hear any better with one ear than with the other? If so, we'll test the better ear first; if not, we'll begin with the right ear. Are you ready? Signal when you hear the tone by pushing the button, and hold it down until you cease to hear the tone. Here we go. . . .

Note that the instructions to the patient are given *before* the earphones are placed on the patient's head. The examiner should if necessary use a higher than normal level of speech when speaking to the patient and of course should articulate clearly. It is advisable for the examiner to follow a routine of always putting the earphones on patients in the same way; for example, red (or gray) phone on the right ear, and blue (or black) phone on the left ear. Such habits tend to prevent errors in recording test results for the respective ears. It should be pointed out here that it is not necessary to utilize the patient's signal button and light if this system should, for any reason, seem inadvisable. Sometimes it is difficult for the patient to concentrate on listening and at the same time coordinate muscles to push and release the button at the right moment. Other methods of signaling are permissible, such as having the patient raise a finger when the tone is heard and lower the finger when the tone is no longer heard. Or the patient can be instructed to say "Yes" when the tone is heard and "No" when it can no longer be heard. The tester can soon discover whether or not the button presents a mental or physical hazard for the patient and shift to an easier type of response, if necessary. The advantage of the signal light is that it permits no equivocal responses: The light is either on or off. If the patient is signaling by raising and lowering a finger, it is possible to have the finger only partially raised. The examiner, therefore, has a problem in interpreting the response. Nevertheless, many audiologists prefer to utilize the finger-raising response.

7. As indicated in the instructions, test the better ear first if the patient reports that there is a difference in sensitivity between the two ears. The

reason for this procedure is to alert the audiometrist to the need for masking the better ear so that it will not participate in the test of the poorer ear. Whenever the apparent thresholds of the two ears differ by 40 dB or more, you should suspect that the thresholds obtained for the poorer ear may actually be a "shadow curve" of the better ear's hearing. What happens is that before the tone can be made loud enough to be heard by the poorer ear, it is heard by the ear not under test, probably in large part by transmission through the bones of the skull by bone conduction. Thus, it is advisable to test the better ear first, so that as soon as the test of the poorer ear begins you can tell whether there is sufficient difference between the ears to make masking necessary. More will be said later about masking. If the patient reports that there is no difference between the ears, it is suggested that the right ear be tested first. The reason for this suggestion is merely to establish a routine, because there are fewer chances for error in conducting the test and recording the results if the same procedure is followed in test after test.

8. It is advisable to begin a test at the frequency of 1000 Hz because this frequency is near the center of the most sensitive area of the human ear. Also, it has been demonstrated to have a good test-retest reliability.

9. Throughout this description of testing, it is assumed that the tone is inaudible except when the interrupter switch is depressed. The procedure to follow in testing at 1000 Hz, and at all succeeding frequencies, is to start with the hearing-level control at its minimum reading—either −10 dB or zero dB, depending on the particular instrument you are using—depress the interrupter switch, and gradually increase the intensity until the patient signals that the tone is heard. Increase the intensity of the tone beyond this point by about 20 dB in order to give the patient an opportunity to hear the tone well. If there is evidence that the patient is abnormally sensitive to above-threshold intensities, increase the tone by only 5 to 10 dB, as an increase of 20 dB may make the tone uncomfortably loud.

10. Now decrease the intensity of the tone in a continuous manner until the patient signals that the tone can no longer be heard. Note mentally what the reading of the hearing-level dial is at this point.

11. Immediately reverse the direction of the hearing-level control, increasing intensity of the tone until the patient signals that the tone is heard again. Make a mental note of this hearing-level dial reading. You now have "bracketed" the patient's threshold within 10 to 15 dB by sweeping across it first in a descending fashion and then in an ascending manner.

12. At this point, you have stopped as soon as the patient signaled that the tone was heard. Now cut off the tone completely by releasing the interrupter. The patient should immediately signal that the tone is not heard. While the interrupter switch is off, decrease the setting on the hearing-level dial by 10 dB. Depress the interrupter, and see whether or not the patient signals that the tone is heard. If the patient does not hear the tone, skip the next step and proceed to step 14.

13. If the patient signals that the tone is heard again, release the inter-

rupter switch and lower the intensity by another 10 dB. This time, when you depress the interrupter, the patient should not hear the tone, provided that steps 10 and 11 have been performed properly.

14. With the tone off again, this time *increase* the intensity by 5 dB, and then depress the interrupter. If the patient does not hear the tone, repeat this step until the tone is heard again.

15. When the patient signals that the tone is heard, release the interrupter briefly and decrease the intensity by 10 dB. The patient should signal that the tone is not heard. If the patient signals that the tone is heard, repeat this step until it is no longer heard.

16. Increase the intensity by 5 dB and depress the interrupter briefly. If the patient does not respond, increase the intensity by 5 dB again and depress the interrupter. Continue in this manner until the patient responds. Then, drop the intensity by 10 dB again and repeat the procedure of presenting brief bursts of tone at 5-dB steps of increasing intensity until the patient responds. Each time a response occurs, decrease the intensity and repeat this procedure, until the patient has responded at least four times. For audiometric purposes, the patient's threshold is defined as the lowest hearing level at which a response is obtained to the tone at least 50 percent of the time. Suppose, for example, that in step 14 the minimum hearing level at which the patient responds is 40 dB. In step 15, you present the tone at 30 dB, and the patient does not respond. In step 16, you present the tone at 35 dB, and the patient responds. You decrease the intensity to 25 dB, and there is no response. Again, as you present the tone in 5-dB steps of increasing intensity, the patient does not respond until the level of 40 dB is reached. Once more you decrease the intensity by 10 dB and then increase it in 5-dB steps, and the patient first responds at 35 dB. A response has occurred twice at a minimum level of 40 dB and twice at 35 dB. You record the threshold as being 35 dB, since this is the minimum hearing level at which the patient responded correctly to the presence of the tone for at least 50 percent of the trials. When there is doubt that the patient is responding appropriately 50 percent of the time, the tester should record the next higher 5-dB step as the patient's threshold. If no consistent picture emerges from steps 14, 15, and 16, you had better start all over with step 9. The patient may have become confused about what to listen for, and it may be necessary for you to present a clearly audible sound before trying again. In a later section of this chapter, there will be further discussion of the term *threshold*.

17. Assuming that you have succeeded in getting a consistent threshold picture at 1000 Hz, change the frequency control to 500 Hz and start again at step 9. Next test at 250 Hz. It is not necessary to test at 125 Hz, because a patient's threshold at 125 Hz is likely to be the same as the threshold at 250 Hz. Moreover, in order to ensure accuracy of test results at 125 Hz the test room must be exceptionally quiet. The lower a frequency is, the more subject it is to masking by ambient noise. Many audiologists advocate testing the frequencies

higher than 1000 Hz before testing those lower. The authors' preference for testing the lower frequencies first is based on the fact that most patients will have better hearing at 500 and 250 Hz than at 2000 Hz and higher frequencies. Some patients will hear nothing at maximum hearing levels available at the higher frequencies. It seems to the authors to be better practice to determine thresholds for the frequencies the patient can hear relatively well before testing for the frequencies not heard so well or not heard at all. Record each threshold on the audiogram as it is obtained.

18. Having obtained thresholds for the frequencies below 1000 Hz, test again at 1000 Hz. Pay no attention to the previous threshold obtained at this frequency until you have completed the steps necessary to obtain another threshold measurement. Then compare the second with the first threshold obtained. If they agree exactly, or differ by no more than 5 dB in either direction, you can be satisfied that the reliability of your test is adequate. You should then proceed to obtain threshold measurements for frequencies above 1000 Hz. Acceptable test reliability is considered to be ± 5 dB at any frequency. If the reliability of the first threshold measure is within acceptable limits, the assumption is that other threshold measures will be equally reliable. If, on the other hand, there is a difference of 10 dB or more between your first and second threshold measurements at 1000 Hz, the reliability of the test is in doubt, and it would be advisable to repeat from the beginning, even to restating your instructions to the patient.

19. Ordinarily, one would test only the octaves above and below 1000 Hz, except that frequently 6000 Hz would be the highest frequency tested. If the loss pattern at the octave intervals is uneven, it may be desirable to obtain thresholds at other mid-octave intervals: 750, 1500, and 3000 Hz. For example, if the patient's hearing threshold levels (HTLs) were 20 dB at 1000 Hz and 50 dB at 2000 Hz, one should test at 1500 Hz to see if the HTL at the mid-octave frequency is closer to that at 1000 Hz or to that at 2000 Hz. It is necessary to consider the patient's fatigue, however, in the testing situation. As the patient tires, the reliability of your test suffers. It would be better to obtain accurate measures of the patient's hearing at octave intervals than to have a complete test of all frequencies with questionable accuracy. Then, too, it is always possible to perform additional testing on the patient after an interval of rest or even on another day.

20. Special caution must be exercised in testing a patient at 8000 Hz, to make sure that the threshold is not influenced by standing waves. It will be recalled from Chapter 2 that when a pure tone is introduced into a closed pipe of the same length as the wavelength of the tone, the reflected wave from the closed end of the pipe produces a cancellation effect because the original tone and the reflected tone are 180 degrees out of phase. The wave is said to be "standing" because particle movement in the medium is at a standstill. The wavelength of a tone of 8000 Hz frequency is about one and one-half inches. When the diaphragm of an audiometer earphone is approximately one and a

half inches from the eardrum, a standing wave might result, because the external canal and eardrum may be likened to a closed pipe. The cancellation effect of the standing wave thus minimizes the vibration of the eardrum. In other words, the patient may not respond to the test tone because of the standing wave rather than from a hearing loss at this frequency. If a patient presents an apparent hearing loss at 8000 Hz, a slight adjustment of the earphone away from the ear may cause the patient to respond at lower hearing levels. Moving the earphone breaks up the standing wave by altering the distance from the earphone diaphragm to the eardrum. Because of the problem of standing waves and also because audiometer earphones are least stable at very high frequencies, many audiologists prefer not to test at 8000 Hz. Actually, the threshold at 8000 Hz contributes little to the clinical picture.

21. After completing the measurements on the first ear, switch the output selector to the opposite earphone and proceed in the same manner to obtain HTLs on the other ear.

22. If the HTLs of the second ear tested appear to differ by 40 dB or more from those of the first ear, you should repeat the test while masking the better ear in order to rule out its participation. Because in "cross-hearing" the nontest ear is apparently stimulated largely through the mechanism of bone conduction,[1] there may be occasions when the need for masking in air-conduction testing is not apparent until after bone-conduction HTLs have been determined. According to Studebaker, the need for masking is determined by comparing the air-conduction thresholds of the test ear with the bone-conduction thresholds of the contralateral (nontest) ear. Studebaker's rule is to use masking whenever differences between air-conduction HTLs of the test ear and bone-conduction HTLs of the contralateral ear equal or exceed 35 dB at 250 Hz; 40 to 45 dB at 500, 1000, or 2000 Hz; or 50 dB at 4000 Hz.[2] Thus, to cite an example, the difference between the ears in air-conduction HTLs may be only 25 to 30 dB—a magnitude of difference that ordinarily would cause no concern about cross-hearing. Yet the difference between the air-conduction thresholds of the poorer ear and the bone-conduction thresholds of the better ear may be on the order of 45 to 50 dB. In such a circumstance, the air-conduction HTLs of the poorer ear should be measured again while the better ear is masked.

23. If masking is indicated, it is best to explain to the patient that you are going to introduce a noise to the better ear so that you can obtain a more accurate measure of the hearing loss in the poorer ear. Caution the patient not to be distracted by the masking noise but to concentrate on listening for the tone and to signal as before. Then turn on the masking switch of the

[1] Jozef Zwislocki, "Acoustic Attenuation Between the Ears," *Journal of the Acoustical Society of America* 25 (July 1953):752–59.

[2] Gerald A. Studebaker, "Clinical Masking of Air- and Bone-Conducted Stimuli," *Journal of Speech and Hearing Disorders* 29 (February 1964):24.

audiometer. The selection of the intensity setting on the masking control dial may present a problem. There is no one setting that would be appropriate for all instances of masking. Moreover, it is seldom clear just what intensity values are indicated by the graduations on the masking control—sound-pressure levels, hearing levels, or "effective masking" levels. Although formulas for determining the proper levels of masking have been worked out,[3] they cannot be applied unless the examiner performs considerable experimentation with a given audiometer. The problem is to use sufficient masking intensity to prevent the masked ear from hearing the test tone but not so much intensity that the masking noise affects the sensitivity of the test ear (overmasking). Overmasking is not likely to occur in air-conduction testing because the *interaural attenuation*—the barrier to sound transmission from one ear to the other—in air-conduction testing, plus the amount of hearing loss in the ear under test, combine to protect the test ear from overmasking even at maximum intensity settings of the masking control on most audiometers. To be certain, however, you should experiment by obtaining thresholds in the ear under test while various levels of masking are tried on the contralateral ear. The technique of selecting the correct masking level through experimentation is discussed in the next section of this chapter. In bone-conduction testing, the selection of the "correct" intensity of masking is more critical.

24. If a choice of masking noises is available, it is best to use a narrow-band masker. This is furnished by some audiometer manufacturers as an accessory, and it will provide the most efficient masking of all. A segment of noise having its maximum energy centered on the test frequency makes possible the masking of each frequency with a lesser amount of overall sound energy than is required with a wide-band masker. Thus, in addition to being more efficient, narrow-band masking is more comfortable for the patient.

25. Avoid spending a great deal of time on the test. The beginner usually makes the mistake of spending too much time on each frequency, in an effort to guarantee that the best possible threshold is obtained for the patient. Actually, the tester is probably unconsciously postponing the time when it is necessary to make the decision about what the HTL is because of lack of confidence on the part of the examiner. By prolonging the test, however, accuracy is compromised since patients tire quickly in the testing situation, especially when they have to listen for any length of time to tones that are close to threshold levels. It is preferable, therefore, in the interest of accuracy, to proceed through a test rather quickly. For the average patient, no more than ten to fifteen minutes should be required to obtain air-conduction measurements for both ears.

26. Make sure, in operating the interrupter, that you do not fall into "rhythm patterns" that the patient can follow, even though the test tone may

[3] Ibid., p. 29.

not be heard. The pattern of tonal presentations should be irregular; that is, one time the interrupter switch should be off for several seconds, and the next time it should be depressed almost immediately after it has been released. In any event, the patient should not be able to predict what the length of time of the next interruption will be.

27. Some ears *adapt* rapidly to a tone; that is, a steady tone becomes inaudible in a very short time. The purpose in seeking threshold by means of short bursts of tone is to avoid producing adaptation, which, of course, would result in erroneous threshold determinations. It is best to limit the bursts of tone to durations of no more than one to two seconds. The silent intervals between tonal presentations permit recovery from any adaptation that might occur. Information about the validity of the responses is obtained by noticing how promptly the patient becomes aware of the presence of the tone, and also how promptly the tone becomes inaudible. Some audiometers provide for automatic pulsing of the tone, so that every time the interrupter is depressed the tone goes "beep-beep-beep . . ." for as long as the interrupter is held down. For many patients the pulsed tone is easier to hear at near threshold levels. Of course, the examiner can pulse a tone manually as well. On some audiometers, there is provision for warbling a tone, that is, modulating its frequency over a range of several Hz. A warbled tone is easier to distinguish than a tone of fixed frequency, especially for the patient who confuses a test stimulus with tinnitus. Sometimes a patient will continue to signal that the tone is heard after you have released the interrupter. On the other hand, the tone may be heard for only a fraction of the time that it is presented; that is, the patient may push the button and release it immediately before you have released the interrupter. If the patient's responses are inconsistent in either of these ways, it may be necessary to repeat the instructions to the patient to signal as soon as the presence of the tone is detected and to keep signaling as long as the tone is present. Even with the repetition of these instructions, there will be some patients whose responses pose a problem in interpretation for the tester. In such cases, the tester must exercise judgment in determining threshold and should note on the audiogram that the patient's responses were not consistent.

28. The method of threshold determination recommended here is based on the suggestions of Carhart and Jerger that determining threshold by an ascending method, that is, proceeding from inaudibility to audibility, is preferable to using a descending technique (proceeding from suprathreshold levels to inaudibility) or a combination of ascending and descending procedures.[4] Carhart and Jerger urge that all audiologists follow the same method for determining threshold so that test results will not be influenced by differences in procedure. They suggest that the ascending technique, originally

---

[4] Raymond Carhart and James F. Jerger, "Preferred Method for Clinical Determination of Pure-Tone Thresholds," *Journal of Speech and Hearing Disorders* 24 (November 1959):330–45.

ascribed to Hughson and Westlake,[5] be used in preference to other techniques because of its long history and general acceptability to otologists and audiologists. Guidelines for pure-tone audiometric procedures have been proposed by the American Speech-Language-Hearing Association (ASHA).[6]

BONE-CONDUCTION TESTING

After the air-conduction tests, it is standard practice to administer bone-conduction tests on each ear. Of course, if the air-conduction tests disclose no hearing loss, it would be useless to subject the patient to bone-conduction tests, for you know already that hearing is normal. The purpose of bone-conduction testing is to determine whether the loss detected in air-conduction testing is due to conductive or sensori-neural factors, or perhaps to a combination of the two. If the bone-conduction thresholds obtained are essentially normal, the loss is of the conductive type. On the other hand, if the bone-conduction measurements show losses that are equal to those obtained by air-conduction testing, the loss is of the sensori-neural type. If there is some loss by bone conduction, but not as much as by air conduction, the loss is a mixed one.

Bone-conduction testing is performed with a small hearing-aid type of bone-conduction vibrator that is attached to a metal headband. The traditional method of testing bone conduction is to place the vibrator on the mastoid process of the temporal bone behind the pinna of the ear to be tested. Other techniques have been suggested and will be discussed at the conclusion of this section. The method to be described here in detail is the one involving mastoid placement of the vibrator because it is the procedure most commonly in use.

Some authorities recommend that masking be utilized routinely in every bone-conduction test in order to prevent the opposite ear from participating in the test. Whereas a difference in sensitivity of 40 to 50 dB between the ears by air conduction is necessary before the tone will be transferred to the opposite ear, a bone-conducted sound may be heard by the opposite ear if the difference is as slight as 10 to 15 dB, or even in some cases when there is no apparent difference between the ears in bone-conduction sensitivity. In other words, the interaural attenuation in bone-conduction testing varies from zero dB at 250 and 500 Hz to a maximum of 15 dB at 4000 Hz with values between zero and 15 dB at 1000 and 2000 Hz. In both air- and bone-conduction testing, the opposite ear is stimulated through the mechanism of bone conduction. An

---

[5] Walter Hughson and Harold Westlake, "Manual for Program Outline for Rehabilitation of Aural Casualties Both Military and Civilian," *Transactions of the American Academy of Ophthalmology and Otolaryngology Supplement* 48 (1944):1–15.

[6] "Guidelines for Manual Pure-Tone Threshold Audiometry," *Asha* 20 (April 1978):297–301.

air-conduction earphone, however, is not as efficient a transducer for bone conduction as is a vibrator that has been specifically designed for this purpose. Hence, in air-conduction testing, the interaural attenuation greatly exceeds that existing in bone-conduction testing.

Although, where there is doubt, masking should be used in bone-conduction testing, it is not always necessary. In fact, sometimes it is sufficient to test only one ear. If a patient presents a bilateral loss pattern by air conduction and an unmasked bone-conduction test of one ear reveals HTLs that are approximately the same as those obtained by air conduction, it is unnecessary to test the bone conduction of the other ear. Because of the minimal interaural attenuation involved, you know that the bone-conduction HTLs of the other ear could not vary from those of the first ear by more than zero to 15 dB. On the other hand, if the initial bone-conduction HTLs indicate that there is a significant air-bone gap, that is, better hearing by bone conduction than by air conduction, it will be necessary to test the bone conduction of both ears, using masking at least on the "better" ear by bone conduction and perhaps on both ears. Even though there are equal air-conduction HTLs in each ear, the bone-conduction sensitivity of the two ears may be markedly different. The unmasked bone-conduction results reflect the ear with the more sensitive bone conduction, regardless of where the vibrator is placed.

The audiometric Weber test can be helpful in determining the need for masking.[7] Place the bone-conduction vibrator on the midline of the forehead and gradually increase the intensity of the tone until the patient reports that it can just barely be heard. Increase the intensity by 10 to 15 dB and then ask if the tone is heard in one ear or the other, or if it seems to be equally loud in each ear, that is, unlocalized. If the tone lateralizes to one ear, masking should be delivered to that ear while the contralateral ear is tested by bone conduction. If no lateralization occurs at any frequency, probably the ears are equal in bone-conduction sensitivity. If the Weber test results are inconclusive or inconsistent, the examiner should employ contralateral masking when testing each ear, although in retrospect it may be determined that the unmasked bone-conduction HTLs were in fact valid. Incidentally, it should be mentioned that any use of masking—either in air-conduction or in bone-conduction testing—even at such low levels of intensity that overmasking is impossible, will result in shifting the threshold of the test ear by 5 or 10 dB at each frequency. This phenomenon is called *central masking*, because it apparently is a function of the central nervous system.[8] Central masking will frequently result in HTLs by bone conduction that are greater than HTLs by air conduction, an occurrence that theoretically should not happen.

---

[7] D. M. Markle, E. P. Fowler, Jr., and H. Molouquet, "The Audiometric Weber Test as a Means for Determining the Need for and the Type of Masking," *Annals of Otology, Rhinology, and Laryngology* 61 (September 1952):888–900.

[8] Studebaker, "Clinical Masking," p. 24.

As stated earlier, various formulas for determining the "correct" amount of masking have been developed, but none has received universal acceptance. The following procedure is suggested as an empirical method that can be applied regardless of how the masking noise is calibrated on a particular audiometer. It is an adaptation of the "plateau" method suggested by Hood[9] and described in detail by Studebaker.[10] The examiner must arbitrarily select a given level of masking with which to begin the testing. For example, suppose that a setting of 60 dB is selected on the masking control dial, regardless of what actual intensity value that setting may be. The examiner then proceeds to obtain a bone-conduction HTL of the ear under test while that level of masking is applied to the opposite ear. The level of the masking noise should then be increased by 10 dB and again a threshold should be obtained on the ear under test. If the HTLs are the same regardless of whether the masking control is set at 60 or at 70 dB, it is assured that the level of the masking noise is not interfering with the ear under test. If, on the other hand, the HTL in the ear under test should increase by 10 dB when 70 dB of masking is applied, there may be two explanations: (1) The contralateral ear was insufficiently masked with 60 dB of masking, so that the threshold obtained with that amount of contralateral masking was underestimating the amount of loss present; or (2) the increase in the level of the masking noise caused an interference with the ear under test, and the threshold obtained with 70 dB of masking was an overestimation of the amount of loss. To determine which explanation is correct, it is necessary for the examiner to continue increasing the level of the masking noise and to obtain a threshold of the ear under test at each 10-dB increase in masking. If the threshold in the ear being tested increases proportionately with the increases in level of the masking noise, the examiner knows that the masking noise is too intense, and was too intense at the point where the threshold began to increase in proportion to increases in the masking level. When the proper level of masking is attained, an increase or decrease of 10 dB in the masking noise will not affect the threshold of the ear under test. In other words, the "plateau" will have been reached, and the bone-conduction threshold of the ear under test should remain stable over a range of at least 20 dB in masking noise. It is the examiner's responsibility, through experimentation, to locate the level of the masking noise within this range. This experimentation must be conducted at each frequency to be tested by bone conduction, as the same level of masking may not be suitable for all the frequencies tested.

In bone-conduction testing, it is important for the room noise to be at a minimum, especially if the patient's air-conduction loss is slight. In a normal ear, it is almost impossible to obtain zero-dB bone-conduction HTLs except in

[9] J. D. Hood, "The Principles and Practice of Bone Conduction Audiometry," *Laryngoscope* 70 (1960):1211–28.

[10] Studebaker, "Clinical Masking," pp. 29–33.

the very quietest of soundproof rooms because any sounds heard by air conduction serve to mask the bone-conducted tones. It may not be feasible,
therefore, to check the calibration of the bone-conduction vibrator on a normal ear. Rather, it should be checked on ears known to have pure sensori-
neural losses, by comparing the obtained air- and bone-conduction HTLs.
With such patients, the differences between the thresholds obtained by air
and by bone should average out to zero.

In routine testing, whenever substantially greater losses are obtained by
bone conduction than by air conduction, the examiner should suspect the
level of room noise, the calibration of the vibrator, or the validity of the patient's responses. Theoretically, it is not possible for a patient to have greater
losses by bone conduction than by air conduction. There are many variables
operating in bone conduction, however, that may combine to give a confusing
picture of the patient's bone-conduction sensitivity. In addition to the factors
of room noise and vibrator calibration, the thickness of the skin and tissue
covering the mastoid process and the degree of *pneumatization* of the mastoid
itself affect the sensitivity of the individual to bone-conducted sound. The
type of bone in the mastoid and the thickness of its covering are factors obviously beyond the control of the examiner. Because bone-conduction vibrators must be calibrated for the "average" mastoid, one must expect variations
both above and below the average. The examiner, therefore, should not be
concerned if, with a given patient, bone-conduction HTLs are obtained that
are greater than air-conduction HTLs by no more than 10 to 15 dB. The examiner should bear in mind also that with a particular patient, bone-
conduction thresholds that are better than air-conduction thresholds by 10 to
15 dB do not necessarily mean that there is an actual air-bone gap signifying
some conductive component.[11]

Bone-conduction vibrators are more limited in their sound-transmission
characteristics than are air-conduction earphones. For this reason, it is not
possible to test by bone conduction all frequencies tested by air. Generally,
audiometers allow bone-conduction testing only from 250 through 4000 Hz.
Many examiners will check bone conduction only at 500, 1000, 2000, and 4000
Hz. At 250 Hz, the patient may respond tactually to the vibrations of the
vibrator without actually hearing the tone. For this reason, bone-conduction
testing at 250 Hz may produce misleading results.

Audiometers are calibrated differently for air-conduction and bone-
conduction testing. More power must be delivered to the bone-conduction
vibrator than to the air-conduction earphone in order to reach the threshold of
the normal ear. Consequently, bone-conduction hearing levels are measured
only up to 65 or 70 dB. Usually a notation will be found on the audiometer indicating the maximum hearing level for bone conduction at each frequency.

[11] Gerald A. Studebaker, "Intertest Variability and the Air-Bone Gap," *Journal of Speech and Hearing Disorders* 32 (February 1967):82–86.

The step-by-step procedures in bone-conduction testing are similar to those detailed for air-conduction testing.

1. Explain to the patient that now you are going to check hearing sensitivity by bone conduction, that is, determine how well sounds conducted through the mastoid process are heard. Explain that the sounds and responses will be the same as those used for air-conduction testing.

2. Theoretically, the better ear should be tested first, as in air-conduction testing, but it is difficult, if not impossible, for a patient to tell which ear is better by bone conduction. It is possible that the ear that is poorer by air conduction may be better by bone conduction, as in a unilateral conductive impairment, for example. Therefore, in order to determine which is the better ear by bone conduction, it may be desirable to perform the audiometric Weber test, as mentioned previously. If neither ear is "better," it makes no difference which is tested first.

3. Place the bone-conduction vibrator carefully, so that it is making good, solid contact with the mastoid process. Avoid having the vibrator touch the pinna or hair. It may be necessary for you to experiment with the placement of the vibrator while the patient listens to a test tone, until you are sure that the vibrator is properly placed for maximum sensitivity.

4. If you are not employing masking during the bone-conduction testing, do *not* cover the opposite ear with an air-conduction earphone. To do so would create a moderate degree of air-conduction loss in the opposite ear and might cause the tone produced by the vibrator to refer to the covered ear, just as a Weber tuning-fork test causes the tone to refer to the ear that has the greater conductive loss. In Europe, it is customary to perform bone-conduction tests with both ears occluded. The thresholds thus obtained are called *absolute* bone-conduction thresholds, as contrasted with *relative* bone-conduction thresholds obtained with the ears uncovered. With normal ears, the difference between absolute and relative bone conduction (the "occlusion effect") exceeds 20 dB at 250 and 500 Hz, amounts to about 15 dB at 1000 Hz, and is negligible (less than 5 dB) at 2000 and 4000 Hz.[12] In this country, it is customary to obtain relative bone-conduction measurements. Therefore, both ears should be uncovered during bone-conduction tests, unless, of course, the opposite ear is being masked.

5. Follow the same routine of testing as was suggested for the air-conduction test: Test first at 1000 Hz; sweep up, down, and up again in intensity, bracketing the threshold; then find the threshold point by means of the interrupter and by changing the intensity of the tone in the manner suggested in air-conduction testing. Next, test the frequency or frequencies below 1000 Hz, recheck 1000 Hz, and then test the frequencies above 1000 Hz. After

[12] Scott N. Reger, "Pure-Tone Audiometry," in *Audiometry: Principles and Practices,* ed. Aram Glorig (Baltimore: Williams & Wilkins, 1965), p. 128.

testing one ear, switch the bone-conduction vibrator to the other mastoid and repeat the procedure. If masking is required, determine the correct amount through experimentation, as described earlier in this section, and in placing the headset on the patient make sure that the pinna of the test ear is not covered by the inactive earphone. Place that earphone on the cheekbone in front of the pinna in order to avoid occluding the test ear.

6. Tell the patient that the test tone may be heard in the ear not being tested, and to inform you if this occurs. Sometimes, even when maximum masking is employed, the patient will insist that the tone is heard in the ear not being tested. Theoretically, the test tone should not be able to be heard in the ear that is being masked, provided, of course, that the masking has an appropriate spectrum and is sufficiently intense. No one can say for certain, however, that the patient is not reporting what is actually happening. In such circumstances, the only thing that the examiner can do is to record the obtained results of the test, with the notation that even with maximum masking the patient reported that the tone was heard in the ear not under test.

Some audiometers are equipped so that bone-conduction testing may be performed in a different fashion. Rainville first suggested a method designed to avoid the problems of lateralization of the bone-conducted signal to the contralateral ear and the difficulties of masking in bone-conduction testing.[13] Rainville suggested that bone-conduction hearing level could be determined by comparing the amount of masking required to mask a pure-tone signal delivered at threshold through an air-conduction earphone when (1) a white noise was delivered through the same air-conduction earphone as the signal, and (2) the masking noise was delivered through a bone-conduction vibrator on the mastoid of the ear receiving the pure-tone signal.

Following Rainville's lead, investigators in this country developed tests in which the masking noise was introduced through the bone-conduction vibrator while the pure-tone signals were delivered through an air-conduction earphone. Jerger and Tillman called their test *SAL* (for sensori-neural acuity level),[14] and Lightfoot[15] called his test *M-R* for Modified-Rainville. Both these methods are similar. There are two main differences between the SAL and M-R tests and the Rainville method: The former utilize the middle of the forehead for vibrator placement, and they determine bone-conduction hearing levels by comparing threshold shifts produced by the bone-conducted

[13] M. J. Rainville, "New Method of Masking for the Determination of Bone Conduction Curves," *Translations of the Beltone Institute for Hearing Research*, no. 11 (July 1959).

[14] James Jerger and Tom Tillman, "A New Method for the Clinical Determination of Sensorineural Acuity Level (SAL)" A.M.A. *Archives of Otolaryngology* 71 (June 1960):948–55.

[15] Charles Lightfoot, "The M-R Test of Bone-Conduction Hearing," *Laryngoscope* 70 (November 1960):1552–59.

masking noise in normal-hearing subjects and in patients. Because the SAL test is the preferred method of assessing bone-conduction hearing, with the masking noise delivered to the bone-conduction vibrator, it will be described here.

The SAL test requires a standard pure-tone audiometer, a noise generator, and a bone-conduction vibrator. The bone-conduction vibrator, connected to the noise generator, is placed on the patient's forehead, and the headset containing the two air-conduction earphones connected to the audiometer is placed on the patient's head. The first step is to obtain the patient's air-conduction thresholds in each ear without any noise delivered to the bone-conduction vibrator. Although the whole range of audiometric frequencies can be tested, Jerger and Tillman suggest that the frequencies between 250 and 4000 Hz are the most useful for purposes of the SAL test.[16] Next, the air-conduction measurements are repeated with the noise turned on. Then, what Jerger and Tillman term the "sensorineural loss" at each frequency in each ear is determined by subtracting the threshold shift produced by the noise from the amount of shift normal-hearing individuals experience under these conditions. In obtaining their norms, Jerger and Tillman sought a noise intensity that would result in threshold shifts of approximately 50 dB for the frequencies from 1000 through 4000 Hz. They determined experimentally that when the noise level resulted in a signal strength of 2 volts across the vibrator, the desirable amount of threshold shift occurred in normal ears. According to their norms, this signal strength of the noise resulted in air-conduction threshold shifts of 20 dB at 250 Hz; 45 dB at 500 Hz; and 50 dB at 1000, 2000, and 4000 Hz. These, then, are the norms from which the threshold shifts obtained with patients at a noise level of 2 volts at the vibrator are subtracted to determine sensori-neural loss (bone-conduction HTLs). Testing an experimental group of patients with pure sensori-neural hearing losses, Jerger and Tillman concluded that the SAL technique is at least as good as conventional bone-conduction audiometry in measuring sensori-neural loss. The principal advantage of the SAL technique over conventional bone-conduction audiometry is that it eliminates the problem of whether or not to mask the contralateral ear and how much masking to use. Both inner ears are stimulated with the vibrator at the midline of the skull, and the ears are isolated by the amount of difference in sensitivity required before an air-conducted signal will cross over from the test ear to the opposite ear (40 to 60 dB). Because masking in conventional bone-conduction audiometry presents problems to so many clinicians, the SAL test offers many advantages for clinical use.

In the years following the description of the SAL technique by Jerger and Tillman, a number of articles appeared, some praising and some criticizing the method. Even Tillman concluded that "the SAL test cannot be viewed

---

[16] Jerger and Tillman, "New Method for Clinical Determination of SAL," p. 950.

as an adequate substitute for properly applied bone-conduction tests."[17] In an effort to resolve the questions concerning its clinical utility, Jerger and Jerger undertook a "systematic evaluation" of the test, which concluded that the original recommended procedure for SAL audiometry produced results that were valid and equivalent to bone-conduction results obtained with both conductive and sensori-neural losses, provided that the conditions for both methods were comparable. Because the SAL technique requires the occlusion of the test ear with an earphone, the results of the test should be compared with conventional bone-conduction thresholds obtained with the test ear occluded, or in other words, with absolute rather than with relative bone-conduction thresholds. If SAL results are compared with relative bone-conduction thresholds, there will be disagreements between the two methods in some instances.[18]

One modification of conventional bone-conduction testing that is gaining increasing acceptance is the use of forehead placement of the bone-conduction vibrator. Because both cochleas are stimulated with almost equal loudness when the vibrator is placed on either mastoid, it seems logical to place the vibrator midway between the ears and eliminate the involvement of the nontest ear through the use of masking, particularly because the frontal bone provides a better surface for the vibrator than the rounded mastoid process. Moreover, the vibrator can be left in place while testing both ears. The disadvantage to forehead placement is that more signal intensity is required to obtain bone-conduction hearing levels at the forehead, so that the range of hearing levels that can be measured is more limited. Several investigators have reported differences between forehead and mastoid bone-conduction HTLs obtained with normal ears. The means of the differences obtained in six studies as reported by Dirks, Malmquist, and Bower are shown in Table 5–1.[19] The values in Table 5–1 represent zero-dB hearing level at each frequency for

TABLE 5–1.   Differences in dB between thresholds of normal ears obtained by forehead and by mastoid placement of the bone-conduction vibrator.

Frequency (Hz)				
250	500	1000	2000	4000
14.6	14.3	9.2	9.5	5.5

[17] Tom W. Tillman, *A Critical View of the SAL Test*, Technical Documentary Report no. SAM-TDR-62-96, School of Aerospace Medicine, Brooks Air Force Base, Texas (August 1962), p. 2.

[18] James Jerger and Susan Jerger, "Critical Evaluation of SAL Audiometry," *Journal of Speech and Hearing Research* 8 (June 1965):103–27.

[19] Donald D. Dirks, Carol W. Malmquist, and Deborah R. Bower, "Toward the Specification of Normal Bone-Conduction Threshold," *Journal of the Acoustical Society of America* 43 (June 1968):1241.

forehead placement when the test ear is not occluded and appropriate masking is applied to the nontest ear. Martin presents a strong case for the routine clinical use of forehead placement of the vibrator and occlusion of both ears with air-conduction earphones. He points out that the occlusion effect compensates for the loss of sensitivity resulting from forehead placement, thus making available the full range of bone-conduction hearing levels present in the traditional mastoid placement of the vibrator.[20]

Studebaker[21] and Dirks and Malmquist[22] report that in testing ears with various conductive impairments, lower (better) bone-conduction HTLs on the average can be obtained with forehead placement of the vibrator than with mastoid placement. Dirks and Malmquist divided their conductively impaired group into subgroups, according to surgically confirmed middle-ear pathology, and compared bone-conduction hearing levels obtained with forehead placement and with mastoid placement in each subgroup. Their results suggest that the differences in bone-conduction sensitivity by the two methods may have diagnostic significance in differentiating the locus of pathology in conductive impairments.

Before leaving the subject of bone-conduction testing with all its complexities of masking, cross-hearing, interaural attenuation, and occlusion effect, some mention should be made of the influence exerted by the earphone and its cushion on audiometric results. Interaural attenuation or its reciprocal—the level at which cross-hearing occurs—is dependent on the area of the head making contact with the earphone cushion. The greater the area of contact, the lower the amount of interaural attenuation and the lower the level at which cross-hearing occurs.[23] The occlusion effect is dependent on the volume of air trapped under the cushion. The greater the volume, the lesser the occlusion of the ear and the lesser the occlusion effect.[24]

The earphone most commonly used in audiometry today is the Telephonics TDH-39 or TDH-49 mounted in an MX41/AR cushion. Such an earphone and cushion combination is called a *supra-aural* phone, because it fits over the ear. The area of the cushion making contact with the head is relatively large, and the volume of air under the cushion is relatively small. The earphone and cushion effectively occlude the ear, and we know that the interaural attenuation they provide is on the order of 40 to 60 dB.

[20] Frederick N. Martin, "Evidence for the Use of Occluded Forehead Bone Conduction," *Journal of Speech and Hearing Disorders* 34 (August 1969):260–66.

[21] Gerald A. Studebaker, "Placement of Vibrator in Bone-Conduction Testing," *Journal of Speech and Hearing Research* 5 (December 1962):321–31.

[22] Donald D. Dirks and Carolyn M. Malmquist, "Comparison of Frontal and Mastoid Bone-Conduction Thresholds in Various Conductive Lesions," *Journal of Speech and Hearing Research* 12 (December 1969):725–46.

[23] Zwislocki, "Acoustic Attenuation," p. 755.

[24] Ralph F. Naunton, "The Measurement of Hearing by Bone Conduction," in *Modern Developments in Audiology*, ed. James Jerger (New York: Academic Press, 1963), p. 21.

Interaural attenuation can be substantially increased by using an insert phone, which is a hearing-aid type of receiver attached to an earpiece that inserts in the meatus. Such a phone is useful for introducing masking to the nontest ear; the chances of overmasking are reduced because of its superior isolation characteristics.

To eliminate or substantially reduce the occlusion effect, an earphone-cushion combination that encloses a large volume of air—on the order of 1500 to 2000 cc—is desirable. Perhaps the most popular such combination is the Pedersen, which has a small loudspeaker mounted in a spherical enclosure. Because the enclosure goes around the ear instead of over it, the Pedersen is called a *circumaural* earphone. When Jerger and Jerger wished to compare SAL results with relative bone-conduction thresholds, they used Pedersen earphones to obtain unmasked and masked air-conduction thresholds.[25]

At present, the use of insert receivers and circumaural earphones is restricted largely to audiological research activities. The standard earphone mounted in an MX41/AR cushion is not likely to be replaced for routine clinical uses.

MAINTENANCE OF THE AUDIOMETER

The accuracy of testing depends on the proper functioning of the audiometric equipment, as well as the skill of the audiometrist and the adequacy of the testing room. Audiometers must be calibrated at regular intervals to insure that the frequency and hearing-level outputs are actually as indicated on the controls. Manufacturers recommend that audiometers given hard usage be sent to the factory for calibration and cleaning every year. Actually, it is not necessary to send the audiometer to the factory until it is apparent that the instrument is not in calibration and unless it is not feasible to correct measurements that are in error. The audiometer can be cleaned by any electronic service.

Intensity calibration usually is accomplished by varying the resistance in the output circuits of the audiometer's oscillators (pure-tone generators) so that the desired output at the earphone is obtained on an artificial ear. An artificial ear couples the earphone from the audiometer through a 6-cc coupler with a sound-level meter. The coupler is so constructed that its cylindrical volume approximates the volume of the external canal and middle ear plus the air between the earphone diaphragm and the opening of the canal.[26] The earphone is positioned on one side of the coupler, and the microphone of the

---

[25] Jerger and Jerger, "Critical Evaluation of SAL," pp. 105–106.

[26] Hallowell Davis, "Audiometry: Pure Tone and Simple Speech Tests," in *Hearing and Deafness*, 4th ed., eds. Hallowell Davis and S. Richard Silverman (New York: Holt, Rinehart and Winston, 1978), p. 196.

sound-level meter is located at the other side. The audiometer being calibrated is set at a prescribed hearing level for a particular frequency, and the oscillator for that frequency is adjusted until the output, as determined by the reading on the sound-level meter, agrees with the specified value for that frequency and hearing-level dial setting. Figure 5–2 illustrates a calibration system which includes a sound-level meter and an artificial ear. Figure 5–3 illustrates one type of artificial ear to be connected to a sound-level meter.

The American National Standards Institute (ANSI) of New York City publishes standards for manufacturers of various kinds of measuring equipment, including audiometers. ANSI was formerly known as the American Standards Association (ASA) and for a brief period as the United States of America Standards Institute (USASI). In a 1951 publication (Z24.5-1951), the association specified the sound-pressure level for audiometric zero at each octave interval on the audiometer, based on the results of hearing tests conducted during a health survey by the U.S. Public Health Service in 1935–1936.[27] These levels, employed by audiometer manufacturers in this country until 1964, were known both as the "American standard" and the "ASA-1951 standard" for audiometric zero. Subsequent hearing surveys of large popula-

FIGURE 5–2. An audiometer calibration system set up to calibrate an audiometer. This set-up is sometimes referred to as an artificial ear. (Reproduced by permission of Quest Electronics, Oconomowoc, Wisc.)

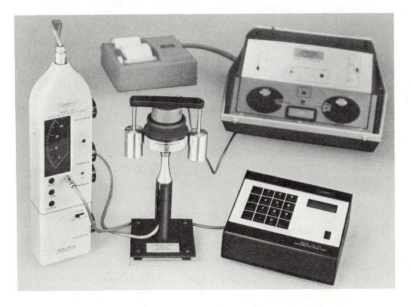

[27] Willis C. Beasley, *National Health Survey (1935–36), Preliminary Reports, Hearing Study Series, Bulletins 1–7* (Washington, D.C.: U.S. Public Health Service, 1938).

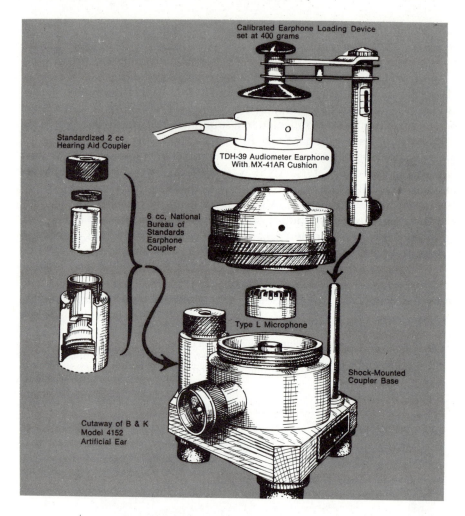

FIGURE 5-3. Details of the artificial ear attachment for a sound-level meter. (Reproduced by permission of Bruel & Kjaer Instruments, Inc., Marlborough, Mass.)

tions conducted at state and world's fairs tended to confirm the adequacy of the Beasley findings as representing "average normal hearing."[28]

Studies that were performed under better-controlled testing conditions, however, in this country and abroad, indicated that average "normal" hearing might be as much as 10 to 15 dB "better" than the ASA-1951 standards for

[28] J. Donald Harris, "Steps Toward an International Audiometric Zero," in "Identification Audiometry," *Journal of Speech and Hearing Disorders*, Monograph Supplement 9 (September 1961):66.

audiometric zero. Many European countries adopted sound-pressure levels for audiometric zero that differed from American standards. For several years, scientists from various countries met under the aegis of the International Standards Organization (ISO) in an effort to agree on the sound-pressure levels to define audiometric zero, or in other words, to write an international standard for audiometer calibration. Finally, this task was accomplished in 1964. The American representatives to the ISO recommended that the international standards be adopted in this country beginning January 1, 1965. Many scientific associations, including the American Speech and Hearing Association, endorsed the new standards—referred to as *ISO-1964* standards—and agreed to implement them immediately.

Between 1964 and 1969, there was much confusion in the audiological world regarding audiometer calibration and audiometric data. It was necessary for manufacturers to indicate to which standards their products were calibrated and for audiologists, otologists, and others reporting test results to specify whether their results were based on ASA-1951 or ISO-1964 standards. Many audiogram forms used in this period contained both ordinates, so the recorded hearing levels could be referred to the ordinate of choice. Some audiogram forms contained instructions concerning the number of decibels to add or subtract to correct one standard to the other. Fortunately, the confusion is now ended because ANSI has published a revised set of standards that replaces the ASA-1951 standards with the ISO-1964 recommendations; now this country is officially in step with the other countries of the world that have accepted the ISO-1964 levels.[29] Table 5–2 contains the new standards and, for comparison's sake, the old American standards and the differences between them.

The calibration of an audiometer and its earphones can be checked at any time by means of the artificial ear, which compares the obtained meter readings with those specified for correct calibration. Portable artificial ears are on the market, so that in many cities the calibration of audiometers can be checked without sending the audiometer to the factory. Some hearing centers possess their own artificial ears and regularly check the calibration of their audiometers. If an audiometer is discovered to be out of calibration, a correction chart must be prepared, the audiometer must be recalibrated by a qualified technician, or it must be sent to a factory-authorized repair station for recalibration.

The results of the calibration check should be recorded on a form such as that shown in Figure 5–4. Checks are made at each frequency at a particular attenuator (hearing-level control) setting. This value should be recorded on the chart for each frequency, so that obtained readings can be compared with specified values and the error at each frequency can be computed. Usually,

[29] "American National Standards Specifications for Audiometers," ANSI S3.6-1969 (New York: American National Standards Institute, Inc., 1970).

TABLE 5–2.   Sound pressure levels in dB re 0.0002 dyne/cm² for audiometric zero according to present and former American standards.

Frequency Hz	Present American Standard (ANSI–1969, same as ISO–1964)	Former American Standard (ASA–1951)	Differences
125	45.5	54.5	9.0
250	24.5	39.5	15.0
500	11.0	25.0	14.0
1000	6.5	16.5	10.0
1500	6.5		
2000	8.5	17.0	8.5
3000	7.5		
4000	9.0	15.0	6.0
6000	8.0		
8000	9.5	21.0	11.5

Values are rounded to the nearest ½ dB.
Adapted from Fred W. Kranz, "Audiometer Principles and History," *Sound* 2 (March–April 1963): 31, and reproduced by permission.

calibration checks are made at each frequency at a hearing-level dial setting of 70 dB in order to avoid any possible interference from room noise or internal noise from the artificial ear. The specified artificial ear meter reading at each frequency will not be exactly 70 plus the ANSI-1969 SPL value in most cases, however, because the earphones furnished with audiometers differ in their response characteristics from the Western Electric 705-A earphone specified in the ANSI-1969 standard. Reference threshold values for various makes of commercially available earphones are based on loudness-balance studies of those particular earphones with the Western Electric 705-A and are given in an appendix to the published ANSI-1969 standard.[30] To the calibration levels specified for a particular make and model of earphone must be applied any sound level meter errors, representing deviations from a flat frequency response. These errors can be read off the frequency response curve furnished by the microphone manufacturer.

The ANSI standard allows for deviations from the specified standard reference threshold sound-pressure levels of ± 3 dB at the frequencies from 250 through 3000 Hz; ± 4 dB at 4000 Hz; and ± 5 dB at 125, 6000, and 8000 Hz. The audiologist should aim to have the audiometer accurate to ± 2.5 dB of the reference value at each frequency. If deviations are within a 2.5 dB range, no corrections are necessary. If, however, one or more frequencies has a deviation between 2.5 and 7.5 dB, a 5-dB correction will have to be applied to

[30] Ibid., p. 21.

AUDIOMETER CALIBRATION

Date: July 25, 1977
Calibration Unit: B & K
Calibrated by: E. Jones

Audiometer: Beltone 10–D 2034
Earphone: TDH–39
Cushion: MX41/AR

EARPHONE OUTPUT CHECK AT 70-dB HEARING LEVEL

Test Frequency	Calibration Level ANSI-1969 for TDH-39	Microphone Error	Corrected Calibration Level	Right Earphone			Left Earphone		
				Measured Level	Error	Correction	Measured Level	Error	Correction
125	115.0	0	115.0	114.2	−0.8	0	114.0	−1.0	0
250	95.5	0	95.5	95.7	+0.2	0	95.5	0.0	0
500	81.5	0	81.5	82.8	+1.3	0	81.8	+0.3	0
1000	77.0	0	77.0	78.8	+1.8	0	79.0	+2.0	0
1500	76.5	0	76.5	77.0	+0.5	0	76.4	−0.1	0
2000	79.0	+0.4	79.4	78.4	−1.0	0	78.8	−0.6	0
3000	80.0	+1.1	81.1	81.3	+0.2	0	81.0	−0.1	0
4000	79.5	+1.8	81.3	80.2	−1.1	0	81.2	−0.1	0
6000	85.5	+2.0	87.5	83.6	−3.9	−5	85.8	−1.7	0
8000	83.0	−3.1	79.9	80.5	+0.6	0	83.2	+3.3	+5

FIGURE 5-4. Recording the results of a calibration check.

an obtained hearing-level reading to indicate the actual HTL. If a deviation between 7.5 and 12.5 dB is found, the correction will be 10 dB. Once the error is determined at each frequency, a correction is needed. Some audiometers allow for changing the level by means of accessible adjusters, which can be manipulated to set the proper level. Alternatively, the corrections can be implemented arithmetically. A correction chart can be prepared, showing arithmetic corrections to apply to hearing-level dial readings, so that the thresholds to be recorded will be correct to the nearest 5-dB step. In order to so correct the dial readings, the correction is applied in the same direction as the error; that is, if there is an error of − 6.3 dB at a particular frequency, meaning that the earphone output is 6.3 dB less than it should be at that hearing-level dial setting, the appropriate correction would be to subtract 5 dB from an obtained hearing level before recording the threshold on the audiogram. A correction chart should be secured to the face of the audiometer, so that anyone using the instrument will know what corrections must be made before recording thresholds. A calibration check must be made on each earphone, and if the audiometer being checked is a two-channel instrument, each earphone must be checked with each channel.

With some artificial ears, it is possible to run checks on the linearity of the attenuator. An attenuator check consists of measuring the changes in voltage that occur in the earphone circuit or the changes in sound-level pressure that occur in the coupler when the hearing-level control is rotated. If the attenuator is functioning properly, the meter on the artificial ear should show exactly 5 dB of change in voltage or sound-pressure level when the hearing-level control is shifted one 5-dB step. The attenuator should be checked over its entire range. The calibration check of the audiometer output at each frequency yields an error value that may apply only at the hearing level at which the check was conducted, usually 70 dB. If there is an attenuator problem, the correction computed on the basis of the output check may not be at all appropriate for other attenuator settings at that frequency. If the attenuator is found to be seriously in error, that is, if some of the intensity steps should be found to differ by more than 2.5 dB from the 5 dB they should be, the audiometer should be returned to the factory for repair or replacement of the attenuator. The ANSI standard specifies that each frequency shall be within 3 percent of the indicated frequency; for example, the allowable tolerance for 1000 Hz would be ± 30 Hz. A frequency counter is required to determine whether an audiometer meets this requirement. The requirement for purity of tone is that any higher harmonic shall be at least 30 dB lower than the sound-pressure level of the fundamental as measured at the maximum hearing level for that frequency.

It is possible for an audiometrist to check on the calibration of the equipment without an artificial ear. Every audiometrist should constantly be aware of the possibility that an audiometer may not be functioning properly. Before giving a test, the examiner should listen to the frequency of 1000 Hz as intensity is decreased to threshold. Every few days, this test should be conducted for all the test frequencies. Because the audiometrist presumably has a known hearing-level pattern, gross deviations can thus be spotted in audiometer output. As mentioned previously, this procedure is called a *biological* check on the calibration of an audiometer.

Another method of checking the calibration requires a second audiometer that is known to be in calibration. The procedure here is for the audiometrist to set the calibrated audiometer at a given frequency and hearing level, set the other audiometer at the same frequency, and then, without looking at the dial setting, adjust the hearing-level control until the loudness of the tones produced by the two audiometers is approximately equal. The hearing-level dial setting on the uncalibrated audiometer is then noted. If the dial setting is different from that of the calibrated audiometer, a correction is indicated. For example, suppose the calibrated instrument is set at 2000 Hz and a hearing level of 70 dB. The audiometrist then sets the other audiometer at 2000 Hz and, without watching the dial setting, adjusts the hearing-level control until the loudness of the tone in the earphone is the same as the loudness of the tone in the earphone of the calibrated instrument. This judgment is made by listening alternately to the earphones from the two audiometers, using only one ear in the process. Let us say in this illustration that the audiometer being checked agrees in loudness with the calibrated audiometer at 2000 Hz when the hearing-level control is set at 75 dB. There is thus a 5-dB difference in output at this frequency. On the correction chart, the audiometrist would indicate that at 2000 Hz, 5 dB should be subtracted from the indicated hearing level. The same procedure would be followed for all frequencies—balancing the loudness of output of the two audiometers, with the calibrated instrument, of course, being the standard.

It should be noted that in this method of calibration, the direction of the correction is apparently opposite that of the error, in contrast to checks with an artificial ear, where the sign of the correction is the same as the sign of the error. Actually, there is no difference in principle between the two methods. In the example just cited, it was necessary to set the hearing-level control of the audiometer being checked to 75 dB to match the loudness of the calibrated audiometer at 70 dB. In other words, the output level of the audiometer being checked was too low at a dial reading of 70 dB. The error measured with an artificial ear would be a minus one, calling for a correction to be subtracted from an obtained hearing level before recording a threshold on an audiogram.

An audiometer may get out of calibration because of changing characteristics of some electronic components (transistors, resistors, or condensers), or as is more likely, the earphones may be damaged through dropping or rough handling, so that they do not respond as they did when the instrument was last calibrated. The earphones are the weakest link in the audiometric chain, and they should always be handled with care. When the audiometer comes from the manufacturer, it has been calibrated to the particular earphones that accompany it. It is not possible to substitute other phones without jeopardizing the calibration because the factory has selected phones that are closely matched in output at all frequencies. From time to time, loudness balance checks should be made with the two earphones, to make sure that they are producing the same output at a given hearing-level setting at all frequencies. If significant differences are found between the two earphones, it is better to send the audiometer to the factory or to an authorized repair service for recalibration with new earphones than to attempt to correct for the errors in either earphone.

Checking the calibration of the audiometer for bone-conduction testing is more difficult than for air-conduction testing. However, artificial mastoids have been developed, so that instrumental checks of bone-conduction vibrator output can be made in a comparable fashion to the artificial-ear measurements of the output of air-conduction earphones. Weiss described the development of an artificial mastoid for the Beltone Company.[31] The Bruel and Kjaer Company has developed an artificial mastoid consisting of a device that replaces the microphone of any of their sound-level meters. An ANSI standard prescribes the mechanical impedance component values for an artificial "headbone" to a vibrator of a given shape and size applied with a given force. Because it will take time to develop calibration equipment and vibrators with characteristics as specified in the standard, an appendix to the standard contains the headbone impedance characteristics of the Beltone artificial mastoid and interim threshold calibration values for mastoid and forehead placement in root-mean-square (rms) force levels in dB re 0.1 dyne.[32]

Because relatively few clinics have access to artificial mastoids, audiometrists themselves must check the calibration of their bone-conduction vibrators. The best way is to have available two or three patients who are known to have pure sensori-neural losses of mild to moderate degree. By definition, then, their bone-conduction HTLs should exactly equal their air-conduction HTLs. If the audiometrist is confident that the audiometer is properly calibrated for air-conduction testing, or if it can be corrected for any known errors in output, only air- and bone-conduction HTLs on a few patients with sensori-neural impairment need to be compared. Because of differences in patients' responses to bone-conducted sounds, owing to the differences in conductivity of skin and bone among different individuals, the HTLs by air and by bone should be averaged for the patients cooperating in the study, and the averages should be compared rather than the individual measures of air and bone conduction for each patient. Thus, if at 500 Hz the average air-

[31] Erwin Weiss, "An Air Damped Artificial Mastoid," *Journal of the Acoustical Society of America* 32 (December 1960):1582–88.

[32] "American National Standard for an Artificial Headbone for the Calibration of Audiometer Bone Vibrators," ANSI S3.13-1972 (New York: American National Standards Institute, Inc.).

conduction HTL for the patients was 25 dB and the average bone-conduction HTL was 30 dB, the audiometrist would conclude that the bone-conduction vibrator was producing a signal at this frequency which was 5 dB too weak. The correction chart would indicate that 5 dB should be subtracted from the obtained bone-conduction HTL at 500 Hz. Naturally, the success of this method depends on the availability of some patients who are definitely known to have pure sensori-neural losses. If there is any doubt about whether their losses are purely sensori-neural, the method should not be adopted. Also, more accurate results can be obtained with eight or ten patients instead of only two or three, because the effect of random errors would be canceled out.

Some audiometrists have the mistaken notion that they should always turn off the power to the audiometer as soon as they have completed a test, apparently on the assumption that the longer the power is on the more wear the audiometer parts receive or in an attempt to conserve electricity. Actually, the wear on the audiometer parts occurs from turning the instrument on and off, and the amount of electricity the audiometer consumes is minimal. When the audiometer is first turned on, power surges through the electronic components, and it is at this time that "weak" parts will fail. If more than one test is to be given during the day, it is better to leave the audiometer turned on throughout the day than it is to turn it on and off for each test. In some television stations, the electronic equipment is kept on twenty-four hours a day because the engineers realize that the components will last longer this way. Of course, in a television station an engineer would be on duty at all hours. It is preferable to turn audiometric equipment off at the end of each day because of the danger of fire when no one is around.

THE AUDIOGRAM

Hearing-test results are recorded in the form of a graph called an *audiogram,* or they may be written in number form on a chart that is also referred to as an audiogram. An audiogram graph has two dimensions: frequency along the abscissa and intensity along the ordinate expressed as dB of hearing level. The patient's HTL at each frequency tested is plotted on the audiogram for each ear separately, both by air conduction and by bone conduction. Standard symbols are used to indicate HTLs for each ear at the appropriate 5-dB step, separate symbols being used for air-conduction and bone-conduction thresholds. Also, different colors can be used to differentiate between the ears, red denoting the right ear and blue the left. Of course, audiograms are not reproduced in color, so the ears must be differentiated by symbols. Figure 5–5 shows a typical audiogram form, the symbols being approved by the American Speech and Hearing Association.[33]

[33] "Guidelines for Audiometric Symbols," *Asha* 16 (May 1974):260–64.

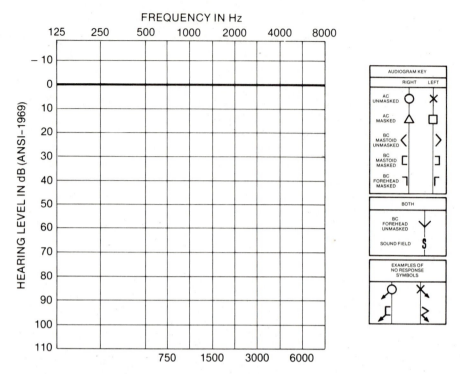

FIGURE 5-5.   A typical audiogram form.

The symbols O and X are used to plot the air-conduction threshold points at each frequency for the right and left ears, respectively. Arrows pointing to the left and right indicate bone-conduction threshold hearing levels for the right and left ears, respectively. The term *threshold* has occurred many times in this book thus far without having been defined. In psychological and physiological work in the field of sensation, *threshold* is defined as the intensity of stimulus required just barely to elicit a sensation in whatever sensory modality is being studied. A subject's threshold at a particular time can be measured in the laboratory with a high degree of precision. In hearing, a subject's threshold is expressed in fractions of a decibel. Sensory thresholds are not absolute; that is, they do not remain constant but tend to fluctuate somewhat as a function of the subject's physical, emotional, and mental state. Nevertheless, at a given moment, the threshold can be established rather precisely.

In clinical hearing testing, in contrast to laboratory measurements, gross increments of sound intensity are employed, generally in steps of 5 dB. The patient's threshold is defined as the lowest level at which the presence of the test tone can be detected at least 50 percent of the time. If the intensity is decreased by another 5 dB, the patient will no longer be able to hear the tone.

Actually, the true threshold may be as much as 4½ dB less than that obtained, but since the audiometer indicates gross steps of intensity, only gross thresholds may be measured—gross, that is, by laboratory standards.

In audiometric work, the terms *above* and *below* threshold and *raised* and *lowered* threshold are frequently confused. The confusion arises from the fact that the lower a patient's audiogram curve appears on the graph, the greater the amount of hearing loss. We tend to think of the terms *above, below, raised,* and *lowered,* therefore, in relation to the position of the patient's curve of hearing sensitivity on the audiogram. Actually, this is just the reverse of the way the terms should be applied. Let's say that a certain amount of intensity is required to reach a patient's threshold at a certain frequency. If we have an intensity less than this amount, that tone is *below* the patient's threshold—it is not sufficiently intense to be heard. If we then increase the intensity beyond the point at which the patient can just barely hear it, we have gone *above* the patient's threshold. If one patient has less hearing loss than another, we say that the threshold for sound is *lower;* that is one patient can respond to a lower intensity of sound than the other. By the same token, if a patient's hearing is improved by an operative procedure or by wearing a hearing aid, we speak of the improvement in hearing as a *lowering* of the threshold—the patient can now respond to sounds of less intensity than formerly. In contrast, if hearing becomes worse, the threshold is *raised*—a greater amount of intensity is now required for a response. We must always remember, then, that the terms *above, below, raise,* and *lower,* when applied to thresholds, have no reference to the position of the audiogram curve, because a *lowered* threshold actually means a *higher* position of the curve on the audiogram.

Customarily, the Os and Xs which mark the points of hearing threshold level across the audiogram are connected by solid lines of the appropriate color, red for the Os and blue for the Xs. Thus, the contour of the hearing loss by air conduction can be seen for each ear at a glance. Usually, the bone-conduction threshold levels are not connected by lines, although some audiometrists prefer to connect them by dashed lines, which contrast with the solid lines connecting the air-conduction threshold hearing levels. If masking is used during the test, appropriate symbols serve to indicate that fact. These symbols are the triangle for the right ear and the square for the left ear, for air conduction, and brackets to the left or right of the frequency line for bone conduction. Sometimes, it is desirable to record thresholds obtained both without and with masking, and then all the symbols would be needed. If the patient does not respond by air conduction to the maximum hearing level at a given frequency, an arrow is drawn pointing downward from the appropriate symbol at that hearing level.

It should be mentioned here that there is not universal agreement concerning the symbols to represent bone-conduction results. Many audiologists, including the authors, believe that the direction of the arrows should be reversed from the way they appear on the sample audiogram in Figure 5–5. In other words, they contend that for right-ear bone conduction, the arrows should appear to the right of the frequency line and point to the right, as they did in previous editions of this book. The majority opinion of 214 audiologists surveyed by Martin and Kopra was in agreement.[34] However, the ASHA Committee on Audiometric Evaluation, which was responsible for generating the guidelines for symbols adopted by ASHA (American Speech and Hearing Association), opted for the arrow or bracket heading to the left for the right ear and to the right for the left ear, largely "in deference to the preferences expressed by representatives of the American Academy of Ophthalmology and Otolaryngology."[35] The logic for this "backward" use of symbols is that the arrow or bracket represents the pinna of the patient and that as the patient sits facing you, the right pinna is to your left; therefore, the symbol for the right ear should be to the left of the frequency line on the audiogram. Apparently, this method of notation is common in medical usage and so for years has been advocated for use on audiograms by otolaryngologists.[36] Of course, this logic falls apart if patients sit with their back to the examiner, as is sometimes the case in hearing testing. Because it is desirable to have uniformity in the use of symbols to avoid confusion, the system approved by ASHA will be used in this book.

Fortunately, there has been agreement for years among otologists and audiologists about how air-conduction thresholds should be recorded on the audiogram. Some clinicians, however, prefer forms that have separate audiograms for the right and left ears appearing side by side. Figure 5–6 shows such an audiogram with a simplified system of symbols suggested by Jerger, because with separate audiograms for the two ears the same symbols can be used for both ears.[37] In addition to symbols for air and bone conduction, this system provides symbols for designating the results of the SAL test and thresholds of the acoustic reflex. A separate audiogram for each ear does avoid the kind of cluttering that occurs when air and bone HTLs for both right and left ears are about the same values. In the next section of this chapter, sample audiograms will illustrate different types and degrees of hearing loss, and the reader can see how the various symbols are employed.

For some purposes, it is preferable to record hearing levels in numbers rather than on an audiogram form. If, for example, one is keeping a cumulative record of hearing tests on a particular patient, the use of such a form as that shown in Figure 5–7 makes it possible to determine at a glance how hearing levels might have changed from test to test.

[34] Frederick N. Martin and Lennart L. Kopra, "Symbols in Pure-tone Audiometry," *Asha* 12 (April 1970):182–85.

[35] "Guidelines for Audiometric Symbols," p. 261.

[36] E. P. Fowler, "Signs, Emblems and Symbols of Choice in Plotting Threshold Audiograms," *Archives of Otolaryngology* 53 (1951):129–33.

[37] James Jerger, "A Proposed Audiometric Symbol System for Scholarly Publications," *Archives of Otolaryngology* 102 (January 1976):33–36.

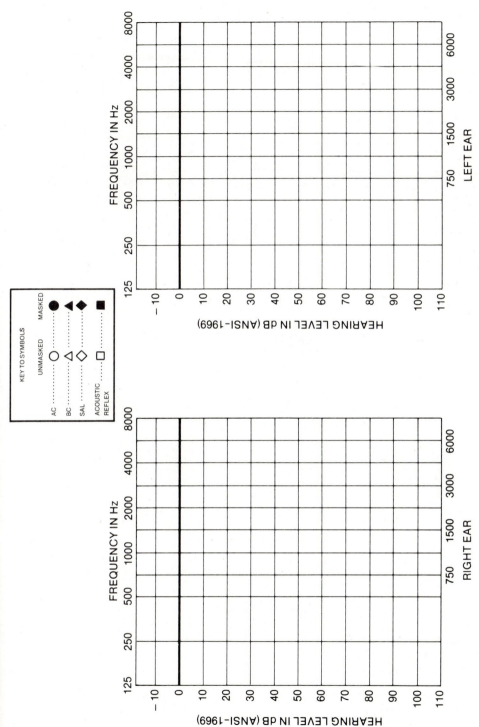

FIGURE 5-6. Separate audiogram for each ear with simplified symbols suitable for use with both ears, as suggested by Jerger.

149

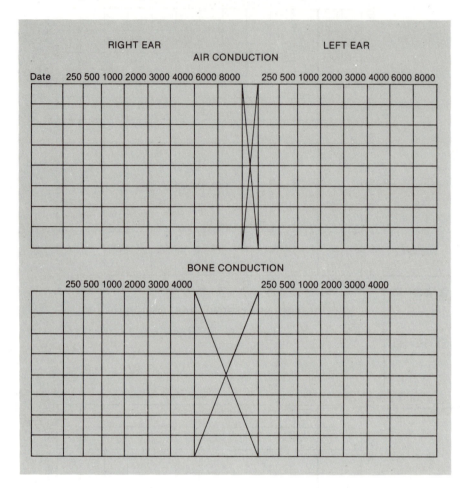

FIGURE 5-7.   Form for recording hearing threshold levels in numbers for serial hearing tests.

INTERPRETING THE AUDIOGRAM

The purpose of hearing tests is twofold: first, to provide information that will assist the otologist in a diagnosis of the hearing impairment; and, second, to indicate what the patient's needs for aural rehabilitation might be. For both purposes, the audiogram requires expert interpretation.

As Aid to Diagnosis

To the otologist, the audiogram is useful for the information it yields on the comparative sensitivity of the patient's air and bone conduction. Such information enables the otologist to diagnose the hearing impairment as conductive, sensori-neural, or mixed in type. The course of treatment prescribed will be based on this diagnosis. Naturally, the diagnosis depends not only on the hearing-test results but also on the results of the physical examination and the patient's medical history.

By definition, a "pure" conductive loss results from pathology or malfunctioning of the outer or middle ear with a normal inner ear. That is, a patient with a conductive loss should present an audiogram showing losses by air conduction but normal hearing by bone conduction. Figure 5–8 illustrates a typical audiogram of a patient with conductive loss.

Although a diagnosis of conductive impairment can be made only by comparing the air- and bone-conduction losses, it is possible to make some generalizations concerning the appearance of the air-conduction curve alone. Generally, in a conductive impairment, the air-conduction losses will be fairly equal at all frequencies, with perhaps slightly greater loss for the lower frequencies. Reference to Figure 5–8 will demonstrate this observation. Yet, to reiterate, diagnosis cannot be made from the air-conduction curve alone because sensori-neural losses may also be fairly uniform at all frequencies. Also, some instances of conductive loss show poorer hearing for the high frequencies.

The cause of a particular conductive loss cannot be ascertained from the

FIGURE 5-8.   Typical conductive impairment.

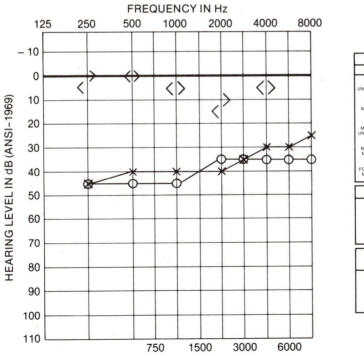
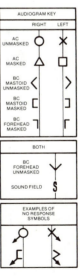

audiogram. There are some differences in the audiometric pictures of otitis media and otosclerosis, but these can be learned only through experience. Tympanometry yields additional information that aids in diagnosing conductive impairments, as we shall see in Chapter 7. No statements concerning etiology can be made, however, without the additional information derived from the physical examination and the medical history. Incidentally, it should be stated here that diagnosis of hearing impairment is not the responsibility of the audiologist. Because hearing loss is a medical disability, only a physician is legally qualified to make a diagnosis. The audiologist must be careful not to get into the position of "practicing medicine" or making medical pronouncements on the basis of audiological workups.

Sensori-neural impairments are characterized usually, but not always, by greater losses at the higher frequencies on the audiogram. The audiogram may show normal or close-to-normal hearing at the lower frequencies, with a rapid decrease in hearing sensitivity as the test proceeds through the higher frequencies. Figure 5–9 represents a more or less typical sensori-neural impairment. It will be noticed that the bone-conduction thresholds are approximately the same as the air-conduction thresholds, which of course is the important diagnostic indication of a sensori-neural loss. Because the bone-

FIGURE 5-9.   Typical sensori-neural impairment.

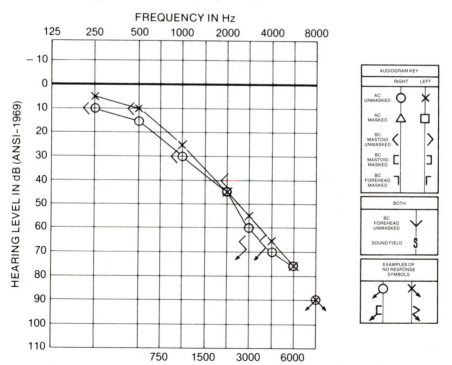

conduction thresholds of the right ear indicated that thresholds by bone were approximately equal to those by air, it was not necessary to test the bone conduction of the left ear. Because of the minimal interaural attenuation for bone conduction, it is obvious that the bone conduction of the left ear cannot differ significantly from that of the right. In this instance, the patient's loss at 8000 Hz exceeded the air-conduction limits of the audiometer. The arrows that point downward at the 90-dB level indicate that the patient did not respond at the maximum hearing level available at 8000 Hz. Likewise, the patient did not respond at the maximum hearing levels available by bone conduction at 3000 and 4000 Hz (65 dB).

The etiology of sensori-neural impairments cannot be determined from the audiogram alone, although certain causes do produce somewhat typical audiometric pictures. Noise-induced hearing loss—exposure to extreme noise for long enough periods to produce permanent hearing loss—usually is reflected in the audiogram by occurrence of the greatest amount of loss around 4000 Hz, with perhaps some recovery at higher frequencies. Figure 5–10 is a typical audiogram of sensori-neural loss caused by exposure to noise.

Sometimes, a patient has extreme losses in one ear whereas the other ear is essentially normal. Where differences of 40 dB or more exist between the

FIGURE 5–10.   Sensori-neural impairment resulting from noise exposure.

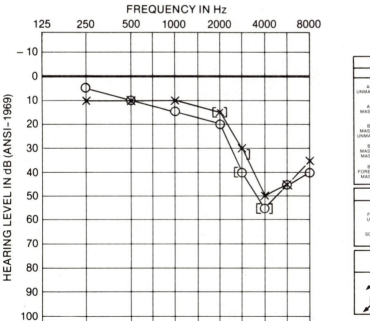
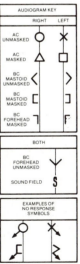

air-conduction curves, or between the air-conduction HTLs of the test ear and the bone-conduction HTLs of the nontest ear, masking should be applied in the better ear in order to obtain an accurate picture of the hearing in the poorer ear. Figure 5–11 is the audiogram of a girl in her twenties who had lost most of the hearing in one ear because of a skull fracture. Both the masked and unmasked HTLs for the left ear are shown on the audiogram. It can be seen that without masking, an entirely false picture of the hearing of the left ear would have been obtained. In this audiogram, the unmasked air-conduction threshold configuration of the left ear is an excellent example of a shadow curve. It mirrors the curve of the right ear because it is actually the right ear that is responding when the signal is being delivered to the left ear. When masking was used in bone-conduction testing, no responses within the intensity limitations of the bone-conduction circuit were obtained.

A mixed impairment will produce an audiogram that shows some loss by bone conduction but a more severe loss by air conduction. Or perhaps the mixed impairment will be manifested by conductive loss in the lower frequencies and sensori-neural loss in the higher frequencies. Figure 5–12 represents a mixed impairment.

FIGURE 5–11.   Comparison of masked and unmasked HTLs in unilateral sensori-neural loss.

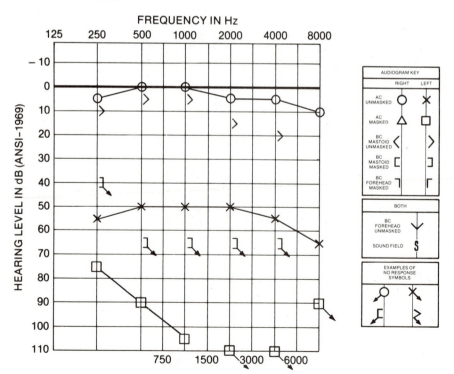

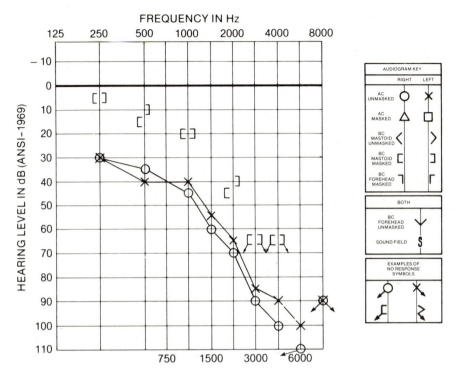

FIGURE 5-12. A mixed impairment.

As Guide to Rehabilitation

The audiogram is useful in pointing to the need for rehabilitative measures, such as a hearing aid, for example, or instruction in speechreading. The audiogram can also serve to some extent to differentiate between children who are deaf, and thus need full-time special education, and children who are hard-of-hearing and can fit into the framework of the regular classroom. Naturally, the audiogram is not the only criterion in making such determinations, as we shall see in Chapter 10, but it is an important guide to rehabilitative needs.

The handicap of a hearing loss is in direct proportion to the effect that the loss has on the patient's communicative ability. Hence, it is important that the audiogram yield some information about how hearing for speech has been impaired. If speech audiometric equipment is available, of course, this information can be obtained directly. Lacking speech-testing equipment, however, an estimate of the effect of the hearing loss on speech can be made from the pure-tone audiogram. In these estimates, two things are important: the amount of loss through the so-called speech frequencies and the configuration of the audiogram curve.

The speech frequencies are 500, 1000, and 2000 Hz, so designated because many studies have shown that there is a high correlation between the average HTL at these three frequencies and the loss for speech as measured directly on a speech audiometer. The HTL for speech in each ear can thus be predicted by adding the levels at each of these frequencies and dividing the sum by three. There is an important exception to this rule: If the shape of the audiogram curve is such that there is an abrupt increase in HTL in proceeding from low to high frequencies, so that the difference in HTL between 500 and 1000 Hz and between 1000 and 2000 Hz equals 20 dB or more, averaging the three frequencies will exaggerate the actual HTL for speech. In such a situation, therefore, the rule is that the HTL for speech can be predicted by disregarding the frequency that shows the greatest loss and averaging the other two speech frequencies. This is called the *two-frequency* method of predicting HTL for speech intelligibility. Fletcher advocates the two-frequency method for predicting the loss for speech regardless of the shape of the air-conduction curve on the audiogram.[38] At the present writing, audiological opinion is divided on this point.

Information concerning a patient's need for a hearing aid can be obtained by inspection of the HTLs at the speech frequencies (500, 1000, and 2000 Hz), although it is no longer advisable to state the minimum hearing levels at which a hearing aid would be indicated. The oft-quoted "rule" that a hearing aid would not be considered unless the hearing loss for speech in the better ear is at least 30 dB no longer applies because there are so many exceptions. Today's hearing aids are easily put on and taken off. They operate quietly, and many patients with only minimal hearing loss for speech find hearing aids helpful to them, even though they may not be used at all times. A hearing aid is usually of little help to a person who has one normal ear, because in most situations speech can be heard adequately with one good ear, but even this type of patient may find some benefit from a hearing aid in certain situations.

Losses for speech up to 80 dB can usually be "corrected" with the amplification of a hearing aid. "Correction" does not mean restoration of the hearing function to normal—or zero hearing level on the audiometer. Rather, it refers to the restoration of the patient's hearing to a useful level. Losses for speech in excess of 80 dB *may* be "corrected" by means of amplification. Each patient must be considered individually, and frequently a decision cannot be made without a period of experimentation with amplification, which may extend over several weeks or months. It is doubtful that any patient whose loss for speech in the better ear is as great as 100 dB can be successfully rehabilitated by means of amplification alone. On the other hand, it cannot be said that such a patient would obtain no benefit from amplification. Here again, experimentation is necessary. The subject of hearing aids and their selection will be discussed more fully in Chapter 10.

[38] Harvey Fletcher, "A Method of Calculating Hearing Loss for Speech from an Audiogram," *Journal of the Acoustical Society of America* 22 (January 1950):1–5.

Before speech audiometry became common as a diagnostic tool, it was necessary to have some means of expressing the amount of handicap produced by a hearing loss, based on the pure-tone audiogram. In medicolegal cases, the amount of compensation for a hearing loss is based on the degree of handicap. The concept of *percentage of hearing loss* was introduced by Fowler and Sabine to meet this need. For a number of years, percentage hearing loss was computed by the Fowler-Sabine procedure, termed the AMA *method,* because it was published under the aegis of the American Medical Association. In this method, only four frequencies on the audiogram were considered: 500, 1000, 2000, and 4000 Hz. These frequencies were weighted in their importance to the total speech-hearing function, as follows: 500 Hz = 15 percent; 1000 Hz = 30 percent; 2000 Hz = 40 percent; and 4000 Hz = 15 percent. Losses in dB at each of these frequencies were assigned percentage values according to a chart used in conjunction with the pure-tone audiogram or sometimes included as part of the audiogram. Losses for each ear were converted to percentages, and a formula was applied for computing the binaural percentage loss.

The disadvantage of the AMA percentage method is that it told little about the patient's ability to communicate. Neither did it shed light on the ability to compensate for the loss by means of a hearing aid. Two patients with very different-appearing audiograms may actually have the same percentage of hearing loss when computed by the AMA system, yet one patient may be considerably more handicapped in communication than the other.

In 1959, a new method for computing percentage hearing impairment was published under the sponsorship of the American Academy of Ophthalmology and Otolaryngology, and hence it is referred to as the AAOO *method.*[39] It has been endorsed by the AMA and thus is also referred to as the AMA *method.* To avoid confusion with the old Fowler-Sabine procedure, we shall refer to it only as the AAOO method. The AAOO method has almost entirely replaced the Fowler-Sabine procedure for determining, on the basis of pure-tone audiometric information, the percentage of impairment. In the AAOO method, only the speech frequencies are assigned any percentage values. Percentage impairment is computed for each ear separately by averaging the air-conduction hearing levels at 500, 1000, and 2000 Hz, subtracting 26 dB from this average, and multiplying the remainder by 1½ percent. The binaural percentage impairment is computed by multiplying the percentage impairment of the *better* ear by five, adding this product to the percentage impairment of the poorer ear, and dividing this sum by six. The AAOO method is illustrated in Figure 5–13.

The rationale of this method is that hearing is "impaired" only when the speech frequencies are affected because the principal use to which hearing is

[39] "Guide for the Evaluation of Hearing Impairment," *Transactions American Academy of Ophthalmology and Otolaryngology* (March–April 1959):235–38. The values in this article were based on ASA-1951 audiometric calibration standards. They have been corrected here to ANSI-1969 calibration standards.

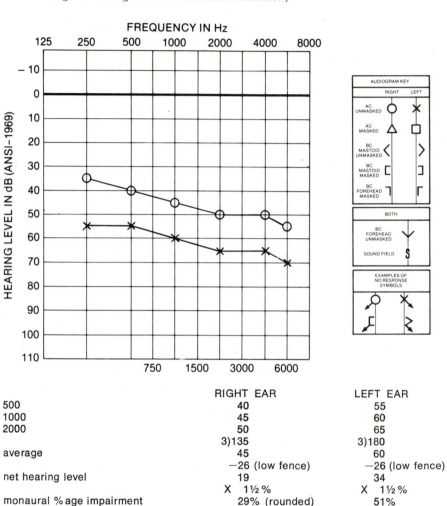

	RIGHT EAR	LEFT EAR
500	40	55
1000	45	60
2000	50	65
	3)135	3)180
average	45	60
	−26 (low fence)	−26 (low fence)
net hearing level	19	34
	X 1½%	X 1½%
monaural % age impairment	29% (rounded)	51%
	X 5 (weighting)	
	145	
impairment poor ear	+ 51	
	6)196	
binaural % age impairment	33% (rounded)	

FIGURE 5–13. Computation of percentage impairment by the AAOO method.

put is in listening to speech. Hearing impairment is confined between two "fences." The "low fence" is an average hearing level through the speech frequencies of 26 dB; until hearing for speech exceeds 26 dB there is no handicapping impairment. Thus, before determining percentage of hearing impairment, 26 dB is subtracted from the average hearing level for the speech frequencies. The "high fence," or 100 percent hearing impairment, is considered to be an average hearing level through the speech frequencies of 93 dB. Subtracting 26 dB (the low fence) from 93 dB (the high fence) leaves a remainder of 67 dB as the span of handicapping hearing loss from 0 to 100 percent. Thus, each dB of this span is worth 1½ percent.

Because a unilateral hearing impairment is not nearly so handicapping as a bilateral impairment, the formula for combining the percentage impairments of the two ears into percentage binaural impairment weights the "better" ear five times the value of the "poorer" ear. The "inflated" percentage impairment of the better ear is then added to the percentage impairment of the poorer ear. Because this sum then contains six parts—five for the better ear and one for the poorer ear—the sum is divided by six. Naturally, because of the weighting, the resulting binaural percentage impairment is much closer to the value assigned to the better ear than it is to the percentage computed for the poorer ear.

The AAOO method is used extensively in medicolegal contexts, as will be seen later in Chapter 9. Although this method of computing percentage hearing impairment represents an improvement over the old AMA method of Fowler and Sabine, it has been severely criticized (1) for having its low fence too high (Kryter, for example, suggests that the low fence should be 16 dB[40]), and (2) for not including higher frequencies in the average of speech frequencies. The importance of 3000 Hz for speech intelligibility under difficult listening conditions has long been acknowledged.[41] Computing hearing impairment as an average of HTLs at 1000, 2000, and 3000 Hz has been proposed by the National Institute for Occupational Safety and Health.[42] Compensation for noise-induced hearing impairment in the State of California is based on percentage of hearing loss computed by averaging HTLs at four frequencies instead of three: 500, 1000, 2000, and 3000 Hz. Working with subjects who had losses only at frequencies above 2000 Hz—or in other words, subjects whose percentage hearing impairment was zero as measured by the AAOO formula—Suter found that averaging HTLs at 1000, 2000, and 4000 Hz correlated well with speech discrimination scores measured in a background of "speech babble" noise varying from 0 to −6 signal-to-noise ratio (noise equal in intensity to speech or up to 6 dB greater intensity).[43] It can be anticipated that future formulas for predicting degree of hearing impairment or handicap

---

[40] Karl D. Kryter, "Impairment to Hearing from Exposure to Noise," *Journal of the Acoustical Society of America* 53 (May 1973):1219.

[41] J. Donald Harris, H. L. Haines, and C. K. Myers, "The Importance of Hearing at 3 Kc for Understanding Speeded Speech," *Laryngoscope* 70 (February 1960):131–46.

[42] National Institute for Occupational Safety and Health, *Criteria for a Recommended Standard . . . Occupational Exposure to Noise* (Washington, D.C.: U.S. Department of Health, Education, and Welfare, Health Services and Mental Health Administration, 1972), p. VI–16.

[43] Alice H. Suter, "The Ability of Mildly Hearing-Impaired Individuals to Discriminate Speech in Noise," unpublished Ph.D. dissertation, University of Maryland, 1977.

will include either 3000 or 4000 Hz (or both) and, at least for noise-induced hearing impairment, eliminate 500 Hz. For example, the A.M.A. has adopted a new formula[44] based on the efforts of the American Academy of Otolaryngology (AAO), a new organization derived when Ophthalmology separated from the old AAOO, and the American Council of Otolaryngology (ACO). This new formula which we will refer to as the AAO-ACO method is identical to the AAOO method except that it incorporates the threshold at 3000 Hz. The audiometric data in Figure 5–13 would result in 30% impairment for the right ear and 35% impairment for the left ear with the AAO-ACO method. At the present time there is no widespread acceptance of this new formula nor of others which have been proposed.[45] No method based on the pure-tone audiogram alone could be as satisfactory a means of representing a communicative handicap as the results of clinical speech audiometry, as we shall see in the next chapter.

In this discussion so far we have considered only the extent of loss. The shape or configuration of the audiometric air-conduction curve and the type of hearing impairment are also important. The patient with a steeply sloping curve (greater losses for the higher frequencies) will usually present more difficult rehabilitation problems than the patient whose audiometric configuration is relatively "flat," that is, approximately equal at all frequencies. The flatness or slope of the curve is important primarily in the area of the speech frequencies—from 500 through 2000 Hz. If the losses at 1000 and 2000 Hz are markedly greater than at 500 hz, the patient may confuse many consonants whose distinguishing characteristics are primarily in the higher frequencies. These consonants are generally the voiceless ones, such as *p, k, s, t, f, sh, ch,* and the voiceless *th.*

The patient who has a flat loss throughout the speech frequencies can usually make good use of amplification, because all speech sounds will be amplified equally. The handicap lies only in the inability to hear speech well. As speech is made louder through amplification, the handicap is diminished.

A flat audiogram curve does not guarantee good performance with a hearing aid, however. Some patients with flat sensori-neural losses show very poor understanding of speech with amplification. On the other hand, the patient whose curve slopes steeply through the speech frequencies will not receive as much benefit from amplification because even with amplification the response to different frequencies will be unequal. In theory, the principle of selective amplification, that is, amplifying only the frequencies for which sensitivity is diminished and by an amount equal to the extent of the loss at

[44] American Academy of Otolaryngology, Committee on Hearing and Equilibrium and the American Council of Otolaryngology, Committee on the Medical Aspects of Noise: Guide for the evaluation of hearing handicap. *Journal of the American Medical Association* 241 (1979):2055–59.

[45] Junius C. McElveen, Jr., "Noise Induced Hearing Loss—How Much Is It Worth," *Hearing Instruments* 32 (March, 1981):14B–15.

those frequencies, should operate to provide usable amplified speech. Unfortunately, in practice, selective amplification has not always been found to be effective. Modifications of the earpiece that connects the receiver of the aid with the ear may be helpful in reducing the distortion of amplified speech for patients with sloping audiograms, however, as we shall see in Chapter 10.

Although the audiogram yields important information concerning the rehabilitative needs of patients, it is most valuable when the information it conveys is combined with the results of clinical speech audiometric tests, which measure directly a patient's ability to hear and understand speech. After all, the measure of the handicap of a hearing loss is how one's communicative ability is affected. Whereas predictions of how communication is affected can be made from the pure-tone audiogram with some confidence, actual measures of the communicative ability can be derived through speech audiometry.

CAUTIONS FOR THE EXAMINER

Before moving into the subject of speech audiometry, we should mention two items of caution for the examiner—one concerning possible misinterpretation of test results, and the other concerning earphone hygiene.

Collapsed Canal

Some patients have very small or slitlike external canals that will seal shut with the relatively slight pressure exerted by the earphones. Because the blocked canals prevent the effective transmission of the airborne sound wave to the eardrum, the patient will present the diagnostic indication of a conductive or mixed loss—an air-bone gap—when in fact no gap exists, or the hearing may even be normal. Whenever the test results reveal an air-bone gap, the examiner should inspect the patient's ears to see if the canals seal shut when pressure is applied to the pinnas. If so, a short length of hollow tubing can be inserted in the canal while the air-conduction test is repeated. The tubing prevents the canal from collapsing under the pressure of the earphone. Air-conduction threshold improvements of from 15 to 30 dB have been reported when this retest procedure was followed.[46]

---

[46] Ira Ventry, Joseph B. Chaiklin, and William F. Boyle, "Collapse of the Ear Canal During Audiometry," A.M.A. *Archives of Otolaryngology* 73 (1961):727–31; Victor H. Hildyard and Milton A. Valentine, "Collapse of the Ear Canal During Audiometry," A.M.A. *Archives of Otolaryngology* 75 (1962):422–23; Mark Ross and C. A. Tucker, "A Case Study of Collapse of the Ear Canal During Audiometry," *Laryngoscope* 75 (1965):65–67; Earl W. Stark, "Collapse of the Ear Canal During Audiometry: A Case Report," *Journal of Speech and Hearing Disorders* 31 (November 1966):374–76.

Earphone Contamination

Talbott has directed attention to the danger of spreading infection from earphone cushions.[47] He found that the MX-41/AR cushions used in routine testing in a hospital audiology clinic contained numerous colonies of bacteria of the type associated with otitis media and otitis externa. Athough he presented no evidence of patients incurring infections from the cushions, he concluded that the potential for infection was present. He reported that irradiation of the cushions with ultraviolet light for a period of five minutes eliminated 90 percent of the bacteria.

The most common way to disinfect earphone cushions is to wipe them off with an ethanol sponge. There is no information available concerning the relative effectiveness of this method of disinfecting the cushions and ultraviolet irradiation. The use of any disinfection liquid, however, can be potentially harmful to the cushions—or to the earphone itself if the liquid reaches the diaphragm of the phone. Alcohol or other disinfecting agents are probably more readily available to the average audiology clinic, however, than the proper kind of ultraviolet irradiation.

It is probably true that most clinics make no attempt to disinfect earphone cushions after each patient's use, and it is also probably true that in most cases no harm results. If a patient is referred with an active otitis media, or with an external otitis, however, the audiologist should take every possible precaution to protect following patients from infection by cleansing the cushions with whatever antibacterial agents are available. An added precaution in testing patients with known infections is to cover the patient's pinna with sterile gauze pads before putting the earphones in place. Of course the best procedure would be to disinfect the cushions after every patient. Incidentally, although the chances are remote that patients will be harmed in any way through audiological procedures, audiologists should protect themselves by carrying malpractice insurance—or making sure that they are covered under blanket policies issued to institutions where they work.

[47] Richard E. Talbott, "Bacteriology of Earphone Contamination," *Journal of Speech and Hearing Research* 12 (June 1969):326–29.

CHAPTER SIX
TESTING
THE HEARING FUNCTION:
SPEECH AUDIOMETRY

EQUIPMENT REQUIRED

Speech audiometers have been produced commercially only since the early 1950s. Before that time, it was necessary to have speech audiometers custom designed and built. Several companies build speech-testing equipment today, usually as part of a console that incorporates pure-tone circuitry as well. Because most of these "clinical audiometers" provide two channels and a variety of inputs and outputs, they constitute extremely flexible (and expensive) instruments with which the most sophisticated pure-tone and speech tests may be performed. Thus, since the first standards for speech audiometers were published in 1953, speech-testing equipment has advanced from a simple turntable, an amplifier and attenuator, and a headset of two air-conduction earphones to the complex circuitry of a modern console. The standards for speech audiometers are now incorporated into the standards for pure-tone diagnostic and screening audiometers.[1]

Speech audiometry requires a two-room suite. The test room ideally should be at least 8 feet square (inside dimensions), constructed so that it is

[1] "American National Standard Specifications for Audiometers," ANSI S3.6-1969 (New York: American National Standards Institute, 1970).

isolated acoustically from surrounding space. The test room should be joined with the control room by a double- or triple-paned window (for acoustic insulation purposes) through which the tester may observe the patient. Access to the test room should be through a specially designed acoustic door. The dimensions of the control room are unimportant, as long as there is sufficient room for the equipment and the examiner. It is not necessary to have the control room acoustically isolated unless the adjacent spaces are particularly noisy, or unless the noises emanating from the control room might disturb others working nearby. It is usually more satisfactory to make use of prefabricated sound-isolated rooms than to attempt to build one's own test suite. Single- or double-walled prefabricated panels, depending on the amount of attenuation required, can be combined to provide any size room desired.

Assuming the desirability of combining pure-tone and speech audiometric equipment, the audiometer used in a two-room suite should provide at least the following:

1. Inputs
   a. Microphone
   b. Turntable
   c. Stereo tape deck with delayed auditory feedback feature (cassette or reel-to-reel)
   d. Pure-tone generator (preferably two)
   e. Masking noise generators—narrow band for pure tones and white noise or "speech" noise for speech
2. Two input channels
3. Selector switches for choosing inputs for each channel
4. Volume controls for each input
5. VU meter usable with either channel (preferably separate meters for each channel)
6. Amplifiers
7. Attenuators
8. Outputs
   a. Air-conduction earphones
   b. Bone-conduction vibrator
   c. Loudspeaker (preferably two)
9. Output selector switches permitting selection of either or both input channels for any of the outputs
10. Monitoring and patient talk-back system, including microphone for the patient; amplifier, attenuator, and earphone and/or loudspeaker for the examiner
11. Patient signaling device—switch and light

With such equipment, all the standard and special speech tests, including those for functional or nonorganic hearing problems, can be administered. Figure 6–1 is a photograph of the console of a two-channel combined speech and pure-tone audiometer. Figure 6–2 shows this audiometer

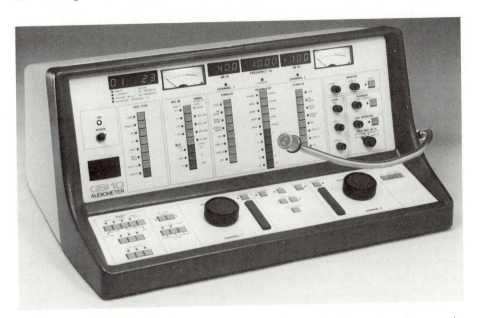

FIGURE 6–1.   Console of a two-channel clinical audiometer. (Reproduced by permission of Grason-Stadler Inc., Littleton, Mass.)

FIGURE 6–2.   A two-channel clinical audiometer with associated peripheral equipment. (Reproduced by permission of Grason-Stadler Inc., Littleton, Mass.)

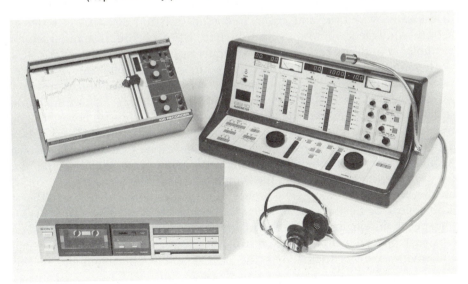

along with an X-Y recorder (for use in Békésy audiometry, to be described in Chapter 7), and a cassette tape deck.

Volume indicator meters (VI meters, or more often VU for "volume units") are needed to enable the examiner to monitor the inputs to the amplifiers. The output of the amplifiers must be calibrated in terms of a specific level of input signal. Once the calibration is established, whatever input is selected must be adjusted to the particular input level that was used in calibration; otherwise the output level will fluctuate with changes in input level. It is customary to monitor all inputs to an average peak reading of zero dB on the VU meter. The input level is controlled by a potentiometer (volume control). The examiner compensates for differences in levels of recording or for differences in vocal intensity in live-voice testing by turning the input volume control until the needle on the VU meter is peaking on the average at zero dB.

The American National Standard calls for the output of speech audiometers to cover a range of at least 100 dB, from 0 to +100 dB in relation to the normal speech HTL in steps of 2.5 dB or less.[2] Actually, most speech audiometers will provide a range of 110 dB or more, with attenuator steps of 1 or 2 dB.

Speech-testing materials may be introduced through either the microphone, which is referred to as monitored live-voice testing, or disc or tape recordings. Both methods have advantages. Live-voice testing is, of course, more flexible, in that the examiner can adapt the manner of testing to suit the particular patient. Thus, with an elderly patient, the examiner can slow down the presentation of test words to a suitable rate. The recorded tests, on the other hand, provide a greater standardization because they can be presented in the same way time and again. Recorded tests are essential in order to achieve equivalence of test results from one clinic or center to another, as, for example, in auditory tests given to veterans for purposes of rating disability. With monitored live-voice tests, the examiner constitutes one source of variability. It is impossible for an examiner, no matter how skillful, to present a list of words two or more times in precisely the same way. For accurate and reliable testing, therefore, recorded speech tests are preferable. There will be times, however, when because of a patient's inability to respond to the standard test materials in recorded form, it will be necessary to adopt the live-voice technique and perhaps to improvise materials and procedures. At such times, the examiner is departing from the standard procedures, and test results must be interpreted accordingly. The beauty of speech audiometric testing is that it is possible to be flexible in approach and thus to obtain some measure of HTL for speech intelligibility for almost any patient who understands spoken language. Special techniques for testing very young children with the speech audiometer will be discussed in the next chapter. The remainder of this

[2] Ibid., p. 16.

chapter will deal with the standard techniques of speech audiometry as applied to adults and older children.

MEASURES SOUGHT

Speech-Reception Threshold

Just as in pure-tone testing we seek to obtain the patient's threshold for individual frequencies, so in speech audiometry we wish to measure the patient's threshold level for speech intelligibility. We want to know how intense simple speech must be before the patient can just understand it. We are not interested at this point in the level at which the patient can barely detect the presence of speech (threshold of speech detectability), but rather in the level at which the patient can repeat simple words or can understand simple running (connected) speech. This level we refer to as the patient's *speech-reception threshold*, abbreviated SRT. The SRT is measured in dB from the level at which the average normal ear's SRT has been established. The sound-pressure level of zero-dB SRT will vary according to the specific test materials employed, the particular methodology used in arriving at threshold, and the "test sophistication" of the listeners. The American National Standard specifies that zero-dB hearing level for speech is a sound-pressure level of 19 dB when normal threshold is based on 50 percent intelligibility of spondee words.[3] When the test earphone is a Telephonics TDH-39 or TDH-49 instead of the Western Electric 705-A employed in the ANSI standard, the sound-pressure level for speech audiometric zero becomes 20 dB instead of 19 dB.[4] The calibration of the speech audiometer is checked by measuring the rms (root-mean-square) level in a 6 cc coupler of a 1000-Hz tone in an earphone that produces a VU meter reading that agrees with the average peaks of the VU meter for the speech signal.[5] The allowable limits for calibration are ±3 dB, or in other words, between 17 and 23 dB SPL (sound-pressure level) for the TDH-39 or TDH-49 earphone.[6] In the past, various investigators have reported sound-pressure levels for zero-dB SRT within these allowable limits.[7]

[3] Ibid., p. 12.

[4] Ibid., p. 21.

[5] Ibid., p. 15.

[6] Ibid., p. 16.

[7] Ira J. Hirsh, Hallowell Davis, S. Richard Silverman, Elizabeth G. Reynolds, Elizabeth Eldert, and Robert W. Benson, "Development of Materials for Speech Audiometry," *Journal of Speech and Hearing Disorders* 17 (September 1952):328; James F. Jerger, Raymond Carhart, Tom W. Tillman, and John L. Peterson, "Some Relations Between Normal Hearing for Pure Tones and for Speech," *Journal of Speech and Hearing Research* 2 (June 1959):126–40; Joseph B. Chaiklin, "The Relation Among Three Selected Auditory Speech Thresholds," *Journal of Speech and Hearing Research* 2 (September 1959):237–43.

In the 1953 American standard for speech audiometers, zero-dB SRT was defined as a sound-pressure level of 22 dB when the speech threshold was determined as the 50 percent intelligibility level of spondee words. Speech audiometric zero was established at 22 dB SPL at that time for two reasons: (1) This was the average of levels reported from laboratory studies of normal-hearing subjects available then; and (2) the assumption was made that the threshold of intelligibility for spondee words should be about 6 dB higher than the normal threshold hearing level for 1000 Hz, which by the ASA-1951 standard was defined as 16.5 dB SPL. It was assumed that establishing zero-dB SRT at 22 dB SPL would result in good agreement between a normal-hearing subject's SRT and the arithmetic average of the HTLs for the "speech frequencies"—500, 1000, and 2000 Hz. Actually, research demonstrated that for normal-hearing subjects the threshold of intelligibility for spondee words was on the average of 13 dB higher in sound-pressure level than the HTL at 1000 Hz.[8] So in order to secure agreement between the average HTL for the speech frequencies and the SRT, it was necessary to peg zero-dB SRT at a sound-pressure level of 29 dB (about 13 dB higher than the ASA-1951 standard of 16.5 dB SPL for 1000 Hz).

Until the ISO-1964 standard for calibration of pure-tone audiometers was generally adopted, there was confusion regarding the sound-pressure level of zero-dB SRT. Some audiometer manufacturers followed the reasoning of Jerger et al. and set zero-dB SRT at 29 dB SPL, whereas others continued to adhere to the 1953 standard of 22 dB SPL. The ISO-1964 standard defined audiometric zero for 1000 Hz as 6.5 dB SPL. Now, adding 13 dB to the normal HTL for 1000 Hz resulted in a sound-pressure level of 19.5 dB (rounded to 20 dB) for the theoretically valid zero-dB SRT. This is exactly the value specified (for the Telephonics TDH-39 or TDH-49 earphone) in the ANSI-1969 standard.

Although a variety of speech materials are suitable for arriving at the SRT, one test is used almost exclusively. This consists of lists of two-syllable words, referred to as *spondees,* although most of these words would normally not be pronounced with equal stress on both syllables. They are words such as *doorway, footstool, airplane,* and *armchair.* Two recorded forms of the spondee test are available: Auditory Tests W-1 and W-2.[9] Test W-1 consists of lists of thirty-six spondaic words which have been recorded at a constant level. The audiometrist introduces as much attenuation as needed in the course of the test to arrive at the patient's SRT. Test W-2 consists of the same lists of words but with attenuation at an average of 1 dB per word built into the recording. For most speech audiometric installations, Test W-1 is preferable.

[8] Jerger et al., "Some Relations," p. 138.

[9] These tests were adapted by Central Institute for the Deaf from Auditory Test No. 9, originated by the Psycho-Acoustic Laboratory, Harvard University. Records and tape cassettes containing these tests are manufactured and distributed by Technisonic Studios, 1201 South Brentwood Blvd., Richmond Heights, Missouri 63117.

The SRT by spondees is defined as the hearing level at which the patient can repeat 50 percent of the words correctly. It is not always practical to follow this definition literally. The tester must sometimes estimate the point at which the patient is right approximately half the time. The test is administered monaurally (to each ear separately) through earphones and then again, if the occasion requires it, through the loudspeaker. Loudspeaker testing is referred to as *sound-field* testing, because the sound is not confined, as it is in an earphone, but circulates in a field about the head of the patient. Unless we are talking over the telephone, or for some reason listening through earphones, all our listening throughout the day is of the sound-field type. It is to judge how the patient hears in a typical, sound-field listening situation that we give speech tests through a loudspeaker.

The method of administering the test is to start the record (or the delivery of the words by live voice) at a level above the patient's presumed threshold. As the patient repeats two or three words successfully, decrease the intensity by a few dB. After two or three more words have been repeated correctly at this new level, decrease the intensity further. Continue in this way until the patient misses some words. Then by following the procedure described later in this chapter, determine the level at which the patient is correct about half the time. This is the SRT by spondees, or the *spondee threshold* (ST), as some audiologists prefer to call it. (The W-1 spondee word lists appear in the appendix to this book.)

Most Comfortable Loudness

A second measure sometimes sought in speech audiometry is the hearing level at which speech is most comfortable for the patient. This measure and the next one to be described have significance in determining the limits of amplification suitable for the patient who is a candidate for a hearing aid. The patient's most comfortable loudness, abbreviated MCL, is measured by means of *running speech* (connected discourse). This is usually recorded informative speech, or it can be delivered by live voice. The patient is instructed to signal when the speech is most comfortably loud as the examiner varies the intensity at suprathreshold levels. The MCL is measured in dB above zero SRT monaurally and if desired by sound-field.

Tolerance Level

The tolerance level, sometimes called the threshold of discomfort (TD), or the uncomfortable loudness level (UCL), is the hearing level at which speech becomes uncomfortably loud. The purpose of this measure is to find the upper limit of the patient's range of hearing for speech, so that the tests that follow can be given at lower levels. Also, the tolerance level represents the maximum amplification that the patient can accept in training or in a hearing aid. Tolerance level is expressed in dB above zero SRT. The normal ear should be able to tolerate speech at hearing levels of 90 to 100 dB without discomfort. It should be remembered that according to the American National Standard, zero SRT is 20 dB (for the TDH-39 earphone) above the standard reference pressure of 0.0002 dyne/cm², so that a hearing level of 100 dB would be a sound-pressure level of 120 dB. It will be recalled from the discussion in Chapter 2 that the average threshold of discomfort is at a sound-pressure level of 120 dB.

The same running speech for measuring MCL can be used to determine the tolerance level. The intensity of the running speech is increased gradually above the MCL until the patient signals that it is uncomfortably loud. This hearing level is then recorded as the patient's tolerance level. The test is performed monaurally and also may be presented by sound-field. The patient should be instructed not to signal until the speech becomes so loud that it actually causes physiological discomfort in the ear, as if a further increase would be unbearable.

Dynamic Range for Speech

The patient's dynamic range for speech is computed by subtracting the SRT from the tolerance level. The dynamic range represents the limits of useful hearing that the patient has in each ear and by sound-field. This is important in diagnosis and in planning for the patient's rehabilitation, as will be brought out later in this chapter.

Discrimination

In addition to the measures of sensitivity for speech, an indication of the patient's speech-discrimination ability is necessary. The handicap of a hearing loss may consist not only of a decrease in sensitivity to sound but also to an impairment in understanding what is heard. With many patients, the primary difficulty is one of interference with the intelligibility of speech. As we have seen in the previous chapter, speech intelligibility is probably related to the audiometric configuration, the type of pathology, the degree of impairment, and perhaps other factors. The term *articulation* is used audiologically for the function of speech discrimination. In this context, an articulation test is one that examines a patient's ability to discriminate among similar sounds or among words that contain similar sounds. It is unfortunate that the word *articulation* has other connotations for individuals whose orientation is in the field of speech. In this chapter, we shall apply the terms *articulation* and *speech discrimination* interchangeably.

The articulation or discrimination function is usually measured clinically by administering so-called *phonetically balanced* (PB) word lists at levels well above the patient's SRT and recording the percentage of words that are correctly identified. The task is more properly termed a *word-identification task*. However, it has been common clinical practice to refer to all such tests as measures of speech-discrimination ability. Each list contains fifty mono-syllabic words, chosen systematically so that each list will contain samples of speech sounds in approximately the same proportion in which they occur in English running speech. Actually, as Lehiste and Peterson have pointed out, the lists should more properly be designated "phonemically balanced" lists[10] because they were designed to include the various phonemes of the language in correct proportion rather than balancing all the physiological and acoustical properties of speech implied by the term *phonetics.*

The original PB lists were created at the Harvard Psycho-Acoustic Laboratory.[11] The twenty lists, consisting of 1000 words in all, were recorded by Rush Hughes, a radio announcer in St. Louis. These are referred to as the PB-50 lists to differentiate them from the PB word lists developed at Central Institute for the Deaf by Hirsh and his associates.[12] Hirsh et al. developed a list of 200 PB words, of which 180 were taken from the 1000 words in the Psycho-Acoustic Laboratory (PAL) lists. Hirsh himself recorded on magnetic tape the 200 words in four lists of fifty words each. Each list was then "scrambled" six times to give different word orders, so that there are twenty-four lists in all. These PB word lists are available in recorded form as Auditory Test W-22.[13] They may, of course, be delivered by live voice as well, although in the interest of reducing variability in test results, the use of live voice for discrimination testing is discouraged. If the test is given by live voice, the examiner must avoid the temptation to monitor each word to the same point on the VU meter. Because there is a wide difference in the phonetic power of various speech sounds, monitoring the words to the same level can alter the phonemic balance and produce inaccurate discrimination scores. The words should be spoken with equal effort rather than with equal intensity as measured on the meter. Not only are the lists phonemically balanced with English speech, they are also balanced with each other. There should be very little variation in a pa-tient's score from list to list, therefore. Although it is possible to obtain a rough estimate of a patient's discrimination ability by using just twenty-five words of a list, it is advisable to use an entire list of fifty words for each discrimination test because the first half of a list has not been balanced with the second half. (The twenty-four W-22 lists are reproduced in the appendix to this book.)

A great deal of research has been done with both the Harvard PB-50 and W-22 PB lists in defining what has been termed the *articulation function.* The research has been with normal ears, as well as with impaired ears of all types. "Articulation curves" have been constructed, showing how the scores on PB

[10] Ilse Lehiste and Gordon E. Peterson, "Linguistic Considerations in the Study of Speech Intelligibility," *Journal of the Acoustical Society of America* 31 (March 1959):281.

[11] J. P. Egan, "Articulation Testing Methods," *Laryngoscope* 58 (1948):955–91.

[12] Hirsh et al., "Development of Materials."

[13] Records and cassette tapes are manufactured and distributed by Technisonic Studios, 1201 South Brentwood Blvd., Richmond Heights, Missouri 63117.

tests for normal and impaired ears are affected by the intensity at which the word lists are presented. As the intensity is increased above the individual's threshold for speech, scores on the tests increase rapidly until the intensity at which the PB words are presented reaches a level of 35 to 40 dB greater than the individual's SRT. At this point, the articulation curve flattens out. With increasing intensity above this point, there is a negligible increase in the discrimination score or even a slight decrease. It is important, in administering the PB tests clinically, to present them at a level that will result in obtaining the patient's maximum discrimination score—referred to as *PB-Max*. Usually, but not always, the patient's PB-Max will be found at a sensation level of 40 dB. As we shall see in the next chapter, one of the recommended procedures in defining the site of lesion in auditory disorders is to note how the discrimination score is affected by the sensation level at which PB words are presented. A patient's articulation function is defined graphically by giving three or four—and in some cases more—PB tests at increasingly higher suprathreshold levels. Jerger refers to this procedure as a study of the performance versus intensity (PI) function. With some ear pathologies, the discrimination score will increase with increased sensation level until a maximum is reached. Then, with increasing sensation level of test presentation, the discrimination score will decrease markedly, a phenomenon called *rollover*.[14]

The best method of administering the PB tests is to have the patient write the responses on a paper with fifty numbered blank spaces. In this way, there can be little doubt about whether or not the patient has heard the words correctly, and there is the added advantage that a permanent record of the patient's responses is available for analysis of the discrimination errors. If you have the patient repeat the words to you while you listen over the talkback earphones or loudspeaker, you are testing your own discrimination for the patient's speech. Of course, sometimes there will be no alternative but to have the patient repeat the words because writing is impossible or difficult for some patients. In this situation, if it is feasible to do so, it is a good idea to have the patient spell each word as it is heard, rather than repeat it, in order to reduce the chances of error in scoring the test.

The discrimination tests are scored in terms of the percentage of words heard correctly. Because there are fifty words to a list, the percentage correct can easily be computed by counting the number of correct responses and multiplying by two. The percentage of correct responses is the patient's discrimination score. As is true of the previously described measures, the discrimination tests may be administered both monaurally and by sound-field.

Part of the motivation for developing the CID W-22 test was that the Hughes recordings of the PB-50 words were considered to be too difficult and were poor in the "equivalence" of one list to another. In other words, an individual's discrimination score might vary over a range of from 10 to 16 per-

[14] James Jerger, "Diagnostic Audiometry," in *Modern Developments in Audiology,* 2nd ed., ed. James Jerger (New York: Academic Press, 1973), chap. 3, p. 80.

cent depending on the particular recorded list employed. In part, this variability was due to the speaker's inconsistent articulation and in part to poor recording techniques. The criticism of the W-22 tests is that they are too easy and thus do not differentiate well among ears with varying degrees of impairment. Since the incorporation of the W-22 tests into standard clinical procedures, there have been many attempts to develop "improved" tests of speech discrimination that would be more sensitive to slight changes in degree and configuration of pure-tone loss. Some of these tests are *open-response-set* tests such as the PB-50 and the W-22, where the patient has unlimited response possibilities. Others are *closed-response-set* tests, so-called because the patient's responses are limited, as in a multiple-choice test. Fairbanks[15] devised the Rhyme Test, which is a completion test requiring the subject to supply the initial consonant to a "stem." The subject has a list of fifty stems and is instructed to write in the missing letter as the words are pronounced by the speaker. There are at least five rhyming choices the subject can make for each word. Thus for the stem–*ame*, some choices would be *tame, same, lame, came, name, dame.* With this test, it is easy to categorize the constant errors the subject makes.

House et al.[16] developed a closed-response-set discrimination test that has come to be known as the Modified Rhyme Test (MRT). The authors supply the subject with six rhyming words for each of fifty stimulus items. The subject must then draw a line through the word which was heard. The MRT consists of twenty-five items that differ only in the initial consonant (*sip, rip, tip, dip, hip, lip*) and twenty-five items that are differentiated by the final consonant (*map, mat, math, man, mass, mad*). To make the listening task sufficiently difficult, both the Rhyme Test and MRT are administered in the presence of a broad-band noise.

The MRT was developed originally to differentiate communication systems, although its authors recognized its possibilities as a clinical tool. Kreul et al.[17] refined the MRT by changing some items and prepared tape recordings of the test to be used in the clinical assessment of speech discrimination. The recordings are furnished with both male and female speakers and with three signal-to-noise ratios (S/N).

Because they were dissatisfied with the PB words as a discrimination test to be used in research, Lehiste and Peterson[18] constructed ten lists of fifty monosyllabic words each (500 different words) that are more rigorously

[15] Grant Fairbanks, "Test of Phonemic Differentiation: The Rhyme Test," *Journal of the Acoustical Society of America* 30 (July 1958):596–600.

[16] Arthur S. House, Carl E. Williams, Michael H. L. Hecker, and K. D. Kryter, "Articulation Testing Methods: Consonantal Differentiation with a Closed-Response Set," *Journal of the Acoustical Society of America* 37 (January 1965):158–66.

[17] E. James Kreul, James C. Nixon, Karl D. Kryter, Donald W. Bell, Janna S. Lang, and Earl D. Schubert, "A Proposed Clinical Test of Speech Discrimination," *Journal of Speech and Hearing Research* 11 (September 1968):536–52.

[18] Lehiste and Peterson, "Linguistic Considerations," pp. 280–86.

phonemically balanced and more carefully selected on the basis of frequency of occurrence in American English. They referred to their lists as CNC lists (consonant-nucleus-consonant). Later, the authors revised the lists by eliminating some rare and literary words and suggested that the revised lists would be useful in both auditory research and clinical testing of speech discrimination.[19] These revised CNC lists have been recorded at the University of Maryland's Biocommunications Laboratory and have had extensive experimental clinical use in various Veterans Administration audiology clinics, primarily in hearing-aid evaluations. (The ten revised CNC lists are reproduced in the appendix to this book.)

From the original list of over 1200 CNC words from which Peterson and Lehiste selected their test words, Tillman, Carhart, and Wilber created two fifty-word lists recorded by a male speaker and designated Northwestern University Auditory Test No. 4.[20] Later, these two lists and two additional fifty-word lists selected from the Peterson-Lehiste pool were recorded with a different male speaker and also with a female speaker. The version with the male speaker was termed Northwestern University Auditory Test No. 6-M, and the female version was termed No. 6-F.[21]

Attempts have been made also to develop speech-discrimination tests based on sentences rather than single words, on the theory that a sentence is more analogous to everyday listening than isolated words and thus a more valid test of an individual's discrimination abilities. Davis[22] discusses sentence tests and reproduces some of them, including a list devised at Central Institute for the Deaf to represent "everyday American speech." This list of CID sentences has also been recorded at the University of Maryland's Biocommunications Laboratory and is available on tape cassettes. Experience with the sentence test is that even when it is presented with a competing noise at an S/N of –10 dB, it is an easy test and thus not very useful as a diagnostic test of speech discrimination.[23] Speaks and Jerger[24] constructed a test consisting of

[19] Gordon E. Peterson and Isle Lehiste, "Revised CNC Lists for Auditory Tests," *Journal of Speech and Hearing Disorders* 27 (February 1962):62–70.

[20] Tom W. Tillman, Raymond Carhart, and Laura Wilber, *A Test for Speech Discrimination Composed of CNC Monosyllabic Words, Northwestern University Auditory Test No. 4*, Technical Documentary Report No. SAM-TDR-62-135, USAF School of Aerospace Medicine, Brooks Air Force Base, Texas, 1963.

[21] Tom W. Tillman and Raymond Carhart, *An Expanded Test for Speech Discrimination Utilizing CNC Monosyllabic Words, Northwestern University Auditory Test No. 6*, Technical Report No. SAM-TR-66-55, USAF School of Aerospace Medicine, Brooks Air Force Base, Texas, 1966.

[22] Hallowell Davis, "Audiometry: Pure Tone and Simple Speech Tests," in *Hearing and Deafness*, 4th ed., eds. Hallowell Davis and S. Richard Silverman (New York: Holt, Rinehart and Winston, 1978), pp. 215, 534–38.

[23] Personal communication from Dr. G. Donald Causey.

[24] Charles Speaks and James Jerger, "Method for Measurement of Speech Identification," *Journal of Speech and Hearing Research* 8 (June 1965):185–94.

closed-message sets of "synthetic" or artificial sentences. These sentences do not bear much resemblance to real sentences because they consist of words strung together without regard for syntax or meaning. The listener's task is to select which "sentence" of a set was spoken. The synthetic sentence test was designed primarily for experimental use when the speech signal is filtered, distorted, or masked in various ways.

The various "improvements" on the PB lists have their adherents and no doubt will be used in audiology clinics for clinical as well as research purposes. However, the CID W-22 and the NU-6 recordings continue to be the standard tool for the clinical assessment of speech discrimination.

STEP-BY-STEP PROCEDURE IN SPEECH AUDIOMETRY

The following procedure is designed for adults or older children and for a typical two-room testing area. The assumption is made that recorded tests will be used and that the patient is capable of writing responses where necessary. Instructions to the patient will be covered in the procedure.

1. Inform the patient that the first test will be through earphones, one ear at a time, and will consist of two-syllable words, such as *doorway* and *footstool*. Give the patient an alphabetized list of spondees to read and inform the patient that the test words will all be from the list, and to respond only with words from the list. If the patient for any reason is unable to read, you should read the list aloud, presenting the words at a high enough suprathreshold level so that the patient can hear them as well as possible. Of course, when presented in test form the spondees will not be in alphabetized order. Tell the patient that at the start the words will be fairly loud and will decrease in loudness gradually. The patient is to repeat each word as it is heard, guessing at the word if necessary. Inform the patient that the object of the test is to find the point at which about half of the words are missed and therefore not to become upset or angry if some words are missed.

2. Place the earphones on the patient's head, making sure that they fit snugly and comfortably over each ear. From the pure-tone test that you have already administered, you will know whether masking will be necessary in either ear for the speech tests (if it is necessary, explain to the patient what you are doing and why). Switch the input selector to "tape." Switch the output selector to "earphone," either left or right. Then put on one of the W-2 tapes. Follow the instructions that accompany the tapes for determining the proper setting of the input volume control. This involves adjusting the control until the VU meter registers the correct value for a 1000-Hz calibrating tone that is on the tape. Having set the input control properly, adjust the attenuator to produce an output level that you estimate will be about 15 to 20 dB above the patient's threshold in that ear. After the patient has repeated three or four

consecutive words correctly, decrease the output level by 5 dB. Repeat this procedure until you reach a point at which the patient is missing some words. Then increase the level by 5 or 6 dB to reach an even step on the attenuator. At this level, present three spondee words. If the patient repeats them correctly, decrease the level by 2 dB and present more spondee words. If the patient misses one or more of the three words presented, continue with spondee words at the same level until a maximum of six words have been presented. If the patient misses four of the six words, increase the level by 2 dB and present up to six additional words. As soon as the patient gets three words of a series correctly, decrease the level by 2 dB and start another series. Thus, at each even step on the hearing-level dial, at least three and up to six words will be presented, depending on the patient's responses. You are seeking the minimum hearing level (in even numbers of decibels) at which the patient can repeat three spondee words correctly. Continue decreasing the hearing level in 2 dB steps until the patient misses at least four out of six words at three consecutive decrements of intensity. This step is a precaution against premature acceptance of too high an SRT. The threshold criterion to be applied is a 50 percent level of correct response, that is, at least three out of six words repeated correctly. Record the lowest hearing level at which the patient achieved this 50 percent criterion as the SRT by spondees for the ear being tested.[25] Although the method just described will yield the patient's SRT to the nearest 2-dB step on the hearing-level control, it is faster and—according to Chaiklin and Ventry—just as valid to use 5-dB steps in arriving at SRT and to express the patient's SRT to the nearest 5-dB step on the hearing-level control.[26] In testing veterans for compensation purposes, however, it is necessary to find the SRT to the nearest 2-dB step. The ASHA Committee on Audiometric Evaluation has developed guidelines for determining the spondee threshold. The method is based on an ascending technique, that is, proceeding from inaudibility to audibility in the manner of arriving at the HTL for pure tones (as described in the preceding chapter.)[27] The authors believe that in establishing the spondee threshold, a descending technique is to be preferred, starting from a point of good audibility and proceeding gradually to the level of 50 percent correct repetitions. It is frustrating to a patient to know that words are being presented and not be able to hear them. Incidentally, some patients will have such poor speech discrimination that they will not be able to repeat 50 percent of the spondee words correctly at any level, even after reading over the words that comprise the test. If this is the

[25] The technique for arriving at SRT by spondees described here is adapted from Chaiklin, "Relation Among Three Speech Thresholds," p. 240.

[26] Joseph B. Chaiklin and Ira M. Ventry, "Spondee Threshold Measurement: A Comparison of 2- and 5-dB Methods," *Journal of Speech and Hearing Disorders* 29 (February 1964):47–59.

[27] "Guidelines for Determining the Threshold Level for Speech," *Asha* 21 (May 1979):353–56.

case, record CNT for "could not test" in the space on the audiogram form for the spondee threshold, and indicate under "Remarks" that the reason the SRT for spondees could not be determined was the patient's poor speech discrimination.

With the W-1 records, on which the calibrating tone and carrier phrase "You will say . . ." have been recorded at a level of 10 dB greater intensity than the test words, you must be careful to record the correct hearing level as the patient's SRT. Speech audiometers are calibrated to zero dB as the average, normal speech-reception threshold for *test words,* not the carrier phrase. In other words, assuming that audiometric zero equals a sound-pressure level re 0.0002 dyne/cm² of 20 dB, the output of the amplifier is set so that when the attenuator dial reads zero, the average normal ear can just understand approximately 50 percent of the spondee words when the *words* are monitored to zero on the VU meter. When the W-1 records are used, the VU meter is set to zero for the calibrating tone and carrier phrase, and the spondee words themselves will peak an average 10 dB below zero on the meter. This means that the output level of the spondee words will be 10 dB less than the indicated hearing level on the attenuator dial. It will be necessary for you, when using the W-1 records, to subtract 10 dB from the obtained SRT in order to arrive at the actual SRT. It is awkward to have to make this correction every time a recorded spondee test is administered. With the situation that pertains currently, it is much simpler to secure the SRT for spondees by means of live voice, monitoring the level of the spondees with the input volume control and the VU meter. Some audiologists prefer to make their own recordings of spondee words on magnetic tape. If you make your own recordings, the carrier phrase and test words can be recorded at the same level, thus obviating the need for any correction.

3. Now switch the output selector to the opposite ear, turn up the level until the spondees are being delivered at about 15 to 20 dB above the patient's supposed threshold in that ear, and proceed to determine the SRT by spondees in the same manner as in step 2. Record this result.

4. Switch the input selector to "microphone" and increase the level to the point that the patient can hear you easily. Inform the patient that now a recording of running speech will be played and to let you know when the speech is at a level that is "most comfortable" to listen to. To be sure that the selected level is the most comfortable, make the speech louder and softer two or three times until the patient is certain of the decision.

5. Switch back to "tape," and put on the running-speech tape. Adjust the input volume control until the speech is peaking at zero dB on the VU meter; then gradually increase the output level of the speech until the patient signals that it is most comfortably loud. Repeat this process until you are sure that the most comfortable level has been found. Record this hearing level as the patient's MCL. Switch to the other ear, and repeat the procedure.

6. Switching back to "microphone," explain to the patient that now you

are going to make the running speech louder still to find out whether it gets so loud that it causes discomfort in the ear. Explain that you want to find out if it causes physiological discomfort, such as a tickling sensation, in the ear. Point out that the patient's signaling switch will illuminate a light on your control panel to signal you immediately to turn off the loud speech.

7. Switch back to "tape," and put on the running-speech tape again. Gradually increase the intensity of the speech, watching the patient through the window. It is a good idea to keep your hand on the channel on-off switch while you are increasing the output. As soon as the patient signals that the speech is uncomfortably loud, immediately turn the signal off without disturbing the setting of the output attenuator. Note what the hearing-level reading is, and record this figure as the patient's tolerance level for that ear. Switch the output selector to the other ear, and repeat the procedure.

8. Subtract the patient's SRT from the tolerance level in each ear and record the difference as the dynamic range.

9. Switching back to "microphone," explain to the patient that now you are going to put on a recording of a man speaking one-syllable words and that there will be no difficulty in hearing the words because you will make them loud enough to be heard easily. Explain that although each word will be preceded by the phrase "You will say . . ." the patient should write the word on the blank rather than repeat it. Explain that there will be fifty words in the list and that when one list has been completed, you will switch to the other ear and present another list. In order to reduce the effect of learning on the test scores, it is advisable to present a practice list of 25 or 50 PB words to the patient before beginning the actual test. The practice list should not be the same one used in the test.

10. Switch the input selector to "tape," and put on one of the W-22 tapes. Adjust the input volume control so that the calibrating tone on the record will peak the needle on the VU meter at zero dB. On the W-22 tapes, the calibrating tone and the carrier phrase are recorded at the same level as the test words. When the input volume control is properly set for the calibrating tone, the carrier phrase will peak consistently at the same place on the VU meter. The PB words will not all peak the same, however, as the words differ in their phonetic power. Once the proper level for the calibrating tone and carrier phrase has been established, the input volume control should not be touched. Adjust the output attenuator so that the output is 40 dB greater than the SRT for the ear being tested, unless adding 40 dB to the SRT will result in an output that equals or exceeds the tolerance level for that ear. In that event, it will be necessary for you to present the PB list at a level less than 40 dB above the SRT, for you cannot present the words at a level that will cause discomfort to the patient. In cases of profound loss, it may be impossible to present the PB words at a sensation level of 40 dB because that would exceed the maximum output level of the audiometer. Note on the audiogram form

the hearing level at which the test was presented, so that anyone reviewing the test results can judge whether or not the obtained discrimination score represents the patient's PB-Max.

11. Switch the output selector to the opposite ear, adjust the attenuator to a level of 40 dB above the SRT in that ear, if that is possible, and put on another W-22 tape.

12. You may wish to determine how well the patient discriminates speech in the presence of competing noise. In Chapter 5, we discussed the effect on speech discrimination of losses above the usual speech frequency range (500 to 2000 Hz). We said that although a patient with good hearing sensitivity through 2000 Hz and a loss at 3000 Hz could understand speech well in quiet, difficulty would occur under unfavorable listening conditions. If you want to obtain a measure of the patient's speech-discrimination ability in noise, present another PB test to each ear while directing a masking noise (preferably speech-spectrum noise or white noise) to the same ear. A good indication of the patient's ability to cope with a competing noise can be obtained by presenting the combined speech and noise at a S/N of +10 dB, that is, with the speech signal at a 10-dB higher level than the noise. Thus, if the PB words are presented at a sensation level of 40 dB in relation to the SRT, the noise would be at a sensation level of 30 dB.

13. You have now completed the monaural tests. Score the PB test papers, and enter the percentage correct for each ear on the speech audiogram under "Discrimination."

14. Remove the earphones from the patient's head. If it is desirable to obtain information about the patient's hearing for speech in a sound-field (as it would be in the case of a hearing-aid evaluation, for example), explain that now you are going to repeat the same series of tests presented with a loudspeaker; that first there will be the two-syllable words and then the running speech, which will be first comfortably loud and then very loud; and that to complete the test there will be an additional list of fifty monosyllabic words to write out.

15. Switch the output selector to "speaker." Then repeat the test procedures as detailed. You will now have sound-field measurements of SRT by spondees, MCL, dynamic range, tolerance level, and speech-discrimination score.

INTERPRETING RESULTS

The results of speech audiometry are recorded on a speech audiogram, a sample of which is shown in Figure 6–3, or they may be recorded in combination with a pure-tone audiogram such as that shown in Figure 6–4.

SPEECH AUDIOMETRIC EXAMINATION

Patient _____   Examiner _____   Date _____

	RIGHT	LEFT	SOUND FIELD
SPONDEE THRESHOLD (dB hearing level)	____	____	____
MOST COMFORTABLE LOUDNESS (dB hearing level)	____	____	____
TOLERANCE LEVEL (dB hearing level)	____	____	____
DYNAMIC RANGE (difference in dB between spondee threshold and tolerance level)	____	____	____
DISCRIMINATION (PB-MAX) (percentage correct at sensation level of 40 dB)	____	____	____

COMMENTS AND RECOMMENDATIONS

FIGURE 6-3. A sample speech audiogram form.

As Aid to Diagnosis

Although the speech audiometric results alone have limited diagnostic value, in combination with the pure-tone audiogram they provide information for a diagnosis about whether an impairment is conductive or sensori-neural in type, and if the latter, whether or not it is cochlear in origin. More will be said concerning the use of speech audiometry in differentiating between cochlear and retrocochlear sensori-neural lesions in the next chapter. Also in the next chapter the contribution of speech audiometry to the diagnosis of functional or nonorganic hearing problems will be discussed.

If the dynamic range is restricted because of a lowered tolerance level, which might be an indication of the presence of recruitment, especially if in addition there are relatively low discrimination scores, the probability is high that the patient has a sensori-neural impairment. On the other hand, if there is no lowering of the tolerance level and the discrimination scores are high, there is no assurance that the patient does not have sensori-neural impairment. Ordinarily, normal tolerance and high discrimination scores would be represen-

AUDIOLOGICAL EXAMINATION

Name: Age: Sex: Telephone: Date:

Referral Source: Audiometer: Examiner:

AIR CONDUCTION

	Right									Left								
	250	500	1000	1500	2000	3000	4000	6000	8000	250	500	1000	1500	2000	3000	4000	6000	8000
Un-masked	45	45	45		35	35	35	35	35	45	40	40		40	35	30	30	25
Masked																		
Mask Level																		

Sp. Freq. Av: RE __42__ LE __40__   Percent Loss: RE __24%__ LE __21%__ Binaural __22%__

BONE CONDUCTION

	Right								Left						
	250	500	1000	1500	2000	3000	4000		250	500	1000	1500	2000	3000	4000
Un-masked	5	0	5		15		5		0	0	5		10		5
Masked															
Mask Level															

Sp. Freq. Av: RE __7__ LE __5__   Audio. Weber: Hz __1000__ RE/LE
                                                           dB __20__ *Midline

SPEECH AUDIOMETRY

	Speech Reception						Discrimination								
	ST	Mask Level	MCL	UCL	Dyn. Range			Unmasked		Masked			Ipsilat. Noise		
								%	Test Level	%	Test Level	Mask Level	%	Test Level	S/N
Right Ear	42		82	108	66		Right Ear	90	82				84	82	+10
Left Ear	42		80	104	62		Left Ear	94	82				86	82	+10
Sound Field	40		76	102	62		Sound Field	96	80				- - -	-DNT-	- - -

COMMENTS:

FIGURE 6-4. Pure-tone and speech audiometric results for the patient whose audiogram was shown in Figure 5-8.

tative of conductive impairment, but there are some patients with sensorineural involvement whose speech audiometric scores would be indistinguishable from those of conductively impaired patients. Thus, it is risky to attempt a diagnosis from speech audiometric results alone as it would be to attempt to delineate the type of impairment from a patient's pure-tone air-conduction curve alone.

Keeping the diagnostic limitations of speech audiometry in mind, let us examine the speech audiometric results that accompany some of the pure-tone audiograms depicted in Chapter 5. For convenience, the information from the graphic audiograms in Chapter 5 has been repeated in number form in Figures 6-4, 6-5, and 6-6. Figure 6-4 shows speech results obtained for the patient whose pure-tone audiogram is shown in Figure 5-8. It can be seen that the obtained SRTs agree well with the predicted loss for speech secured by averaging the HTLs at 500, 1000, and 2000 Hz in each ear. As would be expected because of the flatness of the audiogram curve through the speech frequencies, speech tests reveal high discrimination scores, with minimal decrement from competing noise. Because a conductive impairment is not characterized by recruitment, we would expect the tolerance level or UCL and the dynamic range to be normal, which is borne out by the speech test results.

Figure 6–5 shows speech test results for the patient whose pure-tone audiogram is shown in Figure 5–9. Because this patient has a gradually sloping audiogram curve, rather than an abruptly sloping one, the predicted speech loss is better computed by the three-frequency method than the two-

FIGURE 6-5. Pure-tone and speech audiometric results for the patient whose audiogram was shown in Figure 5–9.

AUDIOLOGICAL EXAMINATION

Name: Age: Sex: Telephone: Date:

Referral Source: Audiometer: Examiner:

AIR CONDUCTION

	Right 250	500	1000	1500	2000	3000	4000	6000	8000	Left 250	500	1000	1500	2000	3000	4000	6000	8000
Un-masked	10	15	30		45	60	70	75	90+	5	10	25		45	55	65	75	90+
Masked																		
Mask Level																		

Sp. Freq. Av: RE 30 LE 27   Percent Loss: RE 6% LE 2% Binaural 3%

BONE CONDUCTION

	Right 250	500	1000	1500	2000	3000	4000	Left 250	500	1000	1500	2000	3000	4000
Un-masked	10	10	30		40	65+	65+							
Masked														
Mask Level														

Sp. Freq. Av: RE 27 LE ____   Audio. Weber: Hz 1000 *RE/LE Midline dB 40

SPEECH AUDIOMETRY

	Speech Reception ST	Mask Level	MCL	UCL	Dyn. Range		Discrimination Unmasked %	Test Level	Masked %	Test Level	Mask Level	Ipsilat. Noise %	Test Level	S/N
Right Ear	28		44	88	60	Right Ear	70	68				54	68	+10
Left Ear	22		40	85	63	Left Ear	74	62				56	62	+10
Sound Field	24	✕	40	82	58	Sound Field	72	64	✕		✕	- -	DNT-	- - -

COMMENTS:

frequency one, and we find that the SRTs obtained in speech audiometry show a fairly close agreement with those predicted. Because the patient has a sensori-neural impairment, there is a possibility that recruitment of loudness might occur. The lowered tolerance level (UCL) in each ear suggests the presence of recruitment. Incidentally, it should be noted that the dynamic range alone cannot be used as an indicator of the presence of recruitment because the patient whose scores are reported in Figure 6–5 has dynamic ranges about on a par with those of the patient with conductive impairment, whose scores are shown in Figure 6–4. The reason for the similarity of their dynamic ranges is that the patient whose scores are depicted in Figure 6–4 has higher SRTs than the patient whose scores are given in Figure 6–5. If both patients had had about the same spondee thresholds, their dynamic ranges would have differed as a function of their differing tolerance levels. It will be noted that the discrimination scores reported in Figure 6–5 are relatively low. Note also that in the presence of competing noise, the patient's discrimination scores drop substantially. The shape of this patient's pure-tone air-conduction curve undoubtedly contributes to speech-discrimination losses in quiet and in noise.

A mixed impairment is represented by the pure-tone audiogram in Figure 5–12. Figure 6–6 shows the speech audiogram for this patient. The obtained SRTs are somewhat better than would be predicted from the audiogram by the three-frequency method. The patient's tolerance levels are slightly reduced, and there is some discrimination loss in each ear, which is probably related to the sensori-neural component and the configuration of the air-conduction curve.

Before we leave the subject of the diagnostic significance of speech audiometry, an additional word should be said concerning the need for masking when there is a difference between the ears. As is true in pure-tone air-conduction audiometry, a speech signal can be heard in the ear not under test when the difference in sensitivity between the ears is on the order of from 40 to 60 dB. To prevent the contralateral ear from participating, it is necessary in such instances to apply a masking noise. The preferred masking noise for speech audiometry is either white noise or a noise "shaped" to resemble the speech spectrum. In speech testing, as in pure-tone air-conduction testing, there is little if any danger that too high a level of masking will be used, that is, so intense a masking noise that the threshold of the ear under test would be affected. Instead, there is danger that the level of the masking signal may not be sufficiently high to rule out the participation of the better ear.

Although the indications for the use of masking during threshold determination are fairly clear, it may not always be apparent that masking should be employed while testing the patient's speech discrimination. If there is sufficient difference in sensitivity between the ears to justify the use of masking while obtaining the SRT, of course masking should be utilized also in the speech-discrimination test of the poorer ear. There are occasions, however,

AUDIOLOGICAL EXAMINATION

Name: Age: Sex: Telephone: Date:

Referral Source: Audiometer: Examiner:

AIR CONDUCTION

	Right									Left								
	250	500	1000	1500	2000	3000	4000	6000	8000	250	500	1000	1500	2000	3000	4000	6000	8000
Un- masked	30	35	45	60	70	90	100	110+	90+	30	40	40	55	65	85	90	100	90+
Masked																		
Mask Level																		

Sp. Freq. Av: RE _50_ LE _48_   Percent Loss: RE _36%_ LE _33%_ Binaural _34%_

BONE CONDUCTION

	Right								Left						
	250	500	1000	1500	2000	3000	4000		250	500	1000	1500	2000	3000	4000
Un- masked															
Masked	5	15	20		45	65+	65+		5	10	20		40	65+	65+
Mask Level	70	80	85		95				70	70	85		95		

Sp. Freq. Av: RE _27_ LE _23_   Audio. Weber: Hz _2000_   RE / LE *Midline
                                                        dB _60_

SPEECH AUDIOMETRY

	Speech Reception						Discrimination								
							Unmasked		Masked			Ipsilat. Noise		
	ST	Mask Level	MCL	UCL	Dyn. Range		%	Test Level	%	Test Level	Mask Level	%	Test Level	S/N
Right Ear	44		60	88	44	Right Ear	80	84				---	DNT-	-	---
Left Ear	42		60	90	48	Left Ear	82	82				---	DNT-	-	---
Sound Field	42	✕	59	86	44	Sound Field	84	82	✕	✕	✕	---	DNT-	-	---

COMMENTS:

FIGURE 6-6. Pure-tone and speech audiometric results for the patient whose audiogram was shown in Figure 5-12.

when threshold differences between the ears are not sufficient to require masking while measuring SRT, and yet masking is required to prevent the participation of the better ear in speech-discrimination testing.

As Guide to Rehabilitation

As a guide to a patient's rehabilitative needs, the speech audiogram is invaluable. It tells us directly how the patient is handicapped in communication by giving information on the degree of loss (the SRT) and the amount of difficulty in understanding what is heard (discrimination or articulation score). In the preceding chapter, suggestions were made concerning how information from the pure-tone audiogram could be applied in determining what the patient needs in the way of rehabilitation. The speech audiogram can be used in the same manner, but with more assurance, because with the pure-tone audiogram only speculation is possible about the effect of the loss on hearing speech, whereas the speech audiogram shows us this effect.

The comments made in the last chapter concerning the utilization of information from the pure-tone audiogram in determining whether or not a patient can benefit from amplification apply here too. The hearing aid should provide enough amplification to reach above the patient's threshold for speech, but at the same time it must not exceed the patient's threshold of discomfort. The dynamic range gives us the limits within which the hearing aid must operate. The MCL tells us at what level of amplification the patient will hear most comfortably.

The speech audiogram yields information about how much difficulty the patient may be expected to have in learning to use the hearing aid effectively. As a rule, a patient who has a poor speech-discrimination score will have much more difficulty with the aid than someone who has a high score. Such a patient needs training in making use of the impaired hearing most effectively (auditory training) and may also need training in speechreading (lipreading). If the patient can learn to take advantage of the minimal sound clues that are received and can learn to distinguish among dissimilar sounds through their appearance on the speaker's mouth, effective communication can occur.

The V.A. employs a method for determining hearing disability for compensation purposes that takes into account both loss of sensitivity for speech (SRT) and the speech-discrimination score (PB-Max). Perhaps in the future, courts of law and compensation boards generally will demand direct evidence of the degree of difficulty in communication a claimant is experiencing, instead of depending on the percentage of pure-tone loss as the sole yardstick for judging disability.

In the next chapter, speech audiometry serving special purposes will be discussed, including techniques in assessing the hearing sensitivity of very young children. The development of speech audiometry has added substantially to the audiologist's armamentarium.

CHAPTER SEVEN
SPECIAL PROBLEMS
IN HEARING TESTING

In the previous two chapters, the emphasis has been on the techniques and procedures of standard pure-tone and speech audiometry. In this chapter, attention will be paid to special problems in clinical audiometry and special tests for particular purposes.

SPECIAL TESTS FOR IDENTIFYING HEARING LOSS
AND SITE OF LESION

Hearing impairments are designated as conductive, sensori-neural, or mixed on the basis of an inspection of air- and bone-conduction hearing threshold levels obtained in routine pure-tone audiometry. Identifying a hearing impairment as conductive tells us only that the problem originates in the outer or the middle ear; it tells us nothing about the pathology producing the impairment. Likewise, identifying an impairment as sensori-neural does not say anything about the pathological condition producing the impairment except that it is not in the outer or the middle ear.

In some cases, standard pure-tone and speech audiometry are not possible because of a wide variety of patient-related phenomena, including age, mental ability, and willingness to cooperate. There has been considerable interest among audiologists and otologists in developing tests that would overcome these problems. Tests based on physiological measures have been developed to identify whether or not a hearing loss exists, and in some cases its magnitude.

Batteries of tests have been designed to differentiate cochlear from VIIIth nerve lesions, sometimes designated *retrocochlear,* although the term refers to lesions anywhere beyond the cochlea and not just VIIIth nerve pathology. The development of immittance measurements and intra-aural muscle-reflex testing has resulted in identification of middle-ear abnormalities, estimates of the magnitude of hearing loss, additional information differentiating cochlear from neural lesions, and identification of the site of central auditory pathology. Because some aspect of immittance testing pervades the whole range of auditory disorders, we shall discuss that mode of testing first.

Acoustic Immittance Measurements

Tympanometry is useful in differentiating conductive impairments and in evaluating Eustachian tube function. Unfortunately, there is not yet standardization of instruments used clinically to obtain tympanograms. Some instruments use only a single probe tone of 220 Hz and derive a tympanogram with the immittance scale in relative (uncalibrated) units; other instruments employ both a 220 and a 660 Hz probe tone and express the immittance in calibrated units. Some instruments are designed to yield measures of acoustic impedance, and others to measure acoustic admittance. In this chapter, we will limit our discussion to the use of an immittance meter manufactured by the Grason-Stadler Company (shown in Figure 7–1).

Complex acoustic admittance (Y_A) is composed of acoustic conductance (G_A) and acoustic susceptance (B_A). In impedance terminology, complex acoustic impedance (Z_A) is composed of acoustic resistance (R_A) and acoustic reactance (X_A). The subscript A used in the preceding symbols stands for "acoustic," which the purist insists on using to differentiate acoustic immittance from mechanical and electrical immittance. Tympanograms obtained from a normal ear at 220 Hz are shown in Figure 7–2. Note the labeling of the three tympanometric tracings: G representing conductance, B representing susceptance, and Y representing admittance. The tympanograms trace conductance, susceptance, and admittance over a range of pressure values in the ear canal. Instantaneous readings of conductance and susceptance can be obtained from a dial on the immittance device.

Static acoustic immittance usually refers to a single value, which represents the immittance at the lateral surface of the tympanic membrane and excludes the immittance of the ear canal itself. The immittance value at the peak of a tympanogram in Figure 7–2 is a combination of the immittance of the canal and the immittance at the lateral surface of the tympanic mem-

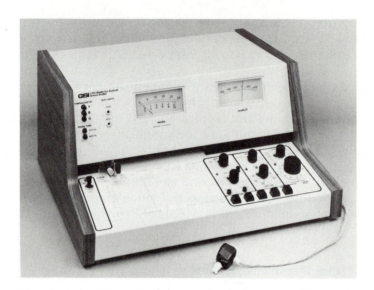

FIGURE 7-1. Grason-Stadler Model 1723 Immittance Meter. (Reproduced by permission of Grason-Stadler Inc., Littleton, Mass.)

brane. At high-negative or high-positive pressures, where the tympanograms become flat, the values represent only the immittance of the canal, since at these air pressures the drum is so tense that little acoustic energy can enter the middle-ear system. Thus, the immittance between the flat portion and the peak of the tympanogram represents the immittance at the lateral surface of

FIGURE 7-2. Tympanograms from a normal ear.

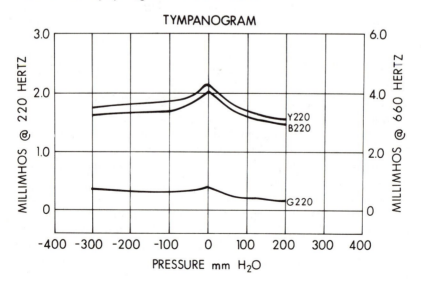

the eardrum and is the static immittance of the ear. For static admittance (Y) subtract the value obtained at + 200 mmH$_2$O from that obtained at the point of maximum amplitude of the curve. Static admittance can also be calculated from the G and B curves. First calculate static G and B the same way as static admittance was calculated. Next, square G and B, add the squares, and then extract the square root of the sum of the squares, yielding static admittance (Y) in acoustic millimhos. Following is the formula for deriving admittance:

$$Y_A = \sqrt{G_A{}^2 + B_A{}^2}$$

Because impedance is the reciprocal of admittance, impedance in acoustic ohms can be calculated by dividing Y into 1. For purposes of illustration, let us calculate static admittance and impedance from the G and B tympanograms of Figure 7–2. G at + 200 mmH$_2$O is 0.20 millimhos, and at maximum amplitude is 0.4 millimhos. B at + 200 mmH$_2$O is 1.50 millimhos, and at maximum amplitude is 2.05 millimhos. Thus, G = 0.20 millimhos (0.40 − 0.20), and B = 0.55 millimhos (2.05 − 1.50). Now we will substitute these values in the formula:

$$Y_A = \sqrt{G_A{}^2 = B_A{}^2} = \sqrt{0.20^2 + 0.55^2} = \sqrt{0.04 + 0.3025} = \sqrt{0.3425}$$
$$Y_A = 0.585 \text{ millimhos} = 0.000585 \text{ mhos}$$
$$Z_A = 1/Y_A = 1/0.000585 \text{ mhos}$$
$$Z_A = 1709 \text{ ohms}$$

Note that the static admittance value determined from the Y tympanogram (Y = 2.20 − 1.60 = 0.60 millimhos) is very close to the value derived from the G and B tympanograms. At 220 Hz, the admittance value (Y) in millimhos is essentially the same as the "compliance" value specified in milliliters of an equivalent volume of air.[1] Thus, the static admittance value of 0.585 millimhos is equal to a static "compliance" of 0.585 ml in equivalent volume units.

In clinical use, the magnitudes of G$_A$, B$_A$, and Y$_A$ are not as important as the determination of whether or not these parameters fall within the normal range. Unfortunately, there is a variability in the normal range as reported by various investigators and even by the same investigator at different times. In 1975, Feldman cited the range of normal impedance (Z$_A$) values obtained with the Grason-Stadler Otoadmittance Meter as being from 1200 to 3000 ohms at 220 Hz and from 200 to 700 ohms at 660 Hz.[2] The reciprocals of these im-

[1] Alan S. Feldman, "Tympanometry—Procedures, Interpretations and Variables," in *Acoustic Impedance & Admittance—The Measurement of Middle Ear Function*, eds. Alan S. Feldman and Laura Ann Wilber (Baltimore: Williams & Wilkins, 1976), chap. 6, p. 105.

[2] Alan S. Feldman, "Acoustic Impedance-Admittance Measurements," in *Physiological Measures of the Audio-Vestibular System*, ed. Larry J. Bradford (New York: Academic Press, 1975), chap. 4, p. 114.

pedance values are the ranges of normal admittances (Y_A): 0.33 to 0.83 millimhos at 220 Hz and 1.43 to 5.0 millimhos at 660 Hz. At 220 Hz, the normal range of static "compliance" in equivalent volume units is then 0.33 to 0.83 ml.

In evaluating tympanograms, one is concerned with static values, the shape of the tympanogram, and the location of the pressure peak. The static values relate to the middle ear independently from the middle-ear air pressure and the size of the external ear canal. The shape of the tympanogram provides additional information concerning the middle ear. Finally, the location of the pressure peak is an estimate of the air pressure within the middle ear, which in turn is dependent on the functioning of the Eustachian tube.

Figure 7–3 shows a flat tympanogram and absence of a pressure peak obtained from a child with middle-ear effusion. A static value cannot be calculated in this case. The fluid-filled middle ear causes an increased impedance of the eardrum. Other conditions which can result in a flat tympanogram include a perforated tympanic membrane, an external ear canal occluded by cerumen, an ear with an open tympanostomy (drainage) tube, cholesteatoma, granuloma, polyps in the middle ear, tympanosclerosis, and glomus jugulare tumors.[3]

FIGURE 7-3.   Fluid-filled middle ear. (Adapted from Alan S. Feldman, "Tympanometry—Procedures, Interpretations and Variables," chap. 6, p. 126, from Alan S. Feldman and Laura Ann Wilber, eds., *Acoustic Impedance & Admittance,* copyright © 1976 by Williams & Wilkins Co. Reprinted by permission.)

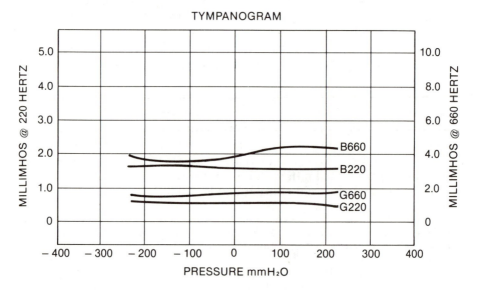

3 Feldman, "Tympanometry," pp. 128–33.

Tympanometry is useful in following the progression of an acute otitis media or the effect of treatment. In Figure 7-4, we see four tympanograms graphed on the same form for convenience, the curves all having the same base line. Over a period of six days, the air pressure in the middle ear changes from $-200\,\text{mmH}_2\text{O}$, as a result of Eustachian tube blockage, to zero as the tube regains patency. Normally, one varies the pressure in the canal from $+200$ to -200 mmH$_2$O while running a tympanogram. If the tympanogram curve shows no peak, it is advisable to decrease the pressure to $-400\,\text{mmH}_2\text{O}$ or even lower, as you may be dealing with a severely retracted eardrum. Positive pressure peaks are generally obtained only in cases of acute otitis media.

Abnormalities of the eardrum result in deviations from the normal shape of the tympanograms, as illustrated in Figure 7-5. A healed perforation results in an eardrum that is highly compliant, as seen in the susceptance (B) curves. The notched B660 curve is typical of a perforated drum that has healed. The 660 Hz probe tone is particularly useful in identifying eardrum abnormalities. According to Feldman, "As the frequency of the probe tone more closely approximates the resonant frequency of the ear, deviations in stiffness and mass influence are disclosed by notching of tympanograms. . . . This dimension of diagnostic information is generally unavailable with the low frequency probe tone."[4]

FIGURE 7-4.   B220 tympanograms showing progress of blocked Eustachian tube over a six-day period. Baselines are arbitrary and the same for each curve. (Adapted from Feldman, "Tympanometry," in Feldman and Wilber, eds., *Acoustic Impedance & Admittance*, p. 123.)

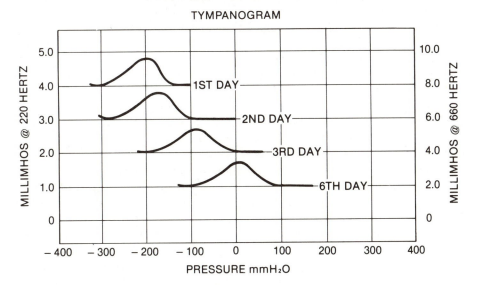

[4] Ibid., p. 111.

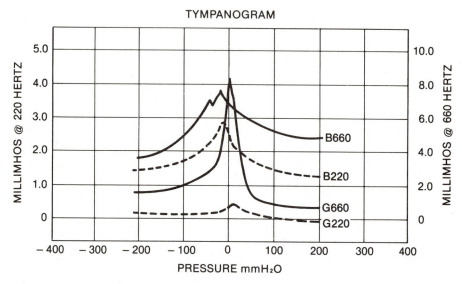

FIGURE 7-5.   Healed perforation of tympanic membrane. (Adapted from *Otoadmittance Handbook 2,* Concord, Mass.: Grason-Stadler Co., Inc., 1973, Figure B-5.)

In Figure 7–6, again there is a deviation from the normal shape of the tympanogram. Ossicular disarticulation results in static susceptance values that may be negative. The center of the susceptance tympanogram tends to be lower than the outer ends of the tympanogram. Deep, multiple notches are typical of tympanograms from ears with ossicular discontinuity.

Otosclerosis and other kinds of ossicular fixation may result in normal middle-ear air-pressure and lower static-admittance values. The resulting tympanogram will show a reduced peak at the normal air pressure, as shown in Figure 7–7, or the static values may be within normal limits.

The results of tympanometry must be viewed in conjunction with audiometric test results. Thus, if a normal-appearing tympanogram is obtained from a patient whose audiogram indicates a conductive loss, it is likely that a fixation of the ossicular chain is present.

Sometimes, tympanograms will show irregularities that coincide with the vascular pulse beat. Figure 7–8 illustrates a case of glomus jugulare tumor. Although only the 220 Hz G and B curves are shown, the vascular perturbations occur in the 660 Hz curves as well.

Tympanometry is useful for assessing Eustachian tube function, knowledge of which contributes to the diagnosis and rehabilitation of middle-ear pathology. Evaluating Eustachian tube functioning may be accomplished directly or indirectly. The indirect method according to Holmquist involves merely noting the pressure peaks of the tympanogram curves. If these peaks

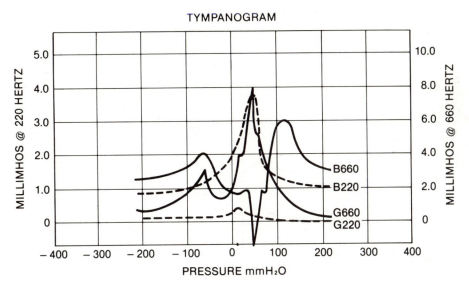

FIGURE 7-6.   Ossicular disarticulation due to degeneration of the stapedial crura. (Adapted from Feldman, "Tympanometry," in Feldman and Wilber, eds., *Acoustic Impedance & Admittance,* p. 141.)

FIGURE 7-7.   Otosclerosis. (Adapted from Feldman, "Tympanometry," in Feldman and Wilber, eds., *Acoustic Impedance & Admittance,* p. 133.)

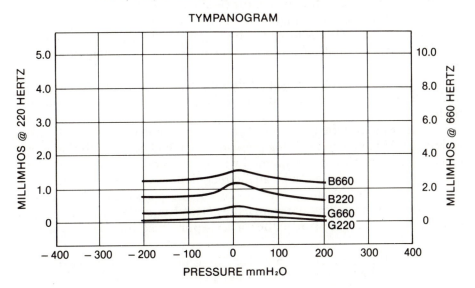

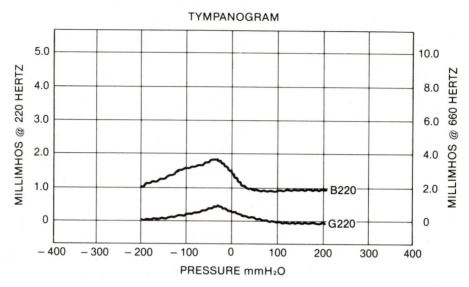

FIGURE 7-8.   G and B curves for 220 Hz showing vascular perturbations resulting from a glomus jugulare tumor. (Adapted from Feldman, "Tympanometry," in Feldman and Wilber, eds., *Acoustic Impedance & Admittance*, p. 150.)

are within ± 25 mmH₂O of zero or atmospheric pressure, the Eustachian tube function is considered to be normal. If the pressure peak is more than ± 25 mmH₂O, the function of the Eustachian tube is regarded as abnormal.[5] Other authors refer to a much wider range of normal. The direct evaluation of Eustachian tube function, according to Holmquist, consists of introducing a negative air pressure in the middle ear (− 200 mmH₂O) by means of the air pump on the immittance equipment and noting whether or not the patient can restore the middle ear to atmospheric pressure by repeated swallowing. The level of the residual air pressure in the middle ear following the swallowing is noted. The same procedure is followed in cases of perforated eardrums or when tympanostomy (drainage) tubes are in place, except that if the induced negative air pressure is unchanged after four swallows the test is discontinued.[6]

Bluestone uses the terms *direct* and *indirect* somewhat differently from Holmquist. He refers to reducing pressure in the middle ear with the immittance equipment by a direct method when a perforated eardrum or a tympanostomy tube is present, or by an indirect method when the eardrum is intact. In the former instance, the pressure in the middle ear is reduced by action of the pump pulling air through the perforation or the tube; in the latter case, the negative air pressure in the ear canal pulls the eardrum outward, thus

[5]Jörgen Holmquist, "Eustachian Tube Evaluation," in *Acoustic Impedance & Admittance*, eds. Feldman and Wilber, chap. 7, p. 166.

[6]Ibid., pp. 167–70.

enlarging the middle-ear space and decreasing the air pressure within it.[7] In the case of a perforated drum or drainage tube, Bluestone introduces $+400$ mmH$_2$O in the middle ear. The patient is instructed to swallow once every twenty seconds until the pressure in the ear returns to normal or until there is no further pressure reduction. Then, the pressure is reduced to -200 mmH$_2$O, and again with successive swallows the patient tries to equilibrate the pressure. If it is impossible to hold any positive or negative air pressure in the middle ear, it indicates that the Eustachian tube is *patulous,* or abnormally open.[8] With an intact eardrum, Bluestone advocates an inflation-deflation procedure that involves first running a tympanogram to determine the pressure peak or the "resting" middle-ear pressure. Next, the pressure in the canal is increased to $+200$ mmH$_2$O, and the patient is instructed to swallow several times, after which a second tympanogram is run. If the Eustachian tube is functioning normally, this second tympanogram will show a slight negative pressure in comparison with the resting pressure. Then, -200 mmH$_2$O is introduced into the canal, and again the patient is instructed to swallow several times, after which a third tympanogram is run. If the tube is patent, a slight positive pressure will be traced in comparison with the resting pressure. The three tympanograms are run on the same form so their pressure peaks can be compared easily.[9]

Williams describes a similar three-tympanogram procedure, except that she introduces 400 mmH$_2$O of both positive and negative pressure. Only a single tympanogram is required to estimate middle-ear air pressure. Williams suggests that the G660 tracing be used. Her procedure is to obtain an initial tympanogram to establish the patient's pressure peak or "resting" pressure as a base line. This tympanogram is labeled 1. Next, she increases the pressure in the canal to $+400$ mmH$_2$O and instructs the patient to swallow several times, letting the patient drink liquid to facilitate swallowing if necessary. Then, another tympanogram is run and labeled 2. All tympanograms are run in the same direction, preferably from positive to negative pressure. After the second tympanogram, the pressure in the canal is returned to the point of peak pressure in the base-line tympanogram and the patient is instructed to swallow "three or four times" to equalize pressure to its original peak value. This step is necessary, according to Williams, to eliminate the effects induced by the $+400$ mmH$_2$O. Finally, the pressure in the canal is reduced to -400 mmH$_2$O, and the patient swallows three or four times, after which a third tympanometric tracing is obtained and labeled 3.[10]

[7] Charles D. Bluestone, "Assessment of Eustachian Tube Function," in *The Handbook of Clinical Impedance Audiometry,* ed. James Jerger (Dobbs Ferry, N.Y.: American Electromedics Corporation, 1975), chap. 6, p. 135.

[8] Ibid., p. 138.

[9] Ibid., p. 140.

[10] Peggy S. Williams, "A Tympanometric Pressure Swallow Test for Assessment of Eustachian-Tube Function," *The Reflex* (Grason-Stadler Company, December 1975), pp. 1–6.

Figure 7-9 shows the results obtained with the Williams procedure with three types of patients. Part (a) illustrates normal Eustachian tube function. Tracing 1 shows a tympanogram with peak pressure within normal limits (± 25 mmH$_2$O). Tracings 2 and 3 demonstrate shifts of pressure peaks following induced pressures of $+400$ and -400 mmH$_2$O, respectively, and swallowing activity. Williams reported that with sixteen normal ears, the mean pressure peak shifts were from 15 to 20 mmH$_2$O. Part (b) of Figure 7-9 illustrates a lack of shift from the base line for tracings 2 and 3 due to inability of the Eustachian tube to open during swallowing. The tracings in part (b) are representative of results obtained with eleven ears having middle-ear disease. Part (c) shows pressure peak shifts of greater than normal extent, which characterized eight ears with healed perforations of the eardrum and no active middle-ear disease. With these ears, the pressure peak shifts averaged 25 to 30

FIGURE 7-9.   Shifts in pressure peaks obtained during the pressure swallow test. (From Peggy S. Williams, "A Tympanometric Pressure Swallow Test for Assessment of Eustachian-Tube Function," *The Reflex,* Grason-Stadler Co., December 1975.)

TYMPANOGRAM

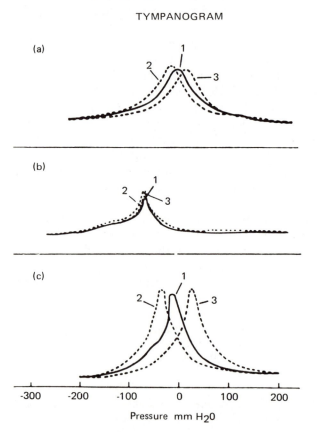

Pressure mm H$_2$0

mmH$_2$O. Williams interprets this result as demonstrating "overly compliant" Eustachian tubes. As was the case with Bluestone's findings, Williams reported that with patent Eustachian tubes, tracing 2 would show a slight negative pressure in comparison with tracing 1, and tracing 3 would show a slight positive pressure—provided that when the Eustachian tube closes after the last swallow at +400 mmH$_2$O the patient does not swallow again until after the second tracing is accomplished, and likewise refrains from swallowing after the last swallow at −400 mmH$_2$O until after the third tympanogram is traced. When air is expelled from the middle ear or drawn into the middle ear by swallowing at high positive or high negative pressures, respectively, in the canal, the peak pressure points of subsequent tympanograms will reflect the lessened air pressure in the middle ear by shifting to negative, and the increased air pressure by shifting to positive. Williams pointed out a finding she could not explain: The amplitude of tracings 2 and 3 tended to be slightly greater than tracing 1 in all instances, as can be seen in Figure 7–9.[11]

Bluestone states that the function of the Eustachian tube should be studied in all patients having "recurrent acute or chronic middle ear effusion." In addition, Eustachian tube studies should be made of patients using tympanostomy tubes. Improvement in Eustachian tube function helps the otologist to decide when to remove the tubes. Inflation-deflation tests are useful in evaluating the adequacy of treatment of nasopharyngeal inflammation and the effects of adenoidectomy and cleft-palate surgery. Finally, Bluestone points out the value of Eustachian tube studies of patients with perforations of the eardrum who are candidates for tympanoplasty procedures. The better the preoperative Eustachian tube function, the better the chances of success in such surgery.[12]

Tests of the acoustic reflex assist the clinician in determining if a conductive impairment exists, and in the case of sensori-neural impairments, if the pathology is cochlear or neural. Also, these tests make possible gross predictions of hearing threshold levels and slope of the audiometric curve. The intra-aural muscles are the tensor tympani, innervated by the Vth (trigeminal) nerve and the stapedius, innervated by the VIIth (facial) nerve. The "acoustic" reflex—that is, the muscle contraction resulting from acoustic stimulation—apparently involves only the stapedius muscle. The tensor tympani contracts as a startle reflex.[13] Of course, a loud sound may also startle an individual, in which case both muscles would contract. Contraction of the stapedius and/or the tensor tympani causes a change in the immittance at the eardrum which can be measured with an immittance meter or other immittance-monitoring device.

[11] Ibid., pp. 4–5.

[12] Bluestone, "Assessment of Eustachian Tube Function," p. 145.

[13] Laura Ann Wilber, "Acoustic Reflex Measurement—Procedures, Interpretations and Variables," in *Acoustic Impedance & Admittance*, eds. Feldman and Wilber, chap. 9, p. 200.

Because the acoustic reflex occurs in both ears, even though only one ear is stimulated, the common practice clinically is to stimulate one ear and monitor the immittance in the other ear, a procedure referred to as a *contralateral stimulation*. Now, because of improvements in equipment design and engineering, it is possible to monitor immittance changes in the stimulated ear, a procedure that is called *ipsilateral stimulation,* or study of the ipsilateral reflex. Comparison of the results of contralateral and ipsilateral stimulation has diagnostic implications.

In the normal ear, the acoustic reflex is elicited by a contralateral or ipsilateral pure-tone stimulus at a sensation level of 70 to 95 dB. As the bandwidth of the stimulus is widened, once a certain bandwidth is exceeded, the intensity of the stimulus required to elicit the acoustic reflex becomes less and less, until for a broad-band noise the reflex threshold may be 20 to 25 dB lower than for a pure tone.[14] If the clinician is interested only in determining whether or not an acoustic reflex is present, white noise would be the preferred stimulus; but if one is concerned with more complete information on the threshold of the acoustic reflex, pure tones should be used as stimuli.[15]

The muscle contraction is generally not detectable in an ear with conductive loss because "conductive loss of any substantial degree will be enough to override the effect of the contraction of the stapedius muscle."[16] In other words the muscle contraction has no observable effect on a tympanic membrane that is immobilized by fluid in the ear or by fixation of the ossicles, or in cases of discontinuity of the ossicular chain or perforation of the eardrum. In the case of a unilateral conductive loss, the muscle contraction may be detected in the contralateral ear if the loss is sufficiently mild that a stimulus at a sensation level of 70 to 95 dB can be presented. With ipsilateral stimulation, the reflex should be absent in the affected ear and present in the normal ear. An audiometrically normal ear may not have a demonstrable reflex by ipsilateral stimulation if there is damage to the VIIth nerve, if there is no stapedial tendon (as sometimes happens), or if there is any middle-ear pathology.

In sensori-neural impairments of cochlear origin, reflex thresholds may be found at sensation levels as low as 20 to 50 dB. Metz first described this phenomenon of lowered reflex thresholds and referred to it as *recruitment of loudness*.[17] Patients with cochlear pathology tend to demonstrate an acoustic

[14] Gerald R. Popelka, Robert H. Margolis, and Terry L. Wiley, "The Effect of Activating Signal Bandwidth on Acoustic Reflex Thresholds," *Journal of the Acoustical Society of America* 59 (1976):153.

[15] Wilber, "Acoustic Reflex Measurement," p. 201.

[16] Ibid., p. 203.

[17] O. Metz, "The Acoustic Impedance Measured on Normal and Pathological Ears," *Acta Otolaryngologica,* supp. 63, 1946; O. Metz, "Threshold of Reflex Contractions of Muscles of the Middle Ear and Recruitment of Loudness," *Archives of Otolaryngology* 55 (1952):536–43.

reflex at the same hearing level as is required by the normal ear; in other words, as their hearing loss increases, the sensation level of the reflex threshold decreases, keeping the HTL of the threshold constant.[18] In the case of unilateral cochlear pathology, with contralateral stimulation the acoustic reflex will be present in the affected ear. If there is sufficient residual hearing in the impaired ear, ipsilateral stimulation will also elicit a reflex.

In the case of unilateral VIIIth nerve pathology, the reflex threshold tends to be at the same sensation level as for the normal ear, which means that if a patient's HTL exceeds 30 to 40 dB, a reflex will not be demonstrated by ipsilateral stimulation. If the reflex is present, it may be characterized by abnormal decay. Abnormal decay exists when a stimulus is presented at a level of 10 dB greater than the reflex threshold and the amplitude of the reflex decreases to less than half its original value in 10 seconds or less. According to Jerger, reflex decay occurs in many normal ears at 2000 and 4000 Hz but rarely occurs at lower frequencies. He suggests testing for abnormal decay, therefore, at 500 and 1000 Hz.[19] Wilber cautions that although other investigators have found that abnormal decay is most prevalent with VIIIth nerve patients, they have also reported observing it with normal ears and ears with cochlear impairment.[20]

The acoustic reflex test has some usefulness in evaluating patients with brain-stem tumors, which may affect the contralateral reflex. In such cases, contralateral stimulation may not elicit a reflex, but ipsilateral stimulation will.[21] With central auditory lesions above the level of the reflex arc, the reflex thresholds should be normal with either contralateral or ipsilateral stimulation.

Jerger et al. developed a procedure for predicting degree of impairment and slope of the audiogram curve by comparing the acoustic reflex thresholds for pure tones and for broad-band noise.[22] As mentioned earlier in this section, the normal ear demonstrates a reflex threshold for broad-band noise that is substantially lower than the reflex threshold for a pure tone. In ears with sensori-neural impairment, the difference between the reflex thresholds for broad-band noise and pure tones narrows in proportion to the severity of the impairment. The procedure of Jerger et al. was a refinement of a method described earlier by Niemeyer and Sesterhenn.[23] Instead of trying to predict dB of impairment as Niemeyer and Sesterhenn did, Jerger et al. placed pa-

[18] Jerger, "Diagnostic Use of Impedance Measures," p. 158.

[19] Ibid., p. 160.

[20] Wilber, "Acoustic Reflex Measurement," p. 209.

[21] Feldman, "Acoustic Impedance-Admittance Measurements," p. 134.

[22] James Jerger, Phillip Burney, Larry Mauldin, and Betsy Crump, "Predicting Hearing Loss from the Acoustic Reflex," *Journal of Speech and Hearing Disorders* 39 (February 1974):11–22.

[23] W. Niemeyer and G. Sesterhenn, "Calculating the Hearing Threshold from the Stapedius Reflex Threshold for Different Sound Stimuli," *Audiology* 13 (1974):421–27.

tients in categories labeled normal, mild-moderate, severe, and profound on the basis of a combination of the difference between reflex thresholds for broad-band noise and pure tones and the SPL of the reflex threshold for the broad-band noise. In general, the less the difference between the reflex thresholds for pure tones and the noise and the higher the SPL of the reflex threshold for the noise, the more severe the predicted hearing loss. With 1156 patients, the predictions were "excellent" in 60 percent of the cases. There was a "moderate" error of prediction (error of one category) in 36 percent of the cases, and a "serious" error (error of two or more categories) in 4 percent. Jerger now calls this procedure *SPAR*, for *sensitivity predictions* from *acoustic reflex*.[24] With a subgroup of 113 patients, Jerger et al. predicted the slope of the audiogram curve between 1000 and 4000 Hz as being flat, gradual, or steep, based on differences between reflex thresholds for a low-pass filtered and a high-pass filtered noise, using 2600 Hz as the upper or lower limit of the filter. If the difference was zero, or if the reflex threshold for the low-pass filtered noise was higher, the prediction was a flat audiometric loss. If the reflex threshold for the high-pass filtered noise was from 1 to 5 dB higher than the reflex threshold for the low-pass filtered noise, the prediction was for a gradually sloping loss pattern. If the difference exceeded 5 dB, the prediction was for a steep slope. The accuracy of the slope prediction was about the same as for the severity of loss prediction.[25] SPAR and prediction of slope have "promise as screening techniques for children who have discernable acoustic reflexes and who cannot be tested in other ways."[26] Several other procedures based on these concepts have been proposed.[27]

If the acoustic reflex cannot be elicited because of the severity of the hearing loss, it may still be possible to evaluate middle-ear function or to check the integrity of the reflex arc by means of the nonacoustic reflex, which is independent of the hearing level in the stimulated ear. Djupesland says,

> It is now well established that the middle ear muscles are activated not only by sound, but also by nonacoustic stimuli. Both in animals and in man the muscles contract during certain movements of the head and neck, during vocalization and on touching or electrical stimulation of the skin in the ear canal.[28]

Djupesland describes two techniques of eliciting the nonacoustic reflex: (1) tactile (cutaneous) stimulation of the skin around or in the external acoustic

[24] Jerger, "Diagnostic Use of Impedance Measures," p. 170.

[25] Jerger et al., "Predicting Hearing Loss," pp. 15–19.

[26] Wilber, "Acoustic Reflex Measurement," p. 214.

[27] Gerald R. Popelka, ed., *Hearing Assessment with the Acoustic Reflex* (New York: Grune & Stratton, 1981).

[28] Gisle Djupesland, "Nonacoustic Reflex Measurement—Procedures, Interpretations and Variables," in *Acoustic Impedance & Admittance*, eds. Feldman and Wilber, chap. 10, p. 217.

meatus with cotton wool twisted around the tip of a metal stick, and (2) lifting both upper eyelids of a patient upward and inward simultaneously with the thumbs. The immittance at the eardrum is monitored with a probe in either ear, although Djupesland believes that ipsilateral cutaneous stimulation produces more immittance change than contralateral stimulation.[29] The cutaneous stimulation apparently causes contraction of the stapedius only; lifting the eyelids causes contraction of both intra-aural muscles, provided the movements of the examiner's thumbs are "forceful and/or surprising," producing a startle or defensive response. If no immittance change occurs from cutaneous stimulation but does occur with lifting the eyelids, the indication is that although the stapedius is not contracting the tensor tympani is, as in the case of Bell's palsy, for example. Information about fixation or disarticulation of the ossicles can be obtained by acoustic and nonacoustic stimuli and by comparing cutaneous stimulation and raising the eyelids.

Although we have discussed static immittance values, tympanometry, and muscle reflex responses separately, the interpretation of test results is made on the basis of the test battery. The results of any single test may be ambiguous when viewed in isolation but fall into a recognizable pattern when studied in conjunction with other tests in the battery. Also, the results of immittance measures must be viewed in the context of the complete audiological examination. Jerger differentiates between "impedance measurement" and "impedance audiometry" as follows:

> ... Impedance measurement is the gathering of data (the tympanogram, the static compliance, etc.). Impedance audiometry, on the other hand, goes beyond mere measurement to include the skilled interpretation of the collective impedance measures in relation to other relevant audiometric data. With a minimum of training almost anyone can carry out impedance measures, but only a person well-trained in audiology can carry out meaningful impedance audiometry.[30]

We shall be making reference to immittance testing in later sections of this chapter and also in Chapter 8.

Evoked Response Audiometry

The electroencephalograph measures the brain-wave activity of the subject. Neurologists and psychiatrists utilize the EEG for evidence of brain pathology or malfunctioning that would be represented by deviations from waves obtained with normal brains. It has been observed that brain-wave activity is subject to variability in the presence of external stimuli. In electroencephalography, the patient is kept as quiet and relaxed as possible, or even in a light sleep, which may require the use of some sedation. Even in this situa-

[29] Ibid., pp. 219–23.
[30] Jerger, "Diagnostic Use of Impedance Measures," p. 172.

tion, the brain-wave pattern will show changes when sound stimuli are introduced at levels above the patient's threshold. Thus, attempts have been made to utilize responses evoked in brain-wave activity as indicators of hearing sensitivity.

There are difficulties in utilizing EEG for auditory measurements. One problem is the length of time required for an examination—usually about one and a half to two hours. Other problems concern the establishment of the optimum degree of wakefulness on the part of the subject and controlling the activity of the subject who is awake. The more active the subject, the more difficult it is to discriminate evoked responses from random brain-wave activity. The development of averaging or summing computers has greatly eased the problem of differentiating EEG responses to auditory stimuli from random brain-wave activity. The computer averages or algebraically sums the responses so that the random activity becomes essentially zero, whereas the nonrandom response remains. The "unusual" brain-wave activity that is associated in time with the introduction of the auditory stimulus thus stands out in contrast to the relatively flat tracing that is the result of the averaging. Since the reports by Lowell et al. of the use of a special-purpose analog computer with EEG auditory evaluations,[31] the literature has reflected the tremendous interest of laboratory and clinical investigators in evoked response audiometry (ERA), or as Davis and Goldstein prefer to call it, electric response audiometry, resulting in the same initials.[32] ERA refers to the use of EEG with an averaging or summing computer. It makes possible the evaluation of small changes in electrical activity of the brain that are present in the waking state, and "except for children less than eighteen months of age and a few older ones who are unruly, electric response audiometry does not require putting the child to sleep," thus simplifying and shortening the procedure.[33]

McCandless and Best demonstrated that reliable summed evoked responses could be obtained with adults within 10 dB of voluntary threshold for clicks, and that evoked responses from children ranging in age from a few weeks to five years could be obtained at hearing levels of 30 dB.[34] Price et al. reported that the mean difference between the averaged evoked response and

[31] Edgar L. Lowell, Carol I. Troffer, Edward A. Warburton, and Georgina M. Rushford, "Temporal Evannation: a New Approach in Diagnostic Audiology," *Journal of Speech and Hearing Disorders* 25 (November 1960):340–45; Edgar L. Lowell, Carol Troffer Williams, Robert M. Ballinger, and Delphi Alvig, "Measurement of Auditory Threshold with a Special Purpose Analog Computer," *Journal of Speech and Hearing Research* 4 (June 1961):105–12.

[32] H. Davis and R. Goldstein, "Audiometry: Other Auditory Tests," in *Hearing and Deafness*, 3rd ed., eds. Hallowell Davis and S. Richard Silverman (New York: Holt, Rinehart and Winston, 1970), p. 244.

[33] Ibid.

[34] Geary A. McCandless and LaVar Best, "Evoked Responses to Auditory Stimuli in Man Using a Summing Computer," *Journal of Speech and Hearing Research* 7 (June 1964):193–202.

the voluntary threshold for eight adults was less than 5 dB.[35] The use of ERA in clinical evaluations of hearing in both children and adults was reported by McCandless. Children over age two could be tested satisfactorily with the technique, but younger children's test results were much more difficult to interpret.[36] McCandless sounds a note of caution regarding the interpretation of ERA data:

> It is safe to assume that appearance of an evoked potential indicates a sound has altered the patient's cortex, but in no way does it imply that the patient can use auditory information meaningfully. The absence of a response, on the other hand, may not mean the child cannot hear, since some children with brain damage respond overtly to sound but give inconsistent and sometimes absent evoked responses. The interpretation of evoked response audiometry, therefore, must be undertaken with extreme caution.[37]

Davis et al. tested all the pupils at Central Institute for the Deaf whose thresholds for the speech frequencies were within the limits of the audiometer. Their conclusion was that ERA was feasible for school-age children. Although the youngest age group (ages four to ten) was more difficult to test, "adequate" ERA results were obtained with every child without the need for drugs, and excellent agreement was obtained between ERA and behavioral test results.[38]

Price reviewed the experimental and clinical work leading to the present state of ERA and cautioned against either placing too much reliance on the technique or being too quick to discard it because of its limitations.[39] Later, in a journal article, Price again urged clinicians to proceed cautiously with the new technique and pointed to the need for further research to improve what already has been demonstrated to be a "clinically useful" tool. He made the point, however, that "evoked response audiometry at present is neither 'the answer' nor 'objective audiometry.' "[40]

Up to this point, we have been using the initials ERA to stand for either "evoked response audiometry" or "electric response audiometry," referring to

[35] Lloyd L. Price, Benjamin Rosenblut, Robert Goldstein, and David C. Shepherd, "The Averaged Evoked Response to Auditory Stimulation," *Journal of Speech and Hearing Research* 9 (September 1966):361–70.

[36] Geary A. McCandless, "Clinical Application of Evoked Response Audiometry," *Journal of Speech and Hearing Research* 10 (September 1967):468–78.

[37] Ibid., p. 477.

[38] Hallowell Davis, Shirley K. Hirsh, Joyce Shelnutt, and Clyde Bowers, "Further Validation of Evoked Response Audiometry," *Journal of Speech and Hearing Research* 10 (December 1967):717–32.

[39] Lloyd L. Price, "Cortical-Evoked Response Audiometry," in *Audiometry for the Retarded,* eds. Robert T. Fulton and Lyle L. Lloyd (Baltimore: Williams & Wilkins, 1969), pp. 210–37.

[40] Lloyd L. Price, "Evoked Response Audiometry: Some Considerations," *Journal of Speech and Hearing Disorders* 34 (May 1969):137–41.

the use of electroencephalography with an averaging or summing computer. At the present time, ERA stands for *electrophysiologic response audiometry*, which includes the recording of action potentials from the VIIIth nerve as well as electrical activity from various levels of the brain in response to auditory stimulation.

The recording and analysis of VIIIth-nerve action potentials is called *electrocochleography* (ECoG). Although the recording of the cochlear microphonic or potential (CP) and the VIIIth-nerve action potential (AP) has been done for years with experimental animals, it is only recently that techniques have been developed for recording and analyzing the AP in human subjects. The CP is not useful in ECoG because when picked up from sites outside the cochlea the CP reflects electrical activity of the hair cells only in the basal turn of the cochlea. In ECoG, the CP is canceled out electrically to keep it from contaminating the AP recording.[41] The AP is most efficiently detected by a needle electrode inserted through the tympanic membrane and making contact with the cochlear promontory in the middle ear, although it is possible to record the AP at a lower amplitude from the external canal, from the annulus of the tympanic membrane, or even from the lobe of the pinna. Generally, a click stimulus is used to generate the AP because it causes many nerve fibers to discharge almost simultaneously. An averaging computer is used in ECoG to decrease the effects of background electrical noise. Figure 7–10 shows nerve action potentials at various sensation levels.

Although there have been some attempts to predict hearing threshold levels from ECoG, the primary clinical use of the technique today is to determine in patients impossible to test otherwise whether or not there is end organ function. Simmons and Glattke say,

> . . . Clearly the cochleogram, in the infancy of its clinical application, is the most powerful electrophysiological index of cochlear integrity yet applied to the damaged ear. In fact, we are aware of no other method by which it is possible to know with reasonable certainty that, when a response is present, there is at least some residual hearing at the end-organ, and that, when there is no response, there is no residual hearing at the frequencies tested. Making that distinction *is* today's clinical application.
>
> Tomorrow's clinical application is equally certain: the not-too-difficult jump to predicting, with perhaps 10-dB accuracy, the contour of the threshold audiogram and some suprathreshold hearing characteristics of damaged ears. The information is present in the wave-form and latencies of the N_1-N_2 action potential. Slightly more sophisticated analysis is capable of extracting it. In fact this is already possible for certain kinds of hearing losses. The number of patients with whom we must resort to any electrophysiological test will, however, be quite limited. Cochleography is not about to replace the audiometer.[42]

---

[41] F. Blair Simmons and Theodore Glattke, "Electrocochleography," in *Physiological Measures*, ed. Bradford, chap. 5, pp. 154–55.

[42] Ibid., p. 173.

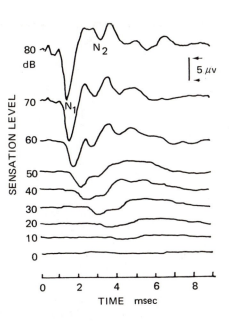

FIGURE 7-10.
Responses of the VIIIth nerve recorded at various sensation levels. Negative (downward) peaks are labeled N_1, N_2, etc. (From Paul Skinner and Theodore J. Glattke, "Electrophysiologic Response Audiometry: State of the Art," *Journal of Speech and Hearing Disorders* 42, May 1977, 183, by permission of the authors and the *Journal of Speech and Hearing Disorders.*)

Because the best cochleograms often are recorded from an electrode on the promontory, which requires anesthetizing the patient to insert the electrode through the tympanic membrane, there is an element of risk and an ethical question for the clinician to face: Is the risk justified in light of the potential benefit to the patient? In an attempt to define the risks, Crowley, Davis, and Beagley sent a questionnaire to "most of the electrocochleographic centers of the world." Replies were received based on 2594 cases, of which 1875 had had a promontory placement of the electrode. The authors report "... that the general risk of electrocochleography is around 0.007 or 0.7%. The risk of serious complication during general anesthesia is 0.005 or 0.5%. The transtympanic promontory electrode entails a risk of 0.001 or 0.1%." The respondents to the questionnaire reported that they had obtained "useful" diagnostic information from 90 percent of the children tested with ECoG.[43]

Skinner and Glattke reviewed recording techniques and clinical findings of ECoG and evoked responses obtained from electrodes placed on the vertex, forehead, and mastoid. The latter responses are categorized as early, middle, late, and very late responses, based on their latency.[44] Table 7-1, adapted from their article, presents the information that characterizes each response. Until recently, most of the work in evoked-response audiometry, including that

[43] David E. Crowley, Hallowell Davis, and Harry Beagley, "Clinical Use of Electrocochleography: A Preliminary Report," in *Electrocochleography*, eds. Robert J. Ruben, Claus Elberling, and Gerhard Salomon (Baltimore: University Park Press, 1976), p. 292.

[44] Skinner and Glattke, "Electrophysiologic Response Audiometry: State of the Art," *Journal of Speech and Hearing Disorders* 42 (May 1977):179-98.

TABLE 7–1.   Characteristics of electrophysiologic responses

Response latency classification	Site of origin	Response waveform	Response latency in msec	Amplitude in μv
ECoG	Auditory nerve	Fast	1 to 5	0.1 –10
Early	Brain stem	Fast	4 to 8	0.01– 1
Middle	Brain stem/ primary cortical projection	Fast	8 to 50	1.0 – 3
Late	Primary cortical projection and secondary asso- ciation areas	Slow	50 to 300	8.0 –20
Very late	Prefrontal cortex and secondary association areas	Very slow	300 and beyond	20 –30

Adapted from Skinner and Glattke, "Electrophysiologic Response Audiometry," p. 180, with permission of the authors and the *Journal of Speech and Hearing Disorders.*

reported earlier in this section, had been with the late responses. Because the response is not affected by stimulus rise time, it can be evoked by pure tones. It can also be evoked whether the subject is awake, asleep, or sedated, although the responses are different in these conditions. Late responses are useful with adults, and pure-tone thresholds obtained agree well with be-havioral thresholds; however, there are problems in the interpretation of late responses with young children, as we have seen earlier, and so they have limited clinical utility.[45]

What are now called "middle" responses were formerly called "early" until the existence of responses in the 4 to 8 msec (milliseconds) range in humans was reported by Jewett and Williston.[46] Now the "Jewett waves" are called the early responses. Middle responses cannot be evoked by tones because of their slow rise time. Eliciting stimuli must be clicks or tone pips. Although middle responses produce threshold determinations agreeing closely with behavioral thresholds in adults, there is disagreement among researchers about their usefulness with young children.

Early responses appear when click stimuli are presented within 10 dB of a subject's behavioral threshold. At sensation levels of 40 to 60 dB, seven in-dividual waves may be identified as shown in Figure 7–11. These waves have been associated with electrical activity in the brain stem. Thus, the term *brain stem evoked response,* or *BSER,* is often used. Wave V has the greatest amplitude and is the subject of the most attention. The latency of wave V is related to the sensation level of the stimulus, varying from 8 to 9 msec near

[45] Ibid., p. 192.

[46] D. Jewett and J. Williston, "Auditory-Evoked Far Fields Averaged from the Scalp of Humans," *Brain* 94 (1971):681–96.

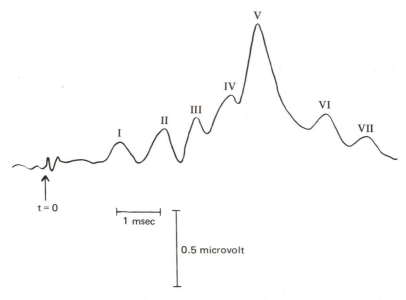

FIGURE 7-11. Early evoked responses from the brain stem showing the seven peaks identified by Jewett and Williston. (From Donald C. Hood, "Evoked Cortical Response Audiometry," chap. 10, p. 351, in Larry J. Bradford, ed., *Physiological Measures of the Audio-Vestibular System*, copyright © 1975 by Academic Press, Inc. Reprinted by permission.)

threshold to 5 to 6 msec at high sensation levels.[47] The main reason for an interest in early responses is to obtain information about both hearing sensitivity and the brain stem.

The threshold hearing level, particularly for the high-frequency region, can be estimated from a series of responses to stimuli presented at several levels. At the present time there is considerable effort in refining the techniques so that more frequency-specific information can be obtained, including threshold information for the low-frequency region. Patients with brain-stem lesions may show missing parts of the early responses or abnormal lateness between peaks in the response. Again there is considerable effort to refine the techniques but this time to improve the ability to locate a particular lesion rather than to estimate hearing sensitivity.

Two very late responses have been found to differ from evoked responses occurring earlier in that "they can be related to specific conditioning stimuli to test certain cognitive or psychological operations in children as well as adults . . . in addition to simple threshold estimation."[48] These very late responses are termed the *expectancy wave* and the *contingent negative variation* (CNV). The presence of the negative variation—a DC shift of negative

---

[47] Skinner and Glattke, "Electrophysiologic Response Audiometry," p. 187.
[48] Ibid., p. 193.

polarity—is contingent upon the pairing of a "conditional" stimulus, for example, a tone, with an "imperative" stimulus that demands a response, for example, a light flash. According to Skinner and Glattke, although the very late responses have been of interest primarily because of "their unique potential to gain information about psychological function . . . the CNV also holds potential to estimate threshold."[49]

Other Physiological Measures

Hogan provided an excellent account of attempts to utilize various physiological responses as indices of auditory sensitivity. He discussed galvanic skin, cardiac, vascular, respiratory, and visual responses to auditory stimulation.[50] We shall take a brief look at galvanic skin, cardiac, and respiratory responses.

Galvanic skin response (GSR).   One of the earliest physiologically based tests in cases of functional hearing loss is the conditioned galvanic skin response test (GSR), frequently referred to also as the *electrodermal response test* (EDR) or *electrodermal audiometry* (EDA). The primary advantage of the test is that it makes possible the measurement of a patient's threshold with a high degree of validity and reliability, provided a careful, systematic methodology is used. The limitation of the test is that it requires the patient to be conditioned to a noxious stimulus (electrical shock), and it is not possible in every case to establish conditioning or to maintain conditioning throughout the test. Investigators with extensive clinical experience in administering the GSR test have reported that it can be successfully administered to about 80 percent of adult male patients.[51] Although the test has usually been given with pure tones as the auditory stimuli, techniques have been suggested for utilizing speech audiometry.

The principle of GSR has been employed for many years in psychological research. Bordley et al.,[52] Doerfler,[53] and Bordley and Hardy[54] made the initial reports on GSR audiometry. The skin of an individual has a resistance to the flow of electric current. As this resistance increases, the

[49] Ibid.

[50] Donald D. Hogan, "Autonomic Responses as Supplementary Hearing Measures," in *Audiometry for the Retarded,* eds. Robert T. Fulton and Lyle L. Lloyd (Baltimore: Williams & Wilkins, 1969), chap. 8, pp. 238–62.

[51] Joseph B. Chaiklin and Ira M. Ventry, "Functional Hearing Loss," in James F. Jerger, ed., *Modern Developments in Audiology,* 1st ed., Chap. 3, p. 106.

[52] John E. Bordley, William G. Hardy, and C. P. Richter, "Audiometry with the Use of Galvanic Skin-resistance Response; a Preliminary Report," *Bulletin of Johns Hopkins Hospital* 82 (1948):569.

[53] Leo G. Doerfler, "Neurophysiological Clues to Auditory Acuity," *Journal of Speech and Hearing Disorders* 13 (September 1948):227–32.

[54] John E. Bordley and William G. Hardy, "A Study in Objective Audiometry with the Use of a Psychogalvanometric Response," *Annals of Otology, Rhinology, and Laryngology* 58 (September 1949):751–60.

amount of current that can flow across the skin decreases, and vice versa. Under circumstances of quiet and relaxation, an individual's skin resistance remains relatively constant. Stimuli that excite any kind of emotional response, however, will cause the resistance of the skin to decrease. The increased flow of current resulting from this resistance drop may be amplified and displayed on a graphic recorder. The technique of utilizing the skin response in hearing testing is to condition the patient to respond to sound as an emotion-producing stimulus. This is done by pairing the test stumulus from an audiometer with a mild electric shock, but one strong enough to produce momentary discomfort. The shock is sufficient to induce an emotional response, which causes a momentary drop in skin resistance. During the conditioning process, a spurt of tone and an almost simultaneous shock are presented to the patient, alternated in a random fashion with presentation of tone alone. When conditioning has been achieved, the presentation of tone alone will cause a drop in skin resistance as the patient anticipates the unpleasantness of the shock that might occur. Once the patient has been satisfactorily conditioned to tones above voluntary thresholds, the "sampling" process begins: attempts to specify the minimum hearing levels at which consistent GSRs can be obtained. Conditioning is maintained by random *reinforcements*, that is, presenting the tone and shock together, as in the conditioning process.

Conditioned GSR audiometry requires carefully controlled procedures at every step if it is to yield valid and reliable results. Without such control, errors in diagnosis may be made, and an examiner's interpretation of the test might be colored by subjective impressions of the patient. At the Veterans Administration Hospital in San Francisco, a set of procedures for administering and interpreting the results of conditioned GSR audiometry with adult patients evolved a number of years ago. These procedures are designed to minimize the factor of subjective evaluation of the test results. They draw on the research results with GSR audiometry reported by Stewart,[55] Doerfler and McClure,[56] Meritser and Doerfler,[57] Aronson et al.,[58] and Hind et al.[59] The pro-

[55] Kenneth C. Stewart, "Some Basic Considerations in Applying the GSR Technique to the Measurement of Auditory Sensitivity," *Journal of Speech and Hearing Disorders* 19 (June 1954):174–83.

[56] Leo G. Doerfler and Catherine T. McClure, "The Measurement of Hearing Loss in Adults by Galvanic Skin Response," *Journal of Speech and Hearing Disorders* 19 (June 1954):184–89.

[57] Clay L. Meritser and Leo G. Doerfler, "The Conditioning Galvanic Skin Response Under Two Modes of Reinforcement," *Journal of Speech and Hearing Disorders* 19 (September 1954):350–59.

[58] A. E. Aronson, J. E. Hind, and J. V. Irwin, "GSR Auditory Threshold Mechanisms: Effect of Tonal Intensity on Amplitude and Latency Under Two Tone-Shock Intervals," *Journal of Speech and Hearing Research* 1 (September 1958):211–19.

[59] J. E. Hind, A. E. Aronson, and J. V. Irwin, "GSR Auditory Threshold Mechanisms: Instrumentation, Spontaneous Response, and Threshold Definition," *Journal of Speech and Hearing Research* 1 (September 1958):220–26.

cedures and rationale originally reported by Chaiklin, Ventry, and Barrett[60] have been described in detail by Ventry.[61]

The equipment used at the San Francisco Veterans Administration Hospital was a Grason-Stadler psychogalvanometer connected with a pure-tone audiometer. The equipment and the examiner are situated outside the test room occupied by the patient, to whom pick-up and shock electrodes have been attached. The two pick-up electrodes are placed on the pads of the index and ring fingers of the left hand, and the two shock electrodes are similarly placed on the right hand. The testing is performed monaurally through earphones, although during the conditioning procedure, tone may be presented binaurally through the phones.

The GSR test is used only on a limited basis, for several reasons. Tests based on other physiologic responses such as the auditory brain-stem response and the acoustic reflex response have become widely available. In addition, there now exist certain restrictions regarding the application of electric current to a patient even if it is part of an accepted clinical procedure. Consequently, GSR testing is not routinely done today. Details of the procedure have been outlined in previous editions of this book.

Cardiac audiometry.   Eisenberg discussed variations in heart rate as an indication of response to sound. She utilized an instrument called the *cardiotachometer*, collecting data primarily from infants under two months of age. As a stimulus, she used a tape-recorded synthetic vowel "ah" presented by sound field at intervals of ninety seconds at a sound-pressure level of 60 dB. Of course at this level of presentation, she was not concerned with threshold estimation but only with an indication of whether or not an infant was seriously impaired for the complex sound patterns of the synthetic vowel. The heartbeat rate decelerates briefly but significantly following the presentation of the speechlike stimulus. Apparently, Eisenberg did not observe this response when pure tones or noise bands were used as stimuli. Eisenberg is not proposing cardiotachometry as a clinical procedure until considerable additional research is accomplished with other stimuli and at levels closer to threshold, although she believes that the real contribution of the technique may lie in suprathreshold testing of "aspects of auditory competence" rather than definition of threshold, for which other procedures are available.[62]

[60] Joseph B. Chaiklin, Ira M. Ventry, and Lyman S. Barrett, "Reliability of Conditioned GSR Pure-Tone Audiometry with Adult Males," *Journal of Speech and Hearing Research* 4 (September 1961):269–80.

[61] Ira M. Ventry, "Conditioned Galvanic Skin Response Audiometry," in *Physiological Measures of the Audio-Vestibular System*, ed. Larry J. Bradford (New York: Academic Press, 1975), chap. 7, pp. 215–47.

[62] Rita B. Eisenberg, "Cardiotachometry," in *Physiological Measures*, ed. Bradford, chap. 9, pp. 319–47.

Respiration audiometry.   Respiration audiometry as described by Brad-ford is geared to determine threshold hearing levels for audiometric tones by using a bellows-actuated photoelectric cell with a two-channel polygraph recorder. The strain gauge is fitted snugly around the chest of the subject. In-spiration causes the marker on one channel to move upward, and expiration causes a downward deflection. The other channel has a marker showing the beginning and duration of the auditory stimulus, which is a 250-msec tone of whatever frequency and hearing level is desired. The stimulus is delivered to the subject through either the earphone or the bone-conduction vibrator of an audiometer. Subjects may be awake, asleep, or mildly sedated. It is necessary for the subject to be sufficiently relaxed so that breathing is regular and stable before testing can begin. After two cycles of normal breathing—called *resting* cycles—have occurred, the tonal stimulus is introduced at the beginning of the next inspiration. Three respiration cycles are examined: the resting cycle immediately preceding the auditory stimulus, the "response" cycle, and the cycle immediately following, called the *recovery* cycle. Response to the auditory stimulus is reflected by one or more of three alterations to the response cycle: (1) a reduction in amplitude; (2) what Bradford calls a "jam-ming" of two cycles together, yielding an M-shaped pattern; or (3) a flattening of the peak of the response cycle.[63] These three alterations, together with three cycles of uninterrupted respiration, are shown in Figure 7–12. Gener-ally, thresholds are obtained for 500, 1000, and 2000 Hz, using an ascending technique. Respiration audiometry has been performed successfully with preschool-age children, with infants, and with neonates. Bradford says that research at the Menninger Foundation over a ten-year period has

FIGURE 7–12.
A = normal vegetative breath-ing cycles showing inspiration (a-d), expiration (d-c), and ampli-tude (b-d). Response cycles, be-tween resting and recovery cy-cles, are modified by tonal stimulus immediately following each resting cycle. B = ampli-tude reduction. C = M-shaped or jamming pattern. D = flat-tening of response peak. (From Larry J. Bradford, "Respiration Audiometry," chap. 8, p. 269, in Larry J. Bradford, ed., *Physio-logical Measures of the Audio-Vestibular System*, copyright © 1975 by Academic Press, Inc. Reprinted by permission.)

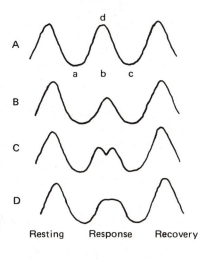

[63] Larry J. Bradford, "Respiration Audiometry," in *Physiological Measures*, ed. Bradford, chap. 8, p. 269.

demonstrated that thresholds obtained with respiration audiometry have agreed with voluntary thresholds where these were obtainable within ± 15 dB in over 90 percent of the subjects.[64] Bradford also reported on the use of the technique to obtain organic thresholds with psychiatric patients who presented psychogenic hearing problems.

Tests for Recruitment

Ever since Dix, Hallpike, and Hood reported that cochlear involvements could be differentiated from retrocochlear pathology on the basis of the presence (cochlear) or absence (retrocochlear) of the recruitment of loudness,[65] there has been a tendency to assume that tests that in any way were indicative of cochlear involvement must be tests of recruitment.

In the late 1940s and early 1950s, considerable interest developed in the use of difference limen for intensity tests as substitutes for binaural and monaural loudness-balance tests, the classic tests for determining the presence of recruitment. Difference limen tests provoked theoretical arguments about whether they measured recruitment of loudness or some other manifestation of cochlear dysfunction that may or may not be related to the recruitment phenomenon.[66] More recently, emphasis has been placed on the development of tests that yield information concerning the site of lesion in cases of sensori-neural impairment, and the question about whether or not a particular test represents the presence of "recruitment" has been considered irrelevant. Jerger sums up this point of view:

> From the standpoint of differential diagnosis the important consideration is not recruitment but site of lesion. Recruitment tests (that is, loudness balance methods) are of value to the extent that they predict site of lesion successfully. The most meaningful criterion to apply to other tests involving other phenomena is not whether they predict recruitment but whether they predict site of lesion. If they do, then they are of value whether they predict recruitment or not.[67]

Regardless of its diagnostic significance—and it seems to be most useful in identifying cases of Ménière's disease and vascular disturbances of the cochlea—the presence of recruitment may be a limiting factor in a patient's ability to benefit from amplification. For example, a patient who has a greatly

[64] Ibid.

[65] M. R. Dix, C. S. Hallpike, and J. D. Hood, "Observations Upon the Loudness Recruitment Phenomenon with Especial Reference to the Differential Diagnosis of Disorders of the Internal Ear and VIIIth Nerve," *Journal of Laryngology and Otology* 62 (November 1948):671–86.

[66] Ira J. Hirsh, T. Palva, and A. Goodman, "Difference Limen and Recruitment," *Archives of Otolaryngology* 60 (November 1954):525–40.

[67] James F. Jerger, "Recruitment and Allied Phenomena in Differential Diagnosis," *Journal of Auditory Research* 2 (1961):151.

compressed dynamic range of hearing may find it impossible to utilize a hearing aid because when the aid's volume control is turned to the point where speech can be heard, the intensity peaks of speech may be uncomfortably loud. Thus, from the standpoint of planning for rehabilitative procedures, if not for purposes of medical diagnosis, it is important to ascertain whether or not a patient with a sensori-neural type impairment does have recruitment.

Alternate binaural loudness balance. The ABLB test was first described by Fowler.[68] Briefly, the test consists of comparing the hearing levels at which a pure tone sounds equally loud to both ears of a patient, and it is useful only when there is a monaural impairment or when a patient presents a picture of one relatively normal ear and one ear with some degree of sensori-neural impairment. The test requires an audiometer with which the examiner can present pulses of a tone of the same frequency but different hearing level to each ear. If such an audiometer is not available, a separate audiometer may be used with each ear. The test is performed, of course, through earphones.

The method of administering the test is as follows. Threshold measurements are obtained for both ears at all frequencies. The frequencies that show at least a 20-dB loss in the poor ear may then be balanced for loudness in the good ear. Choose one frequency at which to begin the loudness balancing. Increase the intensity of this frequency until it is 20 dB above the threshold of the good ear, and present the tone briefly to the good ear. Then, leaving the hearing-level control for the good ear at that setting, change the hearing-level control for the poor ear until an intensity of about 20 dB above the threshold of the poor ear is obtained. Present the tone briefly to the poor ear, and ask the patient to tell you whether the tone in the poor ear is louder or softer than the one heard in the good ear. Switch the tone from good to poor ear several times, changing the intensity in the poor ear as necessary until the patient tells you that the tones are equally loud. In other words, the patient must balance the loudness of the tone in the poor ear to the fixed loudness of the tone that is 20 dB above threshold in the good ear. Some audiometers provide for automatic alternation of the tone from one ear to the other. Note the hearing level of the tone in the poor ear when loudness balance is achieved. Then increase the intensity of the tone in the good ear by another 20 dB, and again vary the intensity of the tone in the poor ear until the patient tells you that the loudness has balanced. Again make note of the hearing level of the tone in the poor ear. Continue in this fashion, increasing the intensity of the tone in the good ear by 20 dB each time and finding the hearing level of the tone in the poor ear necessary to obtain a sensation of equal loudness, until the intensity limits of the audiometer have been reached. The same procedure is then followed for each of the other frequencies to be balanced.

[68] E. P. Fowler, "Marked Deafened Areas in Normal Ears," *Archives of Otolaryngology* 8 (1928):151–55.

Figure 7–13 illustrates the usual manner of recording the results of the binaural loudness-balance test. The points of equal loudness in the good and the poor ear are connected by lines that straddle the frequency being balanced. The points on the audiogram for the good (right) ear appear at intervals 20 dB apart, starting at threshold; the points for the poor ear are marked at whatever hearing level was required to balance loudness. If the lines connecting the points of equal loudness remain essentially parallel throughout the course of the test at a specific frequency, no recruitment has been demonstrated, because an equal increment of intensity results in an equal increment of loudness in each ear. However, if the lines tend to converge on the poor ear, indicating that increments of loudness in the poor ear are not proportional to the increments of increasing intensity, the presence of recruitment is demonstrated. The graph of equal loudness at each frequency is called a *laddergram*. In Figure 7–13, for purposes of illustration, no recruitment is evidenced at the frequency of 500 Hz because the lines connecting the points of loudness balance are parallel throughout. At 1000 Hz, there is some recruitment, although "incomplete," because the sensation of loudness in the poor ear does not ever equal the loudness in the good ear. At 2000 Hz, the recruitment is "complete"; that is, the loudness of the tone in the poor ear equals the loudness in the good ear at maximum intensity levels. The laddergram at 4000

FIGURE 7-13.   Binaural loudness balance at four frequencies.

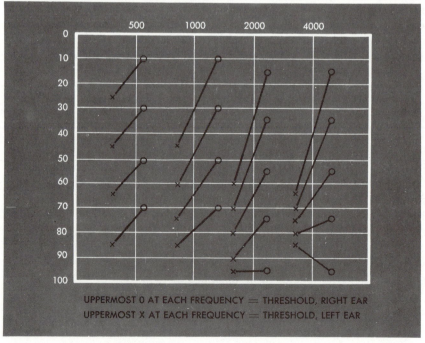

Hz illustrates "hyper-recruitment." As the intensity increases above threshold, a point is reached at which the sensation of loudness in the poor ear exceeds that in the good ear, although a difference of some 50 dB existed between the ears at threshold levels. One must be careful not to make conclusions regarding the presence or absence of recruitment or the differentiation of one degree of recruitment from another, unless the differences in hearing level on which the conclusions are based are greater than the allowable limits of reliability of pure-tone testing, in other words, greater than ± 5 dB.

When administering the binaural loudness-balance test, it is essential that the presentations of tone in each ear are very brief. If the tone is prolonged at above-threshold levels, there is danger of fatiguing the ears, thus invalidating the loudness-balance results. It is best if the tone is alternated between the good and the poor ear with pulses of no longer than one second's duration. In Figure 7–13, the growth of the loudness sensation has been studied at intervals of 20-dB intensity in the good ear. The selection of the interval of intensity is purely arbitrary; it could as well be 10 dB or 30 dB. As a matter of fact, the presence of recruitment can be disclosed by having the patient perform a loudness balance only at maximum intensity at each frequency. Then, only the top and bottom "rungs" of the laddergram would be drawn. Of course, the complete laddergram, as shown in Figure 7–13, gives information concerning the *growth* of the sensation of loudness, which would not be obtained if loudness were balanced only at threshold and at maximum intensity. With some patients, recruitment may be most pronounced at the first step above threshold. With others, there may be a "delayed" recruitment that does not become evident until hearing levels considerably above threshold are reached. Thus, it is important to observe the growth of loudness throughout the patient's range of hearing in the impaired ear.

The procedure for administering the alternate binaural loudness-balance test described here calls for using fixed intensity in the good ear and variable intensity in the poor ear until loudness balance is achieved at any given step on the laddergram. Jerger and Harford administer the test by putting the fixed intensity in the poor ear and varying the intensity in the good ear, but they report that either method yields the same results.[69] Their rationale for reversing the "traditional" procedure is that conclusions regarding the presence or absence of recruitment, or the degree of recruitment found, can be based on fewer judgments because it is seldom possible to exceed the threshold of the poor ear by more than 40 dB—two "steps" in the alternate binaural loudness-balance test. Jerger and Harford also recognize only two degrees of recruitment: partial (incomplete) and complete. Although it may be difficult to rationalize the existence of hyper-recruitment on any theoretical neurological basis, it is a frequent clinical finding in patients with Ménière's disease or a

[69] James F. Jerger and Earl R. Harford, "Alternate and Simultaneous Binaural Balancing of Pure Tones," *Journal of Speech and Hearing Research* 3 (March 1960):20.

vascular disturbance of the cochlea; therefore, the classification "hyper-recruitment" has clinical usefulness.

Monaural loudness balance.   In bilateral sensori-neural impairment in which the higher frequencies are more severely impaired than the lower ones, it is possible to administer a monaural loudness-balance test. In this test, first suggested by Reger,[70] the loudness of tones in the impaired-frequency region is compared with the loudness of tones in a normal region at threshold and at set intervals above threshold. The procedure is the same in principle as for the ABLB test. A standard (test) frequency in the normal region is increased in intensity in 20-dB steps above threshold. The patient is instructed to balance the loudness of the test frequency to the loudness of a tone in the hearing-loss region at each step. The points of equal loudness are then connected to form a laddergram. Each frequency to be evaluated is then compared in this manner with the frequency that has been selected as the standard.

The usefulness of the monaural loudness-balance test is that it is not necessary for the patient to have one good ear with which to compare a poor ear in order to obtain a measure of recruitment. The test can be performed in either ear in the case of a bilateral impairment. Of course, the patient must have normal or relatively normal hearing for at least one frequency, so that this frequency can serve as the standard to which the sensation of loudness at other frequencies is compared. The primary disadvantage of the monaural loudness-balance test is that it is a difficult task for a patient to match the loudness of two tones of different frequency. The greater the separation of the tones in frequency, the more difficult the task becomes. The patient may need considerable practice in balancing loudness at different frequencies before the examiner can place reliance on the results.

Temporal summation or integration.   Psychoacousticians have long been interested in the effects of stimulus duration on auditory sensitivity for pure tones. According to Harris, ". . . for careful studies at threshold, Hughes first showed the regularity of the trading relation between audibility and duration, popularly known as the phenomenon of temporal integration."[71] As the duration of a tonal burst at threshold is decreased from 500 msec to 10 msec, the normal ear requires increased intensity to make the tone audible. At some frequencies, the normal ear's threshold will shift 12 to 13 dB over this range of durations.[72] On the other hand, the recruiting ear will demonstrate signifi-

[70] Scott N. Reger, "Differences in Loudness Response of the Normal and Hard-of-Hearing Ear at Intensity Levels Slightly Above the Threshold," *Annals of Otology, Rhinology, and Laryngology* 45 (December 1936):1029–39.

[71] J. W. Hughes, "The Threshold of Audition for Short Periods of Stimulation," in *Forty Germinal Papers in Human Hearing*, ed. J. Donald Harris (Groton, Conn.: *The Journal of Auditory Research*, 1969), pp. 43–46.

[72] J. Zwislocki, "Theory of Temporal Auditory Summation," *Journal of the Acoustical Society of America* 32 (August 1960):1053.

cantly lesser degrees of threshold shift with decreasing duration.[73] Thus, the measurement of threshold shift obtained by varying duration of the signal holds promise as another clinical technique for determining the presence of recruitment. Wright has proposed a "tracking" technique with the Békésy audiometer (to be described later in this chapter) to evaluate threshold at various short durations and has demonstrated that recruiting ears can be differentiated from normal and from conductively impaired ears by this technique.[74] Wright and Cannella have also shown that in cases of mixed impairment, it is the amount of sensori-neural loss that determines the degree of abnormal threshold-duration function.[75] More recently, Djupesland reported investigations of temporal integration on acoustic reflex thresholds by varying the duration of tonal and noise stimuli. He reported that with normal ears a tenfold increase in stimulus duration results in a reduction in reflex threshold of about 22 to 25 dB. Citing audiometric findings of abnormal temporal integration in ears with cochlear lesions, Djupesland predicts that studying temporal-integration effects on the reflex threshold may lead to objective evidence of the presence of cochlear pathology.[76]

By comparing "time thresholds" and loudness-balance data on ears demonstrating recruitment, Miskolczy-Fodor developed a rationale and method for translating time thresholds into loudness functions and thus measuring degrees of recruitment in terms of variation of time thresholds from normal values. A time threshold is the minimum pulse length in msec that a subject can maintain the audibility of a tone, measured at sensation levels of 1 to 6 dB.[77]

Most comfortable and uncomfortable loudness levels. A simple, although not very reliable, means of determining the presence of recruitment is to obtain two points on the pure-tone audiogram at above-threshold levels. One of these points is termed the patient's *most comfortable loudness level* (MCL), and the other is called the patient's *uncomfortable loudness level* (UCL). These measures can be secured while the patient is being given a stan-

[73] H. N. Wright, "Clinical Measurement of Temporal Auditory Summation," *Journal of Speech and Hearing Research* 11 (March 1968):118–24.

[74] H. N. Wright, "The Effect of Sensori-Neural Hearing Loss on Threshold-Duration Functions," *Journal of Speech and Hearing Research* 11 (December 1968):842–52.

[75] H. N. Wright and F. Cannella, "Differential Effect of Conductive Hearing Loss on the Threshold-Duration Function," *Journal of Speech and Hearing Research* 12 (September 1969):607–15.

[76] Gisle Djupesland, "Advanced Reflex Considerations," in *Handbook of Clinical Impedance Audiometry*, ed. Jerger, chap. 5, pp. 98–100.

[77] F. Miskolczy-Fodor, "Relation Between Loudness and Duration of Tonal Pulses. 1. Response of Normal Ears to Pure Tones Longer Than Click-Pitch Threshold," *Journal of the Acoustical Society of America* 31 (August 1959):1128–34; "III. Response in Cases of Abnormal Loudness Function," ibid. 32 (April 1960):486–92.

dard pure-tone audiometric test. If the patient has a sensori-neural loss, the examiner can ask the patient to indicate at which point, as the intensity of a tone is increased, the patient finds it most comfortable to listen, and again the examiner can find the point at which the tone becomes uncomfortably loud for the patient as the intensity is increased. For each frequency thus tested, there will be three points marked on the audiogram: first, the patient's threshold for that tone; second, the level at which the patient reported that the tone was most comfortable to listen to; and, third, the level at which the tone became intolerably loud. These points will tend to be relatively close together for the patient who presents recruitment, whereas with the patient with no recruitment the points may be spread far apart. As a matter of fact, the patient who has no recruitment should be able to tolerate the full intensity at each frequency without physiological discomfort.

The range from threshold to MCL to UCL may vary at different frequencies. A patient who has a typical sensori-neural loss, showing greater losses for the higher frequencies, would be expected to show the presence of recruitment at the higher frequencies where the loss is greatest. At the lower frequencies, where hearing is more normal, the recruitment should be negligible or absent. The interpretation of the degree of recruitment present by this method requires the examiner to have examined many audiograms of patients both with and without recruitment. There is no quantification of results; the examiner must rely on clinical experience to judge the severity of the recruitment. Also, the judgment of most comfortable loudness of a pure tone is a difficult one for a patient to make reliably. A number of trials may show a wide spread of judgments. It is best to average the results of several trials, some with ascending intensity and some with descending intensity. The method of comparing threshold, MCL, and UCL is useful as a gross indication of the presence of recruitment.

Where speech audiometric equipment is available, the MCL and UCL for speech may be obtained in the same manner as with pure tones. As was mentioned in Chapter 6, the MCL is obtained by asking the patient to report the point above threshold at which speech is most comfortably loud. Although spondee words may be used for this determination, it is preferable to use running speech. The UCL for speech is obtained in the tolerance test, as the highest level of speech that the patient can tolerate. A patient who is unable to tolerate speech at a hearing level of 90 dB or less may have some degree of recruitment. The presence of recruitment may be indicated also when the patient's SRT, MCL, and tolerance level for speech are relatively close together, or in other words, when the dynamic range is compressed. The speech audiogram form in Figure 6–3 has space for recording MCL and dynamic range. A patient will have difficulty in making reliable judgments of MCL for speech as well as for pure tones. Determining the presence of recruitment from an evaluation of speech audiometric results requires considerable clinical experience, and at best only general observations of the patient's loudness function can be obtained.

SISI Test

As was mentioned earlier in this section, there was a period during the late 1940s and early 1950s when tests of the difference limen became popular as a means for determining the presence or absence of recruitment. Many psychological experiments in the field of sensation and perception have been performed to measure *difference limens* or *limena*. A difference limen (DL) in any sensory process is defined as a *just noticeable difference* (jnd) in whatever aspect of the sensation is under investigation. Thus, so far as hearing is concerned, the DL for frequency is the amount of change in frequency required to produce a jnd in pitch, or the DL for intensity is the amount of change in intensity required to produce a jnd in loudness. Most of the work with DLs in clinical hearing tests has been concerned with measuring the size of the DL for intensity.

Lüscher and Zwislocki described a DL test administered at a sensation level of 40 dB. It involved the presentation of a tone that "wobbulates" in intensity, that is, varies in intensity so the patient hears intensity beats. The examiner then reduces the wobbulation gradually until the patient reports that the tone sounds "steady." The amount of intensity variation occurring at the point at which the patient signals the tone is no longer fluctuating is the DL. An "abnormal" DL is one that is smaller than the minimum value within the range of the norms established by Lüscher and Zwislocki.[78]

Denes and Naunton developed a test that compares the size of a patient's DLs at sensation levels of 4 and 44 dB. In determining the size of the DL at each sensation level, they use two separate tones of the same frequency, one tone held constant in intensity and the other varied. These tones are presented to the patient's ear alternately. In the beginning, the tones are of equal intensity, but as the test progresses one tone is varied until the patient reports a difference in intensity between the tones. The amount by which the intensity of the variable tone differs from the tone of constant intensity at this point is the patient's DL. Denes and Naunton were not interested in the absolute size of a patient's DLs, but only in the *difference* in the value of the DLs at the two sensation levels. They determined that normal ears had fairly wide differences, the DL at 4 dB sensation level being greater than the DL at 44 dB; whereas the ear with abnormal DL functioning was able to detect about as

---

[78] E. Lüscher and J. Zwislocki, "A Simple Method for Indirect Monaural Determination of the Recruitment Phenomenon (Difference Limen in Intensity in Different Types of Deafness)," *Acta Otolaryngologica*, supp. 78 (1949):156–68.

small increments of intensity at 4 dB as at 44 dB. Denes and Naunton reported a range of norms for DL differences.[79]

Jerger experimented with two different tests based on the DL for intensity. He first employed a technique similar to that described by Lüscher and Zwislocki, except that he presented the tone at a sensation level of 15 dB, and he started with a steady tone, gradually introducing intensity changes until the patient reported that the tone was fluctuating in intensity.[80] Later, Jerger developed a difference-limen-difference (DLD) test similar to that described by Denes and Naunton. He compared the size of a patient's DL at sensation levels of 10 and 40 dB and used a single wobbulating tone for determining the size of the DLs.[81]

Because the results of DL tests could not always be correlated with the presence or absence of recruitment as determined with loudness-balance techniques, and because of apparent lack of reliability (repeatability of results) in DL testing, little emphasis was placed on the clinical significance of "abnormal" DLs until Jerger and his coworkers reported in 1959 a new procedure that was satisfactorily reliable and could be administered with a greater degree of objectivity than was previously possible. By this time, Jerger was interested in test results that shed light on the site of lesion, instead of attempting to develop a different technique for assessing the presence or absence of recruitment. The new test was christened *SISI* for the words, *short-increment sensitivity index*.[82]

The SISI test consists of superimposing brief bursts of 1-dB intensity increments on a sustained tone presented at a sensation level of 20 dB at each frequency to be tested. The test is administered monaurally through earphones. The patient is instructed to report any "jumps in loudness" that are detected while listening to the sustained tone for a period of about two minutes. The apparatus used makes possible the presentation of an intensity increment every five seconds. Each increment has a rise time of 50 msec, a duration at full strength of 200 msec, and a decay time of 50 msec. The size of the increment can be zero dB, 1 dB, or 5 dB, depending on the choice of the examiner, although the test is scored only on the percentage of 1-dB increments correctly identified by the patient. During the test, twenty 1-dB increments are presented. If the patient pushes the signal button for five of the

[79] P. Denes and R. F. Naunton, "The Clinical Detection of Auditory Recruitment," *Journal of Laryngology and Otology* 64 (July 1950):375–98.

[80] James F. Jerger, "A Difference Limen Recruitment Test and Its Diagnostic Significance," *Laryngoscope* 62 (December 1952):1316–32.

[81] James F. Jerger, "DL Difference Test: Improved Method for Clinical Measurement of Recruitment," *Archives of Otolaryngology* 57 (May 1953):490–500.

[82] James Jerger, Joyce Lassman Shedd, and Earl Harford, "On the Detection of Extremely Small Changes in Sound Intensity," *Archives of Otolaryngology* 69 (February 1959):200–11.

twenty 1-dB increments, the sensitivity index is 25 percent. In all, twenty-eight increments are presented in a series. The first five increments presented are 5 dB in size in order to give the patient a noticeably intense increment to which to respond. The next five increments are 1 dB in size. If the patient responds to three or more of these, the size of the sixth increment is set at zero dB as a "control presentation" for checking on the validity of the test. If the patient responds to two or less of the first five 1-dB increments, the size of the sixth increment is set at 5 dB to enable the patient once again to respond positively. After the tenth and fifteenth presentations of 1-dB increments, the following increment is set either at zero dB or 5 dB, depending on whether or not the patient responded to the majority of the preceding five 1-dB increments. As mentioned before, only the responses to the twenty 1-dB increments are scored. If the patient signals during a control presentation (increment of zero dB), the examiner discards the test as being invalid. In such a case, the patient is probably responding to the rhythmic presentation of increments instead of to an increase in intensity. If the patient does not respond to a 5-dB increment, it is necessary to stop the test and reinstruct the patient about the task, because a 5-dB increment should be a noticeable increase in intensity for any patient.

The results of the SISI test can be reported as percentages scored at each frequency, or they can be graphed on a "SISI-gram," which has frequency on the abscissa and percentages ascending from 0 to 100 percent on the ordinate. Jerger et al. reported the following ranges of SISI scores (in percentages) at the frequencies of 1000 and 4000 Hz for a group of seventy-five patients with various medical diagnoses:[83]

	No. Cases	1000 Hz	4000 Hz
conductive	21	0–15	0–15
noise-induced	9	0–40	95–100
Ménière's	8	70–100	95–100
presbycusis	34	0–100	0–100
retrocochlear	3	0	0

They have the following comments about their results:

. . . In general, purely conductive losses yield very low scores, while losses presumed to be localized in the sensory structure of the inner ear tend to show very high scores. Values between these extremes are infrequent. When they do occur, they are observed most commonly in presbycusis. . . . Presbycusis appears to be a clinical entity in which the SISI score is quite unpredictable.[84]

[83] Ibid., p. 208.
[84] Ibid., pp. 203–206.

The spread of SISI scores in cases of presbycusis suggested that presbycusis may be either sensory or neural in nature, or it may be due to a combination of sensory and neural factors. In other words, there apparently is no single pathology characteristic of the hearing impairments associated with aging.

Since its first description, the SISI test has been widely used in a number of clinics and is now a valuable part of the test battery used to yield information regarding site of lesion. Almost all clinical audiometers have built-in SISI units. Although some authors have suggested minor variations in test procedure, such as shortening the test to ten presentations or varying the sensation level at which the test is presented, there is agreement that the SISI is useful (although not 100 percent effective) in differentiating cochlear from VIIIth-nerve lesions.[85] Owens suggests that the SISI test reflects recruitment and is duplicative with the ABLB test. He prefers the SISI, however, because it can be used in cases of bilateral impairment; it appears to provide a more precise, objective measure than the ABLB; and it is easier for the patient to perform.[86]

With the development and clinical acceptance of the SISI test, interest in the clinical application of DL tests was rekindled. In a comprehensive survey of the literature and psychophysical experimental data on the loudness-discrimination function, Harris suggests that the variability in test results and lack of reliability from examiner to examiner reported in previous clinical trials of DL for intensity measures may have been due to improper test administration rather than to any inherent defect in the tests themselves. He points out that the examiner must instruct the patient carefully in the task to be performed and must be willing to "train" the patient in taking the test. With careful methodology, the examiner can obtain valid and reliable results in DL testing, according to Harris, who suggests also that the different kinds of psychophysical judgments required of patients in the Lüscher and Zwislocki test and in the Denes-Naunton test may be getting at different kinds of aural pathologies.[87] Whether or not these and other tests of the DL for intensity are revived for clinical use, the SISI test is a quick and reliable way to obtain information of diagnostic significance.

[85] Phillip A. Yantis and Robert L. Decker, "On the Short Increment Sensitivity Index (SISI Test)", *Journal of Speech and Hearing Disorders* 29 (August 1964):231–46; Elmer Owens, "The SISI Test and VIIIth Nerve Versus Cochlear Involvement," *Journal of Speech and Hearing Disorders* 30 (August 1965):252–62; Earl R. Harford, "Clinical Application and Significance of the SISI Test," in *Sensorineural Hearing Processes and Disorders*, ed. A. Bruce Graham (Boston: Little, Brown, 1967), pp. 223–33.

[86] Elmer Owens, "The SISI Test and Recruitment of Loudness by Alternate Binaural Loudness Balance," *Journal of Speech and Hearing Disorders* 30 (August 1965):263–68.

[87] J. Donald Harris, "Loudness Discrimination," *Journal of Speech and Hearing Disorders*, Monograph supp. no. 11 (February 1963):24–32.

Békésy Audiometry

Békésy developed and Reger improved and produced an audiometer by means of which patients could administer their own hearing test.[88] This instrument consists of a pure-tone oscillator, the controls of which are driven by small electric motors and chain or gear drives. The frequency selector control covers a range from the lowest frequency to be tested to the highest in a steady progression. The hearing-level control or attenuator is driven by an instantly reversible electric motor, the direction of rotation of which is determined by a push button operated by the patient. When the button is held down, the hearing-level control rotates counterclockwise, decreasing the intensity of the signal. When the button is released, the control rotates in a clockwise direction, thus increasing the intensity. Patients are instructed to push the button when they hear the signal and keep it depressed as long as they continue to hear the signal and then to release it. The audiometer is connected with an X-Y recorder that traces the patient's audiogram as a series of vertical oscillations of the marking pen along the horizontal dimension of frequency. Figure 7–14 shows a conventional Békésy audiogram. Some information regarding the size of the patient's DL at threshold levels can be obtained by an inspection of the vertical excursions of the pen, which, depending on the rate of attenuation (dB change per second) employed, may cover a range of from 8 to 12 dB or more for a normal ear. An abnormal DL for intensity at threshold would be indicated by narrow excursions of the pen, such as those occurring for frequencies above 2000 Hz in Figure 7–14.

In addition to the conventional tracing shown in Figure 7–14, it is also possible to obtain "fixed-frequency" tracings with Békésy audiometers—that is, to sample a patient's threshold at any given frequency for a period of time, usually not exceeding four minutes. In Figure 7–15, fixed-frequency tracings are shown for three frequencies for the same patient whose conventional tracing was shown in Figure 7–14. Colored pens are supplied with the X-Y recorder, so that different-colored tracings may be obtained for the right and left ears. The examiner may choose to present the stimulus as a continuous tone or as a periodically interrupted or pulsing tonal signal. Tracings for continuous and interrupted signals for the same ear can be compared by using one color for continuous and the other for interrupted.

Although the Békésy audiometer yields some information regarding size of the DL for intensity, as we have seen, the primary advantage of the test method as far as determining site of lesion is concerned lies in the comparison of thresholds obtained with continuous versus periodically interrupted signals, both in conventional and in fixed-frequency tracings. The comparison

---

[88] Georg von Békésy, "A New Audiometer," *Acta Otolaryngologica* 35 (1947) :411–22; Scott N. Reger, "A Clinical and Research Version of the Békésy Audiometer," *Laryngoscope* 62 (December 1952):1333–51.

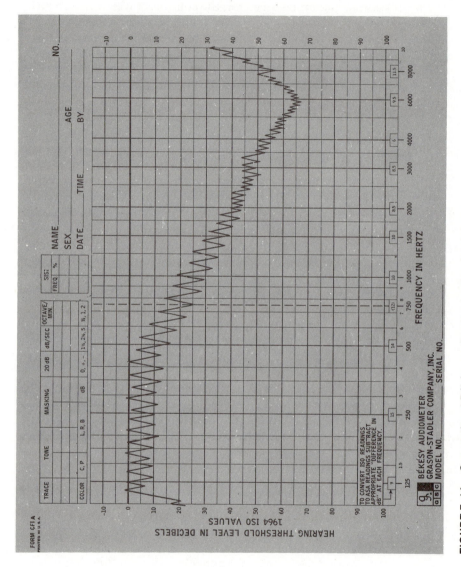

FIGURE 7-14. Conventional Békésy audiogram tracing for one ear.

224

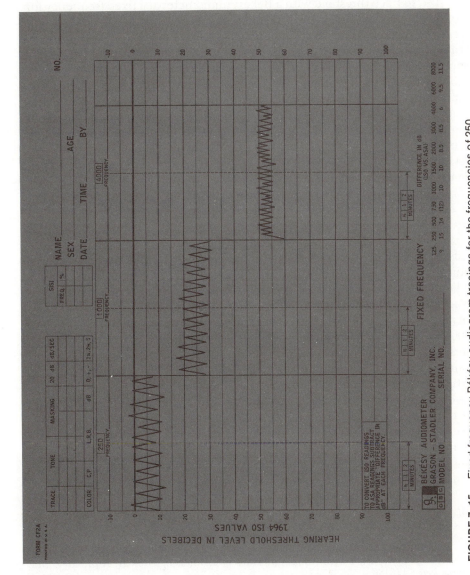

FIGURE 7-15. Fixed-frequency Békésy audiogram tracings for the frequencies of 250, 1000, and 4000 Hz.

of thresholds obtained with continuous versus interrupted tone reveals that some patients demonstrate much higher (poorer) thresholds with the former. Lierle and Reger reported that when a patient who had an acoustic neurinoma was asked to trace threshold with a Békésy audiometer at a fixed frequency for a period of twenty minutes, the threshold steadily became higher; but little difference in threshold occurred when patients with cochlear involvements performed this same task.[89] Jerger, Carhart, and Lassman confirmed the results reported by Lierle and Reger that excessive threshold "adaptation" occurs within a three-minute period in cases of VIIIth-nerve tumors when tonal stimulation at fixed frequencies is continuous, but they reported that the "adaptation" effect was not observed in these patients when the tonal stimulus was pulsed (three interruptions per second). In contrast, patients with sensori-neural losses of cochlear origin showed slight "adaptation" effects that did not increase with time through the three minutes of threshold tracing at fixed frequencies.[90]

Subsequently, Jerger analyzed conventional and fixed-frequency Békésy tracings obtained with continuous and periodically interrupted tones (2 1/2 interruptions per second) on 434 patients seen over a period of three years at the Northwestern Medical School Hearing Clinic. From this analysis, he described four basic types of Békésy audiograms. All but 16 of the 434 audiograms analyzed could be classified as one of the four types.[91] The type I audiogram shows no essential difference in thresholds obtained with continuous versus interrupted tone in either conventional or fixed-frequency tracings. The type II audiogram is the same as the type I for frequencies below 1000 Hz. Above 1000 Hz, the continuous tracing drops below (shows higher thresholds than) the interrupted tracing to a slight degree but usually differs from the interrupted tracing by no more than 20 dB. The tracing narrows in vertical range for the higher frequencies when the tone is continuously presented, but not when it is interrupted. In fixed-frequency presentations, the tracings obtained with continuous and interrupted tones are the same for frequencies below 1000 Hz. At 1000 Hz and at higher frequencies, however, the tracing for continuous tone drops below that for interrupted tone within the first minute by from 5 to 20 dB and then remains stable for the remainder of the three-minute period of stimulation.

In the type III audiogram, the tracing obtained with the continuous tone drops below that for the interrupted tone, beginning with very low frequen-

[89] Dean M. Lierle and Scott N. Reger, "Experimentally Induced Temporary Threshold Shifts in Ears with Impaired Hearing," *Annals of Otology, Rhinology, and Laryngology* 64 (March 1955):263–77.

[90] James Jerger, Raymond Carhart, and Joyce Lassman, "Clinical Observations on Excessive Threshold Adaptation," *A.M.A. Archives of Otolaryngology* 68 (November 1958):617–23.

[91] James Jerger, "Békésy Audiometry in Analysis of Auditory Disorders," *Journal of Speech and Hearing Research* 3 (September 1960):275–87.

cies. As the test with conventional tracing continues, the gap between the thresholds for the continuous and the interrupted tone widens markedly until the maximum intensity limit of the audiometer is reached, perhaps at as low a frequency as 1000 Hz. There is no difference, however, in the vertical range of the tracings for the continuous and the interrupted tone. In the fixed-frequency presentations, the tracing obtained with the interrupted tone remains horizontal for the three-minute period; the tracing for the continuous tone almost immediately begins a sharp decline and descends rapidly to the intensity limit of the audiometer. Fixed-frequency results show this same relationship between the tracings for the continuous and the interrupted tone for all frequencies.

The type IV audiogram resembles type II in that there is a constant difference between the tracings obtained with continuous and with interrupted tone, except that this difference (up to 20 dB) occurs for lower frequencies as well as for 1000 Hz and higher frequencies. There may or may not be some narrowing of vertical range of the tracing for the continuous tone at the higher frequencies. The fixed-frequency tracings demonstrate a constant difference between the tracings for the continuous and for the interrupted tone at all frequencies. So type IV is distinguished from type II in that the difference between the tracing for the continuous and the interrupted tone is noted for frequencies below 1000 Hz, and type IV is distinguished from type III in that there is no increase in the gap between tracings for the continuous and for the interrupted tone with the progress of time.

Jerger compared the Békésy audiogram type—for the 418 patients whose audiograms could be classified—with the otological diagnosis for each patient and drew some conclusions regarding the relationship between the Békésy audiogram type and presumed site of lesion:

> ... In lesions of the middle ear (otosclerosis, otitis media) the type I tracing predominates. In cochlear lesions (Ménière's, noise-induced) the type II tracing predominates although some fall into the type I category. No Ménière's case ever showed a type III tracing. In eighth nerve lesion (acoustic neurinoma) type III and type IV tracings predominate. No acoustic neurinoma ever gave a type II tracing.[92]

Subsequent to the publication of Jerger's 1960 article defining four types of Békésy audiograms, Jerger and Herer described a type V Békésy, which was characterized by poorer threshold hearing levels when the signal was interrupted than when it was continuous—just the opposite result to what would be expected. They suggested that the type V Békésy audiogram might be associated with functional hearing loss.[93] Others have found the type V

---

[92] Ibid., p. 284.

[93] James Jerger and Gilbert Herer, "Unexpected Dividend in Békésy Audiometry," *Journal of Speech and Hearing Disorders* 26 (November 1961):390–91.

Békésy audiogram to be useful as a screening test for nonorganicity, particularly if the interval between pulses is lengthened, as in the LOT test (*lengthened off-time*),[94] and if only separations between tracings for the continuous and interrupted tones in excess of 5 to 6 dB are accepted as indicators of a type V Békésy audiogram.[95]

Owens analyzed Békésy audiogram results with ninety-two patients having cochlear lesions, twenty patients with retrocochlear lesions, and two patients having mixed cochlear and retrocochlear lesions. He feels that the conventional or sweep-frequency definition of the type II Békésy audiogram needs revising, and he suggests the following rewording: "In cochlear lesions the 'C' tracing may drop below 'I' at any point in the frequency range (250–4000 Hz), typically with concomitant narrowing; it then characteristically remains essentially parallel to 'I,' but occasionally may rejoin 'I.' " Broadening Jerger's definition of type II in effect eliminates his type IV, which Owens found was not characteristic of any of the VIIIth-nerve cases in his series. Owens prefers the fixed-frequency Békésy results to the sweep-frequency results. He reported that 23 percent of his patients with cochlear lesions demonstrated type I instead of type II tracings, but generally they were the patients with milder losses. Of the patients with retrocochlear lesions due to VIIIth-nerve tumors, all demonstrated type III tracings. The patients with combined cochlear and retrocochlear involvements yielded type II Békésy tracings and reacted on recruitment and SISI tests in a manner typical of those with cochlear pathology, leading Owens to suggest that the presence of a cochlear lesion may mask the presence of an accompanying VIIIth-nerve lesion.[96]

Jerger and his coworkers have proposed two modifications to the traditional method of administering the Békésy threshold tests that sharpen the tests' ability to identify ears with retrocochlear disorders. One test involves a comparison between forward and backward continuous tracings, "forward" referring to the usual progression from low frequencies to high frequencies and "backward" referring to a progression from high to low frequencies. The ear with an VIIIth-nerve lesion will tend to manifest a discrepancy between the forward and backward continuous tracings. A significant discrepancy was defined as "a separation of more than 10 dB over at least two octaves (not necessarily contiguous), a separation of more than 30 dB over at least one octave, or a separation of more than 50 dB over at least one-half octave."[97] Usu-

[94] Karl W. Hattler, "Lengthened Off-Time: A Self-Recording Screening Device for Nonorganicity," *Journal of Speech and Hearing Disorders* 35 (May 1970):113–22.

[95] Norma Trozzo Hopkinson, "Type V Békésy Audiograms: Specification and Clinical Utility," *Journal of Speech and Hearing Disorders* 30 (August 1965):243–51.

[96] Elmer Owens, "Békésy Tracings and Site of Lesion," *Journal of Speech and Hearing Disorders* 29 (November 1964):456–68.

[97] James F. Jerger, Susan Jerger, and Larry Mauldin, "The Forward-Backward Discrepancy in Békésy Audiometry," *Archives of Otolaryngology* 96 (November 1972):402.

ally, when a discrepancy exists the backward tracing will show a greater loss, but sometimes the reverse is true. The investigators stress that it is the degree of discrepancy that is important, and not whether it is the forward or the backward tracing that shows the greater loss. Jerger, Jerger, and Mauldin reported that a discrepancy between forward and backward continuous tracings was characteristic of patients with functional or nonorganic hearing problems as well as those with VIIIth-nerve disorders.[98] The authors suggest that backward tracing of the continuous tones be incorporated as an integral part of threshold testing with the Békésy audiometer. Not all Békésy audiometers are designed to progress from high to low frequencies, although they may be modified to do so.

The other modification in Békésy procedure proposed by Jerger involves comparing continuous and pulsed tracings at a high suprathreshold level. The patient is instructed to maintain the tone at a comfortable loudness level —neither softer than most comfortable nor so loud that it is uncomfortable. This procedure was termed *BCL* for *Békésy comfort level.* Jerger and Jerger report that they obtained six distinctive Békésy patterns with a series of 164 ears, including normal hearing, conductive impairment, cochlear pathology, and retrocochlear pathology (VIIIth-nerve or brain-stem disorders). Three patterns were termed "negative" and three "positive" on the basis of whether or not they indicated the presence of retrocochlear pathology. In the negative patterns, found in normals, conductive impairments, or cochlear pathology, either there is complete superimposition of the continuous and pulsed tracings, overlapping at very low or very high frequencies, or the continuous tracing is at a lower hearing level than the pulsed tracing. The positive patterns, characteristic of ears with retrocochlear pathology, consist of an abrupt drop of the continuous tracing to the limit of the audiometer, wide separation between the continuous and pulsed tracings at low and middle frequencies only, or wide discrepancy between forward and backward continuous comfort loudness tracings.[99] Although there were some atypical results with individual patients in the nonretrocochlear and retrocochlear groups, the vast majority of patients were properly categorized on the basis of negative or positive BCL results. Jerger and Jerger believe that BCL and acoustic reflex results are the most powerful tests for identifying VIIIth-nerve lesions, with forward versus backward continuous tracings ranking a close second.[100]

Tone Decay Tests

Various investigators have noted that some patients have difficulty maintaining audibility for a tone presented at threshold. In fact, the basis for the recommendation in Chapter 5 that the examiner utilize tonal pulses

[98] Ibid., p. 403.

[99] James Jerger and Susan Jerger, "Diagnostic Value of Békésy Comfortable Loudness Tracings," *Archives of Otolaryngology* 99 (May 1974):351–60.

[100] Ibid., p. 358.

rather than continuous tone for seeking threshold was the recognition that patients might adapt to a steady tone, requiring increases in intensity to keep the tone audible. Hood termed this phenomenon "perstimulatory fatigue."[101] Other terms most frequently used to describe this phenomenon are *abnormal adaptation* and *tone decay*.

Carhart proposed a "tone decay test" and reported that patients with Ménière's syndrome and patients with other types of sensori-neural disorders demonstrated tone decay on this test. Carhart's procedure involved presenting a continuous tone at a patient's previously determined hearing threshold level and checking the patient's response with a stopwatch. If the patient maintains the tone at an audible level for sixty seconds, the test result is negative: There is no tone decay. If the patient "loses" the tone short of sixty seconds, the examiner increases the intensity by one or more 5-dB steps until the patient again signals that the tone is heard. The timing then commences anew. Additional increases in intensity are made if necessary until a hearing level is reached at which the patient can respond to the tone for a full sixty seconds. The amount of tone decay is expressed as the dB change from original threshold to the final hearing level required to meet the sixty-second criterion.[102]

A modification of the tone decay test that shortens the time required for administration was suggested by Rosenberg in a paper read at the 1958 convention of the American Speech and Hearing Association.[103] The patient is presented a tone at threshold, and the examiner starts a stopwatch. When the patient signals that the tone can no longer be heard, the examiner increases the intensity by one or more 5-dB steps, but without stopping the watch. The test is continued for only one minute at each frequency. Tone decay is expressed as the dB shift in threshold that occurred in one minute. Green reported that the degree of threshold shift may be related to the instructions given to the patient. If the patient is instructed to respond only as long as the tone can be heard with its original tonality, considerably more tone decay may be exhibited than if the patient is allowed to respond to any signal heard. In other words, Green believes that in disorders involving the VIIIth nerve, the perception may change from a tone to noise, and unless the patient is specifically instructed to respond only to tone, it may appear that little or no tone decay is present. He calls the test in which the patient is instructed to respond only to tone the *modified tone decay test* (MTDT).[104]

[101] J. D. Hood, "Studies in Fatigue and Auditory Adaptation," *Acta Otolaryngologica*, supp. 92 (1950):26–56.

[102] Raymond Carhart, "Clinical Determination of Abnormal Auditory Adaptation," *Archives of Otolaryngology* 65 (1957):32–39.

[103] David S. Green, "The Modified Tone Decay Test (MTDT) as a Screening Procedure for Eighth Nerve Lesions," *Journal of Speech and Hearing Disorders* 28 (February 1963):31–32.

[104] Ibid., p. 32.

Although abnormal adaptation is characteristic of patients with VIIIth-nerve lesions, patients with cochlear disorders exhibit tone decay as well, which confuses the problem of differential diagnosis. Owens reported tone decay results with fifty-three patients diagnosed as Ménière's cases and eighteen patients with VIIIth-nerve lesions. He employed a test method described by Hood,[105] which permitted the patient to rest for up to sixty seconds after each fading of the tone before the next 5-dB increment was introduced. The test continued until a level was reached at which the patient could sustain the tone for one minute, or until at least four intensity increments had been presented. The test was started at a sensation level of 5 dB instead of at threshold. Owens reported that all but twelve of the fifty-three Ménière's patients showed tone decay at one or more frequencies. The decay was more prevalent at 4000 Hz than at other frequencies. In the VIIIth-nerve group, all but one showed tone decay at two or more frequencies. Owens suggests that the cochlear and VIIIth-nerve groups can be differentiated by the number of frequencies showing decay, and by the rapidity of the decay between intensity increments. Those with cochlear lesions showed a reduced rate of decay as intensity increased, whereas those with VIIIth-nerve lesions showed the same rapid rate of decay at each intensity increment.[106] In a subsequent study, Owens found that patients presenting rapid rate of decay demonstrated Békésy type III tracings, but that patients whose decay rate slowed down with increasing intensity were characterized by Békésy type II tracings. In cases of equivocal tone decay results, the type of Békésy audiogram could be predicted from an ABLB test for recruitment. Patients demonstrating recruitment subsequently yielded type II audiograms. If there was no recruitment, the type III audiogram would occur.[107]

On the basis of their experience with the BCL test and with acoustic reflex testing, Jerger and Jerger hypothesized that VIIIth-nerve pathology is predicted best—and earliest—by tests at the highest testable intensities. Accordingly, they proposed a test for tone decay that involved presenting a sustained tone at an SPL of 110 dB for sixty seconds. If the patient hears the tone for the full sixty seconds, the test result is negative. If the tone is heard for less than sixty seconds, the result is positive. Jerger and Jerger called this test STAT for *suprathreshold adaptation test*. They reported STAT results with seventy-five patients with "presumed cochlear disorder" and twenty patients with "surgically confirmed eighth-nerve disorder." They examined STAT results at various frequencies to determine which combination of frequencies resulted in the least number of "false-positives" (cochlear group showing tone decay)

105 J. D. Hood, "Auditory Fatigue and Adaptation in the Differential Diagnosis of End-Organ Disease," *Annals of Otology, Rhinology and Laryngology* 64 (1955):507–18.

106 Elmer Owens, "Tone Decay in VIIIth Nerve and Cochlear Lesions," *Journal of Speech and Hearing Disorders* 29 (February 1964):14–22.

107 Elmer Owens, "Békésy Tracings, Tone Decay, and Loudness Recruitment," *Journal of Speech and Hearing Disorders* 30 (February 1965):50–57.

and the least number of "false-negatives" (VIIIth-nerve group showing no decay). They found that the best results were obtained by testing at 500, 1000, and 2000 Hz. This combination of frequencies resulted in only 4 percent false positive results but 45 percent false negative results. Confining the test to 500 and 1000 Hz reduced the false positives to zero but increased the false negatives to 55 percent. Adding 4000 Hz to 500, 1000, and 2000 Hz decreased the number of false negatives to 30 percent but increased the false positives to 17 percent.[108]

The advantage of the tone decay test is its simplicity. No special equipment is required other than an audiometer and a stopwatch. The high correlation between the tone decay test results and the comparison of interrupted and continuous tone Békésy tracings suggests that if a Békésy audiometer is unavailable, patients may still be classified according to presumed Békésy types II and III on the basis of tone decay tests, following Owen's criteria of differentiation of cochlear and retrocochlear results and being guided by the ABLB test in cases of equivocal tone decay results.

Other Tests

Comparison of alternate and simultaneous balancing of pure tones. One of the items in the test battery proposed by Jerger and his associates for differentiating between cochlear and retrocochlear sensori-neural involvements is a comparison of intensities required for (1) balancing the loudness of pure tones when the signal is presented alternately to the good and poor ear, and (2) achieving a median-plane localization of the tone when the signal is presented simultaneously to the good and poor ear.[109] In both types of presentation, the duration of the stimulus is one second. We have already discussed the alternate binaural loudness-balance test as a measure for determining the presence of recruitment in unilateral sensori-neural loss. In the simultaneous binaural balance test, the patient's task is to localize the signal in the midline, that is, in the center of the head, by varying the intensity in one ear while keeping the intensity in the opposite ear constant. As mentioned earlier, Jerger and Harford follow the procedure of keeping the signal at constant intensity in the poor ear and varying the intensity in the good ear in performing the alternate binaural loudness-balance test. They follow the same procedure in simultaneous balancing. Without going into the details of Jerger and Harford's findings in various experiments with normal ears, conductively impaired ears, masked normal ears, and ears with unilateral sensori-neural impairment, it can be reported that they found that the two types of balancing procedures do not yield equivalent results. They say, ". . . equal loudness can-

[108] James Jerger and Susan Jerger, "A Simplified Tone Decay Test," *Archives of Otolaryngology* 101 (July 1975):403–407.

[109] Jerger and Harford, "Alternate and Simultaneous Binaural Balancing of Pure Tones."

not be inferred from median-plane localization. The two types of judgment are apparently independent and not interchangeable."[110] Because these two procedures are not interchangeable, it follows that in recruitment testing by binaural loudness balancing, the signal must always be presented alternately to the good and poor ear.

Jerger and Harford noted different relationships between the results of the two types of balancing with "recruiting" and "nonrecruiting" ears with unilateral sensori-neural impairment. With recruiting ears (presumed cochlear involvement) the simultaneous matching procedure results in approximately equal stimulus levels at both ears, whereas with nonrecruiting ears a higher stimulus level is required on the poor ear to achieve a midline localization. With both recruiting and nonrecruiting ears, more intensity at the poor ear is required for the simultaneous match than for the alternate loudness balance. The difference in intensity required at the poor ear for the two kinds of judgments is greater for the nonrecruiting ear than for the recruiting ear. It thus appears that a comparison of the interaural intensity relations required for loudness balancing and for median-plane localization may contribute valuable information regarding the site of lesion in cases of unilateral sensori-neural impairment.

There is some evidence also that patients who have lesions in central auditory pathways will exhibit abnormal interaural intensity relations affecting their ability to perform the loudness-balance task. Median-plane localization may or may not demonstrate an abnormality, apparently depending on the nature and extent of the central nervous system lesion. Cortical or subcortical lesions apparently exert subtle effects on auditory perception that cannot be detected through routine audiological procedures. Thus, a patient with a lesion in one temporal lobe, for example, may have normal pure-tone and speech thresholds and normal speech discrimination ability. It is only when the auditory system is forced to perform difficult tasks that abnormalities become apparent. Unlike unilateral peripheral hearing impairments in which a lesion in the left cochlea or the left auditory nerve produces abnormal test results in the left ear, a unilateral central auditory disorder is manifested by abnormal functioning of the contralateral ear. Thus, a lesion in the left temporal lobe would affect the ability of the right ear to perform complex auditory functions. It will be remembered from Chapter 2 that because of decussations of the ascending auditory pathways at subcortical levels, there is representation of both ears in both temporal lobes. Apparently, this bilateral representation in the auditory cortex is sufficient to enable both ears to respond to simple auditory stimuli even though the auditory pathway or auditory cortex on one side of the brain is damaged. But as the auditory tasks increase in complexity, the presence of the unilateral central nervous system lesion is revealed by an inability of the contralateral ear to perform at the same level as the ipsilateral

[110] Ibid., p. 28.

ear. Also, there may be deficiencies noted in the performance of auditory tasks that demand binaural integration, for example, localizing the source of a sound in space.

Jerger has shown with the alternate binaural loudness-balance test that some patients with central auditory lesions require considerably more intensity in the ear contralateral to the lesion in order to balance loudness with the ipsilateral ear at suprathreshold levels, although the two ears have the same threshold sensitivity for the tonal stimulus.[111]

Speech discrimination tests.   As mentioned in Chapter 6, a study of the PI function (performance versus intensity) may yield information of value in determining site of lesion in the case of a unilateral sensori-neural impairment. Jerger calls this test procedure *PI-PB* when the discrimination task is based on PB words.[112] The procedure is to administer several PB tests at various sensation levels to observe the growth of the PI function, particularly at high suprathreshold levels. Ears with cochlear pathology will show a rise in discrimination score as presentation levels increase until a plateau is reached, representing the patient's maximum discrimination ability (PB-Max). Further increase in presentation level will not result in any higher score. The score will remain the same or may even decline slightly at the highest presentation levels. On the other hand, the ear with VIIIth-nerve pathology will show a marked rollover in the function as presentation levels are increased above the point of PB-Max. Figure 7–16 compares typical PI-PB functions for cochlear and VIIIth-nerve pathologies with that for the normal ear.

The PI-PB function may be useful in pointing to the presence of a central auditory disorder. With central disorders, pure-tone test results generally show no loss of sensitivity. If in the presence of no loss in sensitivity the PI-PB function reveals a difference in speech-discrimination ability between the ears, and particularly if one ear shows rollover, the possibility should be entertained that there is pathology on the side of the brain opposite to the affected ear.[113]

As mentioned earlier, patients with central auditory problems may not demonstrate any impairment in PB word-discrimination tests performed in quiet. Usually, only the more complex psychoacoustic functions are affected. When speech-discrimination tasks are increased in complexity by filtering, by use of masking or competing signals, or by other forms of distortion, the ear contralateral to the central auditory lesion will generally perform more poorly than the ipsilateral ear.

[111] James F. Jerger, "Observations on Auditory Behavior in Lesions of the Central Auditory Pathways," A.M.A. *Archives of Otolaryngology* 71 (May 1960) :797–806.

[112] James Jerger, "Diagnostic Audiometry," in *Modern Developments in Audiology*, 2nd ed., ed. James Jerger (New York: Academic Press, 1973), chap. 3, p. 80.

[113] Ibid., p. 89.

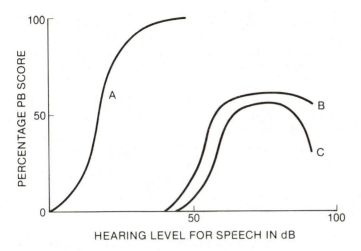

FIGURE 7-16.   PI-PB functions. A = normal ear; B = cochlear pathology; C = VIIIth nerve pathology (note rollover).

Patterning his procedures after those developed in Italy by Bocca and his associates,[114] Jerger developed what he called "distorted speech tests," which consisted of PB word lists recorded on magnetic tape and presented to the patient either through a low-pass filter or at a "faint" level of intensity. The filter passed frequencies below 500 Hz. Filtered PB words were presented to the patient at a sensation level of 45 dB. The "faint" level was established empirically to produce approximately 50 percent correct responses, and it varied, depending on the patient, between sensation levels of 5 and 15 dB. Six distorted speech tests were presented to the patient in the following order:

1. Left ear: low-pass filtered
2. Right ear: faint unfiltered
3. Combined (left ear: low-pass filtered; right ear: faint unfiltered)
4. Right ear: low-pass filtered
5. Left ear: faint unfiltered
6. Combined (right ear: low-pass filtered; left ear: faint unfiltered)[115]

These tests were administered to three patients whose neurological diagnoses were (1) left temporal glioblastoma, (2) left temporal epilepsy, and (3) left frontal meningioma. In routine speech audiometry, the first two patients demonstrated equally good speech-discrimination scores in each ear (88 and

114 E. Bocca, "Clinical Aspects of Cortical Deafness," *Laryngoscope* 68 (March 1958):301–309.

115 J. Jerger, "Observations on Auditory Behavior in Lesions of the Central Auditory Pathways," p. 798.

92 percent for the first patient, and 90 and 98 percent for the second patient). There were marked differences in the scores obtained on the two ears, however, when the speech was distorted by filtering or by making it "faint." The right ear in each case (contralateral to the temporal lobe lesion) performed much more poorly than the left ear. When the distorted conditions were presented binaurally in combination, the speech-discrimination scores were affected equally by conditions 3 and 6. The third patient demonstrated poor discrimination scores in each ear in routine speech audiometry (74 and 60 percent), and both ears were affected equally by low-pass filtering. No data were reported for other conditions of speech distortion. The third patient presumably demonstrated more diffuse central nervous system involvement than the other two patients, although in this case the alternate binaural loudness-balance test revealed disturbed intensity relations in the ear contralateral to the cortical lesion.[116]

In a study of sixteen patients with Parkinsonism, Jerger et al. compared the auditory performance of the patients with age-matched control subjects.[117] In routine pure-tone and speech-audiometric tests, there were essentially no differences in the performance of the experimental and control groups. Two difficult listening tasks were demanded of the subjects, however, that did reveal differences in performance between the patients with Parkinsonism of the postencephalitic and arteriosclerotic types and the control subjects. Five patients whose Parkinsonism was classified as "idiopathic" did not differ in their performance on the difficult listening tasks from their matched controls. The tasks involved, first, listening to low-pass filtered PB words in each ear separately, as in the study by Jerger (referred to in the preceding paragraphs), and second, listening binaurally to PB words while 0.5-second bursts of thermal noise at a level of 20 dB higher than the speech was alternated between the ears. This latter procedure was dubbed the *SWAMI* test (*speech with alternating masking index*). Although differences in performance between right and left ears were not noted for any of the experimental subjects, their mean right and left ear discrimination scores on the filtered-speech test were lower than the mean scores for the control subjects, and their scores on the SWAMI test were likewise lower (by the same amount as on the filtered-speech test) than the scores for the control subjects. Incidentally, although the performance of control subjects was affected by low-pass filtering (although not as much, of course, as for experimental subjects), their performance was relatively unaffected in the SWAMI test. Jerger et al. say,

> ... through either earphone singly the words are virtually unintelligible. The periodic noise bursts effectively mask all or part of most of the words. Listening through both earphones, however, the listener experiences a unique illusion in

116 Ibid., p. 804.

117 J. Jerger, M. Mier, B. Boshes, and G. Canter, "Auditory Behavior in Parkinsonism," *Acta Otolaryngologica* 52 (December 1960):541–50.

which bursts of noise are localized in the ears, but the words are heard in the center of the head. It is as if the brain literally "fuses" the word-fragments from each ear into a single unitary image. As a result, the words are easily understood by normals and the discrimination score is quite good (90–100%).[118]

Bocca and Calearo[119] and Bocca[120] emphasize the advantage of using sentences rather than isolated words in evaluating central auditory disorders. They believe that the effect of a central lesion can best be observed by noting interference with understanding the meaning of sentences, because it is the function of the higher centers to integrate and give form to the acoustic signals processed by the peripheral structures. Under normal conditions of communication, speech messages (sentences) are understood with a minimum of difficulty because of the abundance of neural pathways (intrinsic redundancy) and the multiple cues contained in the speech signal (extrinsic redundancy). Central lesions reduce intrinsic redundancy, but understanding may still occur because of extrinsic redundancy. When extrinsic redundancy is reduced by introducing frequency or time distortions in the speech signal, communication breaks down. Thus, although the reduction of either intrinsic or extrinsic redundancy may not seriously affect the perception of speech, the combined effects of the reduction of both kinds of redundancy may be disastrous. Bocca and Calearo utilize various kinds of distorted speech (sentence) tests: filtered speech, time compressed ("speeded up") speech, swinging speech (alternated between each ear), and interrupted speech. In cases of unilateral central lesions, the ear contralateral to the lesion shows greater involvement; in diffuse central lesions, both ears will demonstrate reduced performance. The authors believe that their tests will differentiate between brain-stem and cortical lesions, because ". . . responses to interrupted and swinging speech are more impaired than those to filtered or time-compressed speech, when brain-stem or midbrain lesions are present, while the contrary is true with cortical pathology."[121]

Instead of using real sentences, Jerger advocates the use of synthetic sentences in testing for central auditory disorders. The SSI (*synthetic sentence identification*) test, devised by Speaks and Jerger,[122] was mentioned in Chapter 6. The sentences are approximations of real sentences in construction, but they are not meaningful sentences. A single list of ten synthetic sentences is

[118] Ibid., p. 547.

[119] E. Bocca and C. Calearo, "Central Hearing Processes," in *Modern Developments in Audiology*, 1st ed., ed. James Jerger (New York: Academic Press, 1963), pp. 337–70.

[120] Ettore Bocca, "Distorted Speech Tests," in *Sensorineural Hearing Processes and Disorders*, ed. A. Bruce Graham (Boston: Little, Brown, 1967), pp. 359–70.

[121] Ibid., p. 366.

[122] Charles Speaks and James Jerger, "Method for Measurement of Speech Identification," *Journal of Speech and Hearing Research* 8 (June 1965) :185–94.

used in testing for central auditory disorders. The listener's task is to select from a printed list of the sentences which one was spoken by pressing a button corresponding to the number of the sentence. The ten sentences may be presented over and over by varying the order of the presentation. Distortion is introduced by presenting a competing message (running speech) first to the ipsilateral ear (the ear receiving the synthetic sentences) and then to the contralateral ear. The signal-to-noise ratio (Jerger calls it MCR for *message-to-competition* ratio) is varied to try to produce a broad range of discrimination scores—from 100 percent to 10 or 20 percent. Jerger reports that patients with brain-stem lesions perform differently from patients with temporal-lobe lesions on the ipsilateral and contralateral competing message conditions. Patients with brain-stem pathology have considerable difficulty with the SSI-ICM (*synthetic sentence identification—ipsilateral competing message*) condition when the synthetic sentences and competing speech are presented to the ear contralateral to the lesion, but they achieve relatively normal scores when the signals are directed to the ear ipsilateral to the lesion. Patients with temporal-lobe lesions may demonstrate some difference in scores for the SSI-ICM when the two ears are compared but not the dramatic difference that occurs with brain-stem patients.

On the other hand, the temporal-lobe patients demonstrate difficulty in the SSI-CCM (*synthetic sentence identification—contralateral competing message*) condition when the ear contralateral to the lesion receives the synthetic sentences and the other ear the competing speech. They will score normally when the signals are reversed and the ear ipsilateral to the lesion is receiving the synthetic sentences. The brain-stem patient is usually relatively unaffected in the SSI-CCM condition, regardless of which ear is receiving the synthetic sentences.[123] The CCM condition is called *dichotic* listening, because the two ears are receiving different messages simultaneously. Thus, according to Jerger, the patient with a temporal lobe lesion has difficulty with dichotic stimulation but not with a difficult monaural listening situation, but the opposite is true of patients with brain-stem lesions. With both types of patients, their performance deteriorates when the ear contralateral to the lesion is subjected to stress.

Another speech test for detecting central auditory dysfunction, but one that utilizes words instead of sentences, is the Staggered Spondaic Word Test (SSW) described by Katz.[124] In this test, the patient is presented with a list of paired tape-recorded spondee words, each pair of which partially overlaps; that is, the second syllable of the first spondee is superimposed on the first syllable of the second spondee. The first spondee is directed to one ear, and the second spondee is directed to the other ear. The superimposition of the

---

[123] Jerger, "Diagnostic Audiometry," pp. 90–92.

[124] Jack Katz, "The Use of Staggered Spondaic Words for Assessing the Integrity of the Central Auditory Nervous System," *Journal of Auditory Research* 2 (1962) :327–37.

two half-spondees constitutes a dichotic listening situation. The presentation is at a sensation level of 50 dB in each ear. The pairs of spondees are chosen so that the first syllable of the first spondee and the second syllable of the second spondee, if combined, would form a third spondee. The paired spondees are spoken with a slight pause between the syllables. The stimulus presentation can be described best in an example:

Time Sequence			
	1	2	3
Right Ear	up	stairs	
Left ear		down	town

The patient is instructed to repeat all the words heard in a group. The "normal" response is to repeat the two basic words—in the preceding example, *upstairs* and *downtown*. If the overlapping syllables interfere with each other, the patient may repeat only the combination word, *uptown*. Or the patient may demonstrate errors in one or both of the competing syllables.

The order in which the ears are stimulated is alternated, so that with every other group the left ear would receive the first syllable of the first word. The examiner keeps track of errors on each syllable and then totals the errors occurring in each of eight conditions: right noncompeting, right competing, left competing, left noncompeting, left noncompeting, left competing, right competing, right noncompeting. In the first four conditions, the right ear was stimulated first; in the second four conditions, the left ear was stimulated first. The raw scores are converted into percentages of errors for deriving an ear score, a condition score, and a total score. Katz has described scores that are characteristic of normal hearing, peripheral disorders, central nonauditory disorders, and central auditory disorders.[125] An analysis of ear performance is apparently most meaningful in pointing to the existence of a central auditory disorder, the presumed lesion being in the cerebral hemisphere contralateral to the ear with the poor score. Scoring procedures are discussed by Brunt.[126]

Interpretations of Test Batteries

In the preceding sections, we have discussed a number of typical individual tests designed to provide information on the site of pathology. This list can be expanded greatly when considering more esoteric procedures such as evoked response measures and magnetic resonance imaging. However, a valid interpretation without these esoteric procedures can be made based on

[125] Jack Katz, "The SSW Test: An Interim Report," *Journal of Speech and Hearing Disorders* 33 (May 1968):132–46.

[126] Michael Brunt, "The Staggered Spondaic Word Test," in *Handbook of Clinical Audiology*, 2nd ed., ed. Jack Katz (Baltimore: Williams & Wilkins, 1978), chap. 23, pp. 262–75.

the results of the more standard tests which are available to the typical clinician. The clinician does not place reliance on any single test that has a certain degree of fallibility but instead administers a battery of tests and seeks to identify meaningful patterns of results that point to conclusions in which some confidence can be attained. In his peripheral test battery, Jerger includes three "primary" tests and three "reserve" tests. The primary tests are immittance measures, Békésy audiometry, and PI-PB functions. His reserve tests are SISI, ABLB, and tone decay. Figure 7–17 represents Jerger's "strategy" in the use of his primary test battery for determining site of lesion in cases of peripheral impairment. Jerger emphasizes that this is a simplified diagram of results that would be obtained ideally for each site of lesion, and every patient cannot be expected to follow the ideal pattern exactly. If this were not so, there would be no need for reserve tests. Further, the scheme is likely to change as new tests become available.

Jerger depends on immittance testing to differentiate conductive from sensori-neural impairment. The pattern of results pointing to a conductive impairment would be an abnormal tympanogram, abnormal static immittance, and absence of the acoustic reflex. On the other hand, a sensori-neural impairment would be characterized by a normal tympanogram and normal static im-

FIGURE 7-17.   Strategy of the peripheral test battery. (From James Jerger, "Diagnostic Audiometry," chap. 3 from James Jerger, ed., *Modern Developments in Audiology,* 2nd ed., New York: Academic Press, 1973, p. 82. Used by permission.)

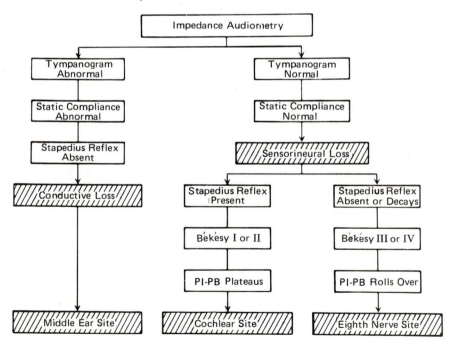

mittance. The differentiation between a cochlear and an VIIIth-nerve site depends on the acoustic reflex, Békésy audiometric type, and PI-PB results. A cochlear site is indicated if there is a reflex in the presence of a hearing loss, if the Békésy tracing is type I or II, and if the PI-PB function shows a plateau or a mild degree of rollover. On the other hand, the results that point to an VIIIth-nerve site are absence or decay of the acoustic reflex; a Békésy tracing type III or IV, obtained frequently with forward-backward tracings at a comfort level; and a marked rollover of the PI-PB function.[127]

Other test results that indicate a cochlear site of a unilateral impairment are the presence of some degree of recruitment of loudness (incomplete, complete, or hyper) as demonstrated by the alternate binaural loudness balance test; positive SISI results (95 to 100 percent at 4000 Hz); slight to moderate tone decay with less decay occurring at higher sensation levels; and approximately equal hearing levels in both ears at the point of simultaneous binaural loudness balance or median-plane localization. The patient with an VIIIth-nerve disorder should demonstrate either no recruitment or decruitment on the ABLB test; a negative SISI result (0 percent at 4000 Hz); marked tone decay, with the rate of decay remaining constant at each sensation level; and a greater hearing level at the poorer ear required to achieve simultaneous binaural balance (median-plane localization).[128]

It must be kept in mind that some sensori-neural impairments are truly combined sensory and neural involvements, and it should be expected that in such cases tests designed to identify *the* site of lesion would yield equivocal results. Shapiro and Naunton[129] agree with Owens[130] that when a patient has both cochlear and VIIIth-nerve pathology the audiologic signs will point to a cochlear lesion. In other words, the cochlear signs seem to dominate the retrocochlear signs so that the presence of the VIIIth-nerve problem may go undetected. Matkin et al., on the other hand, cite two cases of Ménière's disease whose audiologic signs changed from cochlear to retrocochlear immediately following a partial sectioning of the VIIIth-nerve. Of course, in these cases there was no confusion of test results prior to surgery.[131]

We would like to think that audiologic testing can clearly differentiate between cochlear and VIIIth-nerve involvements, and it is true that the more unified the results of a test battery the more confidence the clinician can place in the prediction of site of lesion. Nevertheless, tests—even test batteries

[127] Jerger, "Diagnostic Audiometry," pp. 77–80.

[128] James F. Jerger, "Hearing Tests in Otologic Diagnosis," *Asha* 4 (May 1962) :143.

[129] Irving Shapiro and Ralph F. Naunton, "Audiologic Evaluation of Acoustic Neurinomas," *Journal of Speech and Hearing Disorders* 32 (February 1967):34.

[130] Owens, "Békésy Tracings and Site of Lesion," pp. 466–67.

[131] Noel D. Matkin, William R. Hodgson, R. Carhart, and Tom W. Tillman, "Audiological Manifestations of Acute Neural Lesion in Cases with Ménière's Disease," *Journal of Speech and Hearing Disorders* 30 (November 1965):370–76.

—may be fallible, as Johnson[132] and Shapiro and Naunton[133] have pointed out in discussing misleading and contradictory tests results on patients whose retrocochlear pathology has been confirmed by surgery. One needs reminding occasionally that hearing testing is but only part of the diagnostic process, and one needs to keep searching for ways to make the test batteries more definitive. In the meantime, because both Ménière's syndrome and VIIIth-nerve tumors typically result in unilateral sensori-neural hearing losses and disproportionately poor speech discrimination, the clinician should administer some or all of the site-of-lesion tests to all patients presenting these audiometric symptoms.

Electronystagmography

Because of the intimate association of the auditory and vestibular portions of the inner ear, both systems may be affected by a particular pathology. For example, Ménière's disease consists of increased endolymphatic pressure that produces both cochlear (hearing impairment and tinnitus) and vestibular (vertigo) symptoms. Likewise, tumors may exert pressure on both the auditory and vestibular portions of the VIIIth nerve, causing both auditory and vestibular symptoms. An otologic examination, therefore, frequently includes an investigation of the functioning of the vestibular system, particularly if the patient complains of vertigo.

Within the brain stem, there are connections between the fibers of the vestibular portion of the VIIIth nerve and the nuclei of the IIIrd, IVth, and VIth cranial nerves that innervate muscles producing eye movements, and also the nuclei of nerves controlling muscle movements of the head and neck and of body extremities. These interneural connections enable us to maintain our visual and proprioceptive orientation regardless of our position and to make compensatory bodily adjustments to prevent falling. An examination of the vestibular system includes observing involuntary, repetitive eye movements, called *nystagmus,* produced by controlled stimulation of the semicircular canals. Whereas formerly judgments concerning the presence or absence of nystagmus and the degree of abnormal responses depended on the examiner's subjective impressions, in recent years *electronystagmography* (ENG) has simplified and objectified the observation and analysis of nystagmus. Electrodes placed on the face in the vicinity of the eyes record voltage changes when the eyes move. These voltage changes are amplified and graphically recorded. Thus, very small eye movements can be recorded even if the eyelids are closed. There are two components of nystagmus: a slow

---

[132] E. W. Johnson, "Auditory Test Results in 110 Surgically Confirmed Retrocochlear Lesions," *Journal of Speech and Hearing Disorders* 30 (November 1965) :307–17.

[133] Shapiro and Naunton, "Audiological Evaluation of Acoustic Neurinomas," pp. 29–35.

phase in one direction, and a fast or recovery phase in the other. Nystagmus is identified as being "left-beating" or "right-beating," according to the direction of the fast phase.

The analysis of spontaneous nystagmus—nystagmus that occurs without external stimulation and without regard to head position—and nystagmus that is induced by a particular stimulation can often yield information that together with auditory test results, medical history, and other otological examination findings helps to diagnose a disorder as peripheral or central. Nystagmus can be induced by rapid changing of the head position, by tracking a moving target, by fixing the gaze at various angles to the right and left of straight ahead, and by *caloric* stimulation, that is, by douching the external canal with water that is warm or cold in comparison with body temperature.

It is not within the province of this book to describe the various tests that constitute the ENG battery or to discuss the interpretation of test results. Generally, ENG tests are performed by technicians under the supervision of otolaryngologists, who interpret the results. Some audiologists who work in medical settings, however, are involved in ENG test administration and interpretation. The interested reader is referred to the books by Barber and Stockwell and by Coats listed among the references at the end of this chapter.

PRE- AND POSTOPERATIVE AUDIOMETRY

In all aspects of audiology, the otologist and the audiologist work closely together for the benefit of the hard-of-hearing patient. One of the best examples of the closeness of their teamwork is in the selection of candidates for operative procedures and in the evaluation of the success of an operation in restoring hearing. As was mentioned in Chapter 3, there are a number of operations designed to improve the hearing in patients who manifest a primarily conductive impairment. Perhaps the most common operation is the tonsillectomy and adenoidectomy, usually referred to as a "T and A." The purpose of this operation, when it is performed to improve the hearing, is to restore the patency of the Eustachian tube and thus to correct retraction of the eardrum. The selection of a candidate for the T and A is frequently dependent on a recognition that the hearing is defective in the first place. The otologist turns to the audiologist for information concerning the patient's hearing and the state of the middle ear and Eustachian tube. Comparison of the air-conduction and bone-conduction hearing indicates the amount of conductive impairment. Tympanometry, reflex testing, and tests of Eustachian tube function reveal the state of the middle ear and Eustachian tube. The success of the T and A can be measured by noting the reduction in the air-bone gap and changes in the tympanogram and the patency of the Eustachian tube.

The modified radical mastoidectomy has a dual purpose—the elimination of infection in the middle ear and mastoid process and the improvement of hearing. A tympanoplasty is designed to improve hearing by reconstructive surgery on the eardrum or the middle ear. In both these operations, it is important for the otologist to know the extent of the preoperative hearing loss by air conduction and by bone conduction and as much as possible about the middle ear from tympanometry. Postoperative testing, of course, reveals the amount of improvement in hearing that has occurred and thus measures how successfully the otologist has achieved one of the goals of the operation.

The audiologist can also help the otologist in selecting patients for surgery in cases of otosclerosis and in evaluating the result of that surgery. For many years, the fenestration operation was the only procedure that could effect an improvement in hearing in these cases. Because this is a major operation performed under a general anesthetic, and because in the course of the operation unalterable changes are made in the anatomy of the ear, the proper selection of candidates for this operation assumes tremendous importance. Otologists and audiologists worked together to develop audiometric procedures for the purpose of predicting the results of a fenestration in a specific patient. With careful methods of selection, the "batting average" of the surgeon in fenestration operations rose to the point where eight out of ten suitable candidates could anticipate the achievement of "functional" hearing in the operated ear.

The advent of the stapes mobilization procedure brought a decline in the popularity of the fenestration operation. Then, when stapedectomy was introduced, the stapes mobilization procedure became almost extinct. Because of its simplicity (for the patient) and the potential improvement in hearing to the level of preoperative bone conduction, the stapedectomy is the operation of choice for otosclerosis in almost every case. Occasionally, the fenestration will still be performed when a stapedectomy has been unsuccessful or when in the judgment of the otologist there are contraindications for a stapedectomy.

In two outstanding instances, otologists and audiologists combined their talents to devise methods for predicting postoperative hearing levels on the basis of what were termed "fenestration surveys" performed in the audiology clinic. Davis and Walsh[134] described a method based on a combination of pure-tone and speech audiometric data for predicting the patient's postoperative SRT. Shambaugh and Carhart[135] predicted a patient's postoperative pure-tone air-conduction thresholds on the basis of a comparison of preoperative air-conduction and bone-conduction hearing levels at four frequencies. It was Carhart who reported that preoperative bone-conduction hearing levels could not be measured accurately in otosclerotics because the fixated stapes, in-

[134] Hallowell Davis and Theodore Walsh, "The Limits of Improvement of Hearing Following the Fenestration Operation," *Laryngoscope* 69 (April 1950):273–95.

[135] George E. Shambaugh and Raymond Carhart, "Contributions of Audiology to Fenestration Surgery, Including a Formula for the Precise Prediction of the Hearing Result," A.M.A. *Archives of Otolaryngology* 54 (December 1951):699–712.

terfering with the movement of cochlear fluids, was responsible for producing an "inner ear conductive block." This conductive block resulted in an apparent depression of bone-conduction sensitivity that amounted on the average to 5 dB at 500 and 4000 Hz; 10 dB at 1000 Hz; and 15 dB at 2000 Hz. Thus, a patient whose cochlear function was actually unimpaired would demonstrate preoperatively a depression of the bone-conduction curve that has come to be called the "Carhart notch." In order to obtain a more accurate assessment of an otosclerotic's cochlear function, it was necessary to correct the preoperative bone-conduction hearing levels for the Carhart notch.[136]

In stapes mobilization surgery, operating-room audiometry came into existence. Many otologists found it helpful to have an audiologist in the operating room, so that the progression of the patient's hearing improvement could be monitored audiometrically at various stages in the procedure. Goodhill[137] described the test sequence in operating-room audiometry, and Goodhill and Holcomb devised a graphic means of recording the audiometric results obtained at stages in the operation as a guide to surgeons on the success of their mobilization attempts.[138]

Because both the fenestration and the stapes mobilization operations are largely of only historical interest at the present time, no description will be given of the techniques devised for predicting the outcome or monitoring the progression of the procedures. The student who is interested in reading about these audiological innovations will find a full discussion of them in the first edition of this book (1958).

The selection of candidates for the stapedectomy operation involves making a careful assessment of bone-conduction sensitivity and evaluating middle-ear function through tympanometry. The success of any middle-ear surgery is dependent on the state of the cochlear function because the best result that can be achieved in such surgery is the complete elimination of the air-bone gap on the audiogram. The patient who has preoperative bone-conduction hearing levels of from 40 to 50 dB through the speech-frequency region cannot expect to achieve functional hearing through a stapedectomy operation. On the other hand, such a patient may consider the operation well worthwhile if preoperative air-conduction hearing levels were at the limits of the audiometer, because if the air-bone gap were completely eliminated, a hearing aid could be utilized more effectively following the operation. In assessing a patient's preoperative bone conduction sensitivity, cognizance

[136] Raymond Carhart, "Bone-conduction Advances Following Fenestration Surgery," *Transactions American Academy Ophthalmology and Otolaryngology* 56 (July-August 1952):621–29.

[137] Victor Goodhill, "Surgical Audiometry in Stapedolysis (Stapes Mobilization)," *A.M.A. Archives of Otolaryngology* 62 (November 1955):504–508.

[138] Victor Goodhill and Arthur L. Holcomb, "The Surgical Audiometric Nomograph in Stapedolysis (Stapes Mobilization)," *A.M.A. Archives of Otolaryngology* 63 (April 1956):399–410.

should be taken of the Carhart notch, referred to earlier. Because it is most difficult to rule out the participation of the contralateral ear in measuring bone-conduction hearing levels in cases of extreme conductive impairment, care must be taken to employ proper masking procedures. The Rainville type of bone-conduction testing, as discussed in Chapter 5, will be found to be useful as an adjunct to or perhaps in place of standard bone-conduction methodology.

Holcomb and Goodhill[139] suggested a method for determining the degree of success of an operative procedure on the middle ear that is as useful in stapedectomy as it was in stapes mobilization. The method consists of computing the preoperative air-bone gap by subtracting the "equivalent SRT" by bone conduction from the "equivalent SRT" by air conduction in order to determine the maximum gain that can be achieved by the operation. "Equivalent SRT" is a term coined by Goodhill and Holcomb.[140] It is computed by averaging the two out of three frequencies (500, 1000, and 2000 Hz) in the speech region that show the least amount of loss. This is the Fletcher system for predicting speech loss from the pure-tone audiogram.[141] Following the operation, the air-bone gap in terms of equivalent SRT is computed again. The reduction in air-bone gap achieved by the operation is computed by subtracting the postoperative air-bone gap in terms of equivalent SRT from the preoperative air-bone gap. The percentage of success of the operation is then determined by dividing the preoperative air-bone gap into the reduction in air-bone gap, or what Holcomb and Goodhill refer to as the "air-conduction gain." Thus, if the operation eliminates the air-bone gap completely, it has been 100 percent successful. If half the air-bone gap has been eliminated, the operation is 50 percent successful.

To illustrate the Holcomb and Goodhill method let us assume the following preoperative and postoperative audiometric data for the operated ear.

	Preoperative Hearing levels in dB		Postoperative Hearing levels in dB	
	AC	BC	AC	BC
500	80	20	40	20
1000	85	25	50	20
2000	90	40	55	25
Equivalent SRT	83	23	45	20
Air-bone Gap	60		25	

[139] Arthur Holcomb and Victor Goodhill, "Evaluation of Surgery in Conductive Deafness by 'Per Cent Improvement,'" *A.M.A. Archives of Otolaryngology* 69 (February 1959):163–69.

[140] Goodhill and Holcomb, "Surgical Audiometric Nomograph."

[141] Harvey Fletcher, "A Method of Calculating Hearing Loss for Speech from an Audiogram," *Journal of the Acoustical Society of America* 22 (January 1950):1–5.

The reduction in the air-bone gap in this illustration turns out to be 35 dB (60 − 25). The operation is seen to have been almost 60 percent successful (35/60 = 58%).

It should be emphasized that the Holcomb and Goodhill method of computing the success of an operation tells only how successful the surgeon has been in eliminating the air-bone gap. It was designed as a practical and reasonable way for surgeons to report the success of their particular techniques on a series of patients. Thus, a surgeon might report in a paper or article that with technique A an average of 90 percent success was achieved with a series of 100 patients, whereas with technique B the average success rate with another series of 100 patients was only 84 percent. The success or failure of an operation as far as a particular patient is concerned depends on many factors that cannot be quantified into a formula. If the patient hears appreciably better following the operation, then the operation was a success, and if the patient does not hear appreciably better, the operation was unsuccessful. Of course, in most cases there would be a high correlation between the patient's report of degree of success and the percentage of the air-bone gap that was eliminated, but this would not necessarily be true.

Sometimes, the elimination of the air-bone gap, although resulting in a 100 percent "successful" operation, will have a deleterious effect on a patient's speech discrimination. Rosenberg pointed out this possibility in regard to stapes mobilization surgery, and it is true also for stapedectomy.[142] Consider the following example:

	Preoperative Hearing levels in dB		Postoperative Hearing levels in dB	
	AC	BC	AC	BC
500	60	5	0	0
1000	55	15	10	10
2000	65	60	45	45

It can be seen that the operation in this case was 100 percent successful because the air-bone gap was completely eliminated. But let us compare this patient's preoperative and postoperative speech audiometric results.

	Preoperative	Postoperative
SRT	54 dB	10 dB
Discrimination	96%	80%

Although the operation resulted in an improvement in SRT to within 10 dB of audiometric zero, it *reduced* the discrimination score by 16 percent. So

[142] Philip E. Rosenberg, "Audiometric Considerations in Stapes Mobilization Surgery," *Journal of Speech and Hearing Disorders* 24 (February 1959):21–24.

whereas this patient no longer needs amplification, the patient still has difficulty hearing in the operated ear because of the discrimination loss. The impairment in discrimination has probably resulted from the tilting of the air-conduction curve postoperatively. The patient's preoperative air-conduction curve was flat and discrimination was excellent, at suprathreshold levels of course. It will be recalled from Chapters 5 and 6 that speech discrimination is related to the shape of the air-conduction curve through the speech-frequency region. The more this curve "tilts" toward the high-frequency end, the more speech discrimination is likely to be impaired. Knowing what can happen to speech discrimination following a "successful" operation, the otologist may decide against an operation in a case where the preoperative bone-conduction curve is sharply tilted. At least it should be explained to the patient what is likely to occur with speech discrimination if the air-bone gap is completely eliminated, so that the patient approaches the operation with full realization that a discrimination problem may develop postoperatively.

A patient's preoperative discrimination scores are thought to give a good indication of "cochlear reserve." In considering the suitability of a candidate for surgery in cases of otosclerosis, therefore, discrimination ability as demonstrated in speech audiometry should be evaluated as well as the air-bone gap. Other things being equal, the patient who has a high preoperative discrimination score in the ear to be operated on will probably be more likely to have a "successful" operation—from both the patient's and the surgeon's point of view—than the patient whose preoperative discrimination score is relatively low.

TESTS FOR DETERMINING THE PRESENCE OF FUNCTIONAL OR NONORGANIC HEARING PROBLEMS

Usually, the responses of a patient in testing represent optimal performance, but every audiologist will sooner or later meet a patient who, for some reason, fails to give responses on hearing tests consistent with actual hearing levels. The test results, therefore, reflect a hearing loss that does not exist or exaggerates the seriousness of an actual impairment. It is not surprising, perhaps, that the incidence of functional or nonorganic hearing problems is greatest when the patient is receiving, or may be eligible to receive, some type of monetary payment as compensation for hearing impairment.

The problem of nonorganic or functional hearing loss was discussed in Chapter 3. Reference was made then to the two types of loss that can be termed functional—hysterical, or conversion, deafness and malingering. The first type is marked by the fact that the patient believes that a genuine loss exists or that a moderate loss is really a serious one. The patient is not trying to "fool" anyone and is perfectly willing to cooperate in a test situation. The malingerer, on the other hand, knows the true status of his or her hearing and definitely is trying to deceive the examiner. This patient's attitude during a hearing test may be one of suspicion and belligerence. Nevertheless, "coopera- tion" in the test situation is necessary in order to maintain the role of a hearing-handicapped individual. This type of problem is frequently referred to in the literature as *pseudohypoacusis,* or feigned hearing loss. For the sake of convenience, all hearing problems of a psychological character will be referred to as *functional* losses, to distinguish them from genuine organic impairments.

It is the psychiatrist's and not the audiologist's responsibility to differen- tiate between functional losses due to hysteria or conversion and those that represent malingering. The differentiation is not possible on the basis of test results, in any event. It is the audiologist's responsibility to recognize a func- tional loss, or a functional overlay on an actual loss, and to determine the pa- tient's actual hearing levels. Detection of functional hearing loss requires astute observation of the patient's behavior and speech, correlation of test results to check on their consistency, and administration of special tests designed specifically to disclose the presence of functional factors. The reader who is interested in the psychological profiles of individuals with functional hearing loss as well as otological and audiological evaluations of such in- dividuals is referred to a comprehensive study performed in the San Francisco Veterans Administration Hospital.[143]

Observation of Patient's Behavior

Frequently, clues to functional loss can be detected from observing the patient's behavior before, during, and after the test for its consistency with the amount of hearing impairment that presumably exists. While talking with the patient, note whether any difficulty is experienced in hearing or understanding you. Check to see how closely the patient is watching you as you speak. A person with a genuine hearing loss of serious extent will watch speakers carefully in order to benefit from lipreading. Try talking to the pa- tient occasionally when your head is turned so that your face cannot be seen. At times, speak softly and rapidly, being careful to do so naturally, however.

A patient's own speech is a valuable index to hearing impairment. If a pa- tient claims to be severely or profoundly hard of hearing, yet speaks with a well-controlled voice and good articulation (enunciation), there is reason to be suspicious of the extent of loss. It is possible for a genuinely hard-of-hearing patient to learn control of voice and diction, but as a general rule the presence of a significant hearing impairment is betrayed by its effect on the patient's voice and speech.

Consistency of Test Results

We have seen in previous chapters that a patient's hearing level for speech can be predicted from the pure-tone audiogram by averaging the hear-

---

[143] Ira M. Ventry and Joseph B. Chaiklin, eds., "Multidiscipline Study of Func- tional Hearing Loss," *Journal of Auditory Research* 5 (July 1965):179–272.

ing levels for the frequencies in the speech region. Also, we have seen that the configuration of the pure-tone audiogram gives an indication of the speech-discrimination difficulties that the patient can be expected to demonstrate on the speech tests. Thus, we can examine a patient's pure-tone audiogram and make a rough estimate of performance on the speech test. If the actual speech-test results vary significantly from those that would be predicted from the patient's pure-tone audiogram, there is reason to suspect that functional factors may be operating. For example, suppose that a patient presents a relatively flat sensori-neural loss of approximately 60 dB. You would expect a speech-reception threshold in the neighborhood of 60 dB with perhaps some loss of speech-discrimination ability. Now suppose that this patient instead turns out to have an SRT of only 30 dB and 100 percent discrimination ability. Then it is obvious that factors in addition to organic hearing loss are operating. On the other hand, assume that this patient should present poorer speech-test results than would be predicted from the pure-tone audiogram. Perhaps the SRT turns out to be 80 dB instead of the 60 dB that was predicted, or the discrimination score is close to zero. Again, it is obvious that psychological factors are operating. Before concluding that a patient is demonstrating a functional loss, however, you must make certain that the differences between the predicted and the obtained speech results are not a function of improperly calibrated equipment or of other explainable factors, such as the patient's unfamiliarity with the English language.

One characteristic of functional loss, whether of the conscious or of the unconscious variety, is that the patient may have difficulty in demonstrating the same degree of loss on repeated tests. This is particularly true of the pure-tone tests. Therefore, if a functional loss is suspected, it is wise to administer more than one pure-tone test to the patient and to compare the results. Naturally, the greater the interval between the tests, the more difficulty the patient will have in trying to present a consistent picture. If possible, it is advisable to schedule the patient for tests on different days, rather than giving two or three tests on the same day. As a general rule, if the patient is unable to duplicate test results within ± 10 dB on successive tests, the examiner should suspect the presence of functional loss. It should be emphasized, however, that consistency from test to retest does not, of itself, rule out the possibility that the loss is functional. With practice, a patient may become skilled in selecting the proper loudness level at which to cease responding. If there is other evidence that the patient's response may not be representative of actual hearing levels, the fact that a consistent picture occurs from test to retest should not rule out the possibility of a functional hearing problem.

Another clue to the presence of a functional hearing loss is when a patient who claims to have unilateral impairment fails to demonstrate "shadow hearing" at the expected level. The patient presents a pure-tone air-conduction and bone-conduction picture of normal-hearing in one ear and almost a total loss of sensitivity in the other ear. In the case of an organic unilateral hearing problem, one would expect to obtain a shadow curve by air conduction in the poor ear that would differ from the hearing levels of the good ear by 50 to 60 dB, and without masking, the bone-conduction hearing levels of the poor ear should approach rather closely those of the good ear.

In the preceding example, the lack of a shadow curve, particularly by bone conduction, was a clear indication of a functional hearing loss. If more proof were needed that a patient's ears were in fact both close to normal limits of sensitivity, bone-conduction sensitivity in each ear could be checked while occluding the other ear with an earphone, as suggested by Thompson and Denman.[144] If ears are essentially normal in sensitivity, occluding an ear causes the bone-conducted signal to refer to that ear, as in the Weber test. If a patient's poorer ear were occluded while retesting the better ear by bone conduction, no response for the low frequencies would be given, because the patient would be aware of hearing them in the supposedly impaired ear. On the other hand, if the better ear were occluded while testing bone conduction on the poorer ear, the patient might respond to the low frequencies, because the occlusion would refer them to the good ear. The higher frequencies are of no use in checking the occlusion effect because their thresholds are not affected by occlusion.

Special Tests for Functional Hearing Impairment

The purpose of administering special tests designed to identify functional loss in a patient is to confirm or reject impressions that have been obtained through observation of the patient's behavior and through an examination of the patient's consistency on routine tests. For proper administration, however, most special tests for functional loss require special equipment or at least modifications of standard test equipment. For this reason, the average examiner has to depend primarily on subjective evaluations of the patient's behavior, both in and out of the testing situation, in judging whether or not a functional loss exists. If more complete testing facilities are available in hearing centers or clinics, the audiometrist can refer patients suspected of manifesting functional loss to one of them for the special tests described in the following paragraphs.

These special tests have developed from clinical necessity—the need to identify patients with functional loss or functional overlay. For the most part, these tests evolved from the observations of astute clinicians that patients with functional loss tended to respond in unusual ways to pure-tone and speech stimuli. In 1963, an extensive interdisciplinary research study begun in 1959 was completed at the Veterans Administration Hospital in San Francisco. As a part of this study, various special tests for functional hearing loss

[144] Gary Thompson and Marie Denman, "The Occlusion Effect in Unilateral Functional Hearing Loss," *Journal of Speech and Hearing Research* 13 (March 1970) :37–40.

were evaluated on experimental and control groups. The general findings of this study, including the evaluations of the special tests, have been reported by Chaiklin and Ventry.[145] Before making clinical use of the tests described here, the reader is advised to become familiar with the findings on test validity and efficiency reported by these investigators. In determining whether or not a given patient demonstrates functional hearing loss or a functional overlay on an organic hearing problem, the audiologist must avoid depending too strongly on the results of any single test. Instead, all information obtainable—case history, otological findings, observations of the patient's behavior, results of routine pure-tone and speech audiometric tests, and results of special tests—must be correlated before arriving at a conclusion.

Lombard or voice-reflex test. This test is based on the fact that we monitor our own voices through the sensation of hearing. If we are speaking in a noisy environment, we unconsciously increase the intensity of our voice to compensate for the masking effect of the noise. In the Lombard test, the patient is given some material to read while a masking noise is fed into the earphones. The examiner then observes fluctuations in the intensity of the patient's voice as the level of the masking noise is increased and decreased. The result of the test is positive if the patient's voice does become more intense when the masking is increased. The level of masking at which the patient's voice becomes noticeably more intense should be noted. That level is then compared with the degree of supposed hearing loss the patient has. If voice level is affected when the level of the masking is less than the degree of the supposed hearing loss, it is evident that the patient is actually hearing at lower levels than admitted on routine testing. The result of the Lombard test is negative if the patient's voice remains at the same intensity regardless of the fluctuations in the level of the masking noise within the limits of the supposed hearing loss. The Lombard test is usually administered only in cases of bilateral functional loss.

The limitations of the Lombard test are, first, the test is not standardized to the point where it is known with certainty at just what level of masking in relation to the threshold the voice reflex begins. With this test, therefore, an accurate measure of the patient's true threshold is not assured. The only result obtainable is a gross judgment that the patient's intensity of voice increases when the level of masking reaches a certain point; that point can then be compared with the patient's supposed threshold. If the reflex occurs at levels of intensity less than the supposed threshold, it is apparent that the supposed threshold is in error, but it is not possible to say by how much it is in error. Second, a sophisticated patient, as far as testing is concerned, can learn to control voice intensity even in the presence of an extremely intense masking noise.

[145]Chaiklin and Ventry, "Functional Hearing Loss," in James F. Jerger, ed., 1st ed., Chap. 3, pp. 76–125; Ventry and Chaiklin, "Multidiscipline Study of Functional Hearing Loss."

The Lombard test, then, can be "beaten" by a patient who is aware of its purpose and who knows the expected responses. Attempts have been made to objectify and to quantify the Lombard test,[146] but because other tests are superior in their ability to determine organic thresholds, it is doubtful if the Lombard test will ever be used for more than a rough screening test.

Stenger test.   When both ears are stimulated by a tone of the same frequency but of differing sensation level in each ear, an individual with normal hearing or with an equal bilateral hearing loss is aware of hearing the tone only in the ear in which it is louder. This phenomenon is the basis of the Stenger test, which is useful in determining the genuineness of a patient's claim that one ear is impaired. The test requires either a two-channel audiometer or an audiometer in which the signal can be divided between the ears and its intensity be independently controlled in each ear.

Before the Stenger test is given, measures of the patient's supposed hearing loss should be obtained through standard audiometric techniques. Thus, the examiner has a record of the patient's "thresholds" at each frequency in both the good and the "poor" ear. If the interaural difference between the patient's admitted thresholds at any frequency is at least 20 dB, the use of the Stenger test could be considered. Ventry and Chaiklin report that its efficiency is highest when the admitted thresholds of the patient differ interaurally by more than 40 dB.[147] Suppose, for the sake of illustration, that the patient has yielded threshold measurements at 1000 Hz of 5 dB in the right ear and 50 dB in the left ear. You have reason to believe that the hearing in the left ear is better than the patient has admitted, and you decide to administer the Stenger test. First, you would introduce the 1000-Hz tone to the good ear at a hearing level of 10 or 15 dB. The patient reports that the tone is heard for the patient has previously admitted to a threshold of 5 dB in that ear. Now, without disturbing the level of the tone in the patient's right ear, introduce the tone in the left ear, gradually increasing its intensity until it exceeds the level of the same tone in the right ear. When the sensation level of the tone becomes about 10 dB greater in the left ear than in the right ear, the patient will have the sensation of hearing it only in the left ear. When the patient becomes aware of hearing the tone in the allegedly poor ear at a level lower than the admitted threshold, it will usually be reported that the tone is no longer heard. The patient does not realize that the tone is still present at a suprathreshold level in the good ear. If the patient reports that the tone is no longer heard when it is presented at any level below the admitted threshold of

[146] Daryle L. Waldron, "The Lombard Voice Reflex Test: An Experimental Study," unpublished Ph.D. dissertation, Stanford University, 1960; Clair N. Hanley and Donald G. Harvey, "Quantifying the Lombard Effect," *Journal of Speech and Hearing Disorders* 30 (August 1965):274–77.

[147] Ventry and Chaiklin, "Multidiscipline Study of Functional Hearing Loss," p. 201.

the "poor" ear, the result of the Stenger test is "positive," that is, indicative of a functional loss. The examiner knows that the actual threshold in the "poor" ear is no greater than the hearing level at which the patient ceased responding. On the other hand, if the patient reports that the tone is heard while the level of the signal to the poor ear is being increased up to the point of the admitted threshold, the result of the Stenger test is "negative"; that is, it gives no indication to the examiner that a functional problem is present. It should be noted that methods of administering the Stenger test may differ somewhat from examiner to examiner. Some clinicians will withdraw the signal from the good ear in order to make sure that the patient is responding to the signal in the good ear. If the patient continues to respond after the signal in the good ear has been withdrawn, then obviously the tone is being heard in the "poor" ear. In performing the Stenger test, it is preferable to interupt the signals to the earphones while the hearing-level controls are being adjusted.

Sometimes the Stenger test is ineffective because the patient has pronounced diplacusis; that is, a tone of a given frequency is heard with different pitch in each ear. If this should be so, the patient may be aware of the presence of the tone in the good ear when the level of presentation in the "poor" ear is at a higher sensation level. So even if negative Stenger results have been obtained with pure tones, the test should be repeated with speech stimuli, if the difference in SRT between the ears is at least 20 to 25 dB. When the auditory signal is speech instead of pure tones, the test is called the *modified* or *speech* Stenger test. The manner of administering and interpreting the speech Stenger test is the same as that described for the pure-tone test. Spondee words are used, and the patient is asked to repeat each word. The signal is directed initially only to the good ear at a level at which the words can be repeated with almost 100 percent accuracy (usually 5 to 10 dB sensation level). After the patient has repeated several words correctly, the examiner directs the speech signal also to the "poor" ear and gradually increases its intensity until the hearing level of the signal in the "poor" ear is higher than it is in the good ear. If, as the intensity of the speech signal is increased in the "poor" ear, the patient ceases to repeat the spondee words at any hearing level below the admitted SRT in that ear, the result of the speech Stenger test is positive because the patient is still receiving the speech signal at a suprathreshold level in the good ear. As was the case with the pure-tone Stenger test, the efficiency of the speech Stenger procedure is greater in instances where the apparent interaural difference in sensitivity is large.

Shifting-voice test.   This test is a special modification of the speech Stenger and is useful in disclosing cases of assumed unilateral hearing loss. The examiner keeps talking informally to the patient, asking questions and giving instructions to carry out, while shifting the output of the speech audiometer from one ear to the other. Occasionally, spondees will be inserted that the patient will be asked to repeat. The patient is instructed to indicate in which ear the examiner is speaking by pointing to the appropriate earphone. Johnson, Work, and McCoy suggest that this manner of testing is suitable also in the case of patients with bilateral losses characterized by only a slight difference in admitted threshold between the ears.[148] They suggest starting this procedure with the level slightly above the admitted threshold in the better ear and slightly below in the poorer ear. Pressure is kept on the patient to make immediate responses to the spondee words or to the questions or directions given, so that there is no time to consider in which ear and at what level the spondee occurs. In the course of the testing, the intensity of the signal is independently varied in each ear. Occasionally, a large change in intensity can be made, but usually the changes are slight. The object of this testing method is to confuse the patient so that responses are obtained at levels below those that have been admitted previously. Of course, the patient with an actual hearing loss will be able to respond only when the speech signal is above threshold in either ear, and these responses will be consistent regardless of the manipulations of the examiner; the individual with a functional loss, or a functional overlay on an actual loss, on the other hand, will respond inconsistently on the shifting-voice test.

A similar confusion technique involving pure tones instead of speech has been proposed by Nagel, who calls his method *RRLJ* for *rapid random loudness judgments*.[149] The patient is asked to make rapid judgments concerning the ear in which the tone is heard more loudly, as the examiner skips around frequencies, randomly varying the intensity and the order of tonal presentations to the two ears. Should the patient report that a tone below the admitted threshold is louder, it is evidence of nonorganicity. Both these confusion techniques tax the examiner's manual dexerity and concentration in controlling signal presentations and monitoring the patient's responses.

Delayed auditory feedback test.   In 1950 and 1951, Lee[150] and Black[151] reported that many normal speakers would experience changes in their speech similar to stuttering when they heard themselves through earphones under various conditions of delay. The delay is produced by modifying a tape recorder in such a way that the tape is carried over a spindle and makes a loop between the fixed recording and a movable monitoring head. The spindle is adjustable for different-sized loops, thus producing different amounts of time lag, or delay, between the recording and monitoring heads. The patient's own

[148] Kenneth O. Johnson, Walter P. Work, and Gordon McCoy, "Functional Deafness," *Annals of Otology, Rhinology, and Laryngology* 65 (March 1956):165.

[149] Robert F. Nagel, "RRLJ—A New Technique for the Noncooperative Patient," *Journal of Speech and Hearing Disorders* 29 (November 1964):492–93.

[150] Bernard S. Lee, "Some Effects of Side-Tone Delay," *Journal of the Acoustical Society of America* 22 (September 1950):639–40.

[151] John W. Black, "The Effect of Delayed Side-Tone Upon Vocal Rate and Intensity," *Journal of Speech and Hearing Disorders* 16 (March 1951):56–60.

speech is recorded and played back through earphones. By varying the position of the spindle, and thus the amount of time lag, a critical degree of "delay" in hearing one's speech can be attained that will have distressing effects principally on the rhythm and rate of that speech, but also to some extent on the intensity. For most people who are susceptible to delayed feedback, a delay of 0.1 to 0.2 second has the most devastating effects. The changes that occur in an individual's speech under the influence of the delayed "feedback," or "side-tone," as it is also called, are often quite pronounced.

The delayed-feedback principle can serve as a test for functional loss by providing some means of controlling the intensity of the signal that reaches the patient's earphones. If preliminary speech testing discloses that a patient has a presumed loss of, say, 60 dB, the hearing level of the patient's voice in the earphones in the delayed auditory feedback test would be set at 30 to 40 dB. If the speech deteriorates under the influence of the delayed feedback, this would be evidence that the patient's own voice through the earphones would be heard at a level considerably less than that of the presumed hearing loss.

One change in the patient's speech that can be measured quantitatively in the delayed auditory feedback test is the rate. A patient is given several paragraphs of material to read. The material is read aloud two or three times while wearing the earphones but with no signal in them. Each time that the material is read, the examiner times the reading with a stopwatch. The average time of the reading is then computed when the patient has no signal in the earphones. This is the base for comparing the patient's rate of reading under the conditions of feedback. Then feedback is introduced, and the patient's reading is timed again. Each time a different hearing level of feedback is employed, another timing is obtained. The effect of the feedback is usually to cause a slowing down of the rate of reading, although occasionally a patient will markedly increase the rate, apparently in an attempt to "beat" the test. In either event, the examiner notes the hearing level of the feedback at the point that the patient's rate of reading changes substantially from the base time with no signal in the phones. It has been found that, on the average, delayed feedback affects a person's reading rate when it is heard at a level of 20 to 40 dB above the threshold.[152] Some individuals, however, will be affected when the feedback occurs at a lower sensation level than 20 dB, and some are able to endure feedback at high sensation levels without any observable effects on their speech.

All during the test, the patient's speech is being recorded on the tape, thus providing a permanent record of how the speech has changed owing to the delayed feedback. If the patient actually has a hearing loss the speech patterns will not be changed by a delay in feedback that occurs at any intensity

[152] Clair N. Hanley and William R. Tiffany, "An Investigation into the Use of Electro-Mechanically Delayed Side Tone in Auditory Testing," *Journal of Speech and Hearing Disorders* 19 (September 1954):367–74.

less than the amount of hearing loss, or usually, at any intensity less than 20 dB above threshold. The delayed auditory feedback test can serve as a check for binaural or monaural functional loss. When the feedback is directed to only one ear, the contralateral ear should be masked.

Gibbons and Winchester have reported a technique for administering the delayed auditory feedback test as a screening test for functional hearing loss when voluntary SRTs suggest a unilateral hearing impairment.[153] While the subject reads aloud a passage of simple prose, the delayed feedback is fed to one earphone at a level of 60 dB above the SRT of the better ear, and a complex masking noise is delivered to the other earphone at a level of 80 dB above the SRT of the better ear. The reading is precisely timed with a stopwatch. Next, the signals in the two earphones are reversed, and the subject reads another passage of the same number of syllables while being timed again. If there is a pronounced difference in reading time between the two conditions of the test, the presumption is that there is a real difference in sensitivity between the ears. If, however, the reading times for the two conditions are approximately equal, it would appear that there was no substantial difference in sensitivity between the ears. Norms for this test have been developed at the Audiology and Speech Pathology Service, Veterans Administration Outpatient Clinic, Los Angeles.[154]

Because generally the delayed feedback of speech does not affect an individual at threshold levels of intensity, it cannot be used as a test to determine organic thresholds. Rather, it is useful as a means of detecting the presence of functional loss, although a negative test result does not necessarily rule out the possibility of a functional loss.

Ruhm and Cooper have reported a delayed auditory feedback procedure that can determine thresholds for pure tones within 5 to 10 dB of their actual levels.[155] The subject is asked to tap out a pattern of four taps, pause, and two taps with the index finger on a spring steel key that causes a variation in output voltage of a strain gauge and at the same time triggers a pure-tone signal in a single earphone worn by the subject. The subject keeps repeating the tapping pattern while hearing the pure tone in synchrony with the tapping key. Then a delay circuit is suddenly activated, so that the pure-tone signal in the earphone lags behind the actual key tapping. Under the influence of the delay, the subject's tapping performance deteriorates. The effects can be observed

[153] Edward W. Gibbons and Richard A. Winchester, "A Delayed Sidetone Test for Detecting Uniaural Functional Deafness," *A.M.A. Archives of Otolaryngology* 66 (July 1957):70–78.

[154] "The Unilateral Delayed Sidetone Test," unpublished report (June 1959), Audiology and Speech Pathology Service, Veterans Administration Outpatient Clinic, Los Angeles.

[155] Howard B. Ruhm and William A. Cooper, Jr., "Low Sensation Level Effects of Pure-Tone Delayed Auditory Feedback," *Journal of Speech and Hearing Research* 5 (June 1962):185–193.

and heard by the examiner and can be analyzed more completely on a graphic record of the subject's responses. Ruhm and Cooper validated their test, called *DFA* for *delayed feedback audiometry,* on normals, veterans with organic hearing losses, and veterans with functional components in their hearing losses.[156] There are obvious advantages in this technique as a test for functional hearing loss, provided the instrumentation can be simplified so that it becomes practical for use as a clinical tool.

Doerfler-Stewart test.   One of the earliest tests devised as a screening instrument to detect the presence of functional hearing loss was the Doerfler-Stewart (D-S) test, which was developed at an Army aural rehabilitation center during World War II.[157] This test examines a patient's ability to respond to spondee words in the presence of a masking noise—sawtooth, complex, or "speech" noise. The test is performed binaurally through earphones, and the speech signal and masking noise are mixed and varied in intensity in relation to each other. The theory of the test is that if a patient has a functional loss, the masking noise will interfere with ability to judge the level at which the test material should no longer be "heard." The first step is to obtain a recorded spondee threshold, using an ascending approach. This measure is called SRT_1 Without stopping the test stimuli, set the speech signal at $SRT_1 + 5$ and gradually introduce noise until the level is 20 dB below $SRT_1 + 5$. Then increase the noise in 2-dB steps until the patient stops repeating spondees. The level of the noise at that point is called NIL—*noise interference level.* Continue to increase the level of the noise until it is 15 to 20 dB above the NIL. Then decrease the level of the spondees to 15 dB below SRT_1. The noise level is now gradually reduced to see if the patient begins repeating spondees. If so, you know that SRT_1 was in error by at least 15 dB. Proceed to obtain NIL again, using the new speech threshold plus 5 dB as the level of the speech signal. If no spondees are repeated as the noise level is reduced, fade the noise out completely and proceed to establish a spondee threshold again with an ascending technique. This measure is called SRT_2. Now for the first time, turn off the spondees. The final step is to obtain NDT—noise detection threshold—using a combined ascending-descending technique. This threshold is the lowest hearing level at which the patient reports hearing the noise.

Norms for the test were reported by Doerfler and Epstein and by Hopkinson.[158] Conclusions about whether or not a patient exhibits a func-

[156]Howard B. Ruhm and William A. Cooper, Jr., "Delayed Feedback Audiometry," *Journal of Speech and Hearing Disorders* 29 (November 1964):448–55.

[157]Leo G. Doerfler and Kenneth Stewart, "Malingering and Psychogenic Deafness," *Journal of Speech Disorders* 11 (September 1946) :181–86.

[158]Leo G. Doerfler and Aubrey Epstein, "The Doerfler-Stewart (D-S) Test for Functional Hearing Loss," unpublished monograph submitted to the Veterans Administration, 1956; Norma T. Hopkinson, "Speech Tests for Pseudohypacusis," in *Handbook of Clinical Audiology,* 2nd ed., ed. Jack Katz (Baltimore: Williams & Wilkins, 1978), chap. 25, pp. 291–303.

tional loss are based on (1) comparing SRT_1 and SRT_2—they should agree within ±5 dB; (2) comparing NDT with SRT_1 and SRT_2—NDT should be well below the speech-reception threshold; (3) comparing SRT_1 + 5 and NIL—NIL should be well above the level of SRT_1 + 5; and (4) comparing NDT and NIL—NDT should be considerably lower than NIL. If any of these comparisons result in "unexpected" findings, the result of the test is positive. Doerfler and Epstein recommended that the D-S test be given as an initial screening test for functional hearing loss in all cases involving compensation. If the results of the test are positive, the examiner is then alerted to the possibility that the patient does have a functional hearing loss and should employ other special tests to verify the patient's thresholds.

Other tests.   Any of the physiologically based measures may be used in cases where a nonorganic loss is suspected. The results of measures that provide an estimate of hearing threshold based on a physiological response, such as ERA or GSR, can be compared directly to the behavioral results. Because an acoustic reflex occurs only at suprathreshold levels, reflex testing can be performed with patients presenting profound losses as a check on the organicity of the loss. If a reflex occurs at some level below the patient's voluntary threshold, the examiner knows that the patient's loss has a functional component. Using one of the approaches described in an earlier section of this chapter, an examiner can predict from a comparison of the reflex thresholds for broad-band noise and for pure tones what the patient's approximate threshold should be. The primary value of the acoustic reflex test, however, is as a screening device when a functional impairment is suspected with a patient who apparently has a profound monaural or bilateral loss. The absence of a reflex, of course, is not physiological proof that a profound organic impairment exists.

TESTING CHILDREN

Thus far in the chapters dealing with evaluation of hearing, we have been concerned primarily with patients whose physical and mental maturity make possible their involvement in the test situation as active participants, and except for those individuals who manifest functional hearing problems, the examiner depends on their positive responses to the presence or absence of test stimuli in determining threshold. In other words, the usual test involves a patient who is capable of responding to the test stimuli introduced, whether they be pure tones or speech, who can understand and follow instructions, and who cooperates with the examiner. With such patients, certain standard procedures have evolved to insure test reliability, for example, the ascending method of arriving at threshold in pure-tone audiometry; and certain test materials, such as spondee words and PB word lists, have been agreed upon. When the examiner is confronted by a small child whose hearing must be evaluated, many of the "rules" of hearing testing must be modified or abandoned. The child may or may not be able to understand and follow instructions or may not be capable of responding to auditory stimuli in an adult fashion. Cooperation may be almost completely lacking—at least in the initial stages of the test procedure. Frequently, the examiner must make up the rules of the game and exercise every bit of ingenuity in order to obtain some information concerning the child's hearing. Of course, there are many young children who can be examined easily and accurately with minimum modification of adult testing procedures, but the examiner must be prepared to meet the challenge of assessing the hearing of youngsters who are difficult to test. It is hoped that the suggestions contained in this section will help the examiner meet that challenge successfully.

The Neonate and Infant

With the increasing importance of hearing-conservation programs in the schools (see Chapter 8), there has developed the realization that many children whose hearing impairments are discovered in school testing programs might have been helped medically, educationally, and socially had their hearing problems been identified at an earlier age. At how early an age is it feasible to attempt an assessment of hearing? The answer to this question is that with proper examination methods, some information concerning the integrity of the hearing mechanism can be obtained with infants only a few hours old.

The results of physiologic measures obtained in the very young child cannot be compared directly to normative values obtained from adults. Neonates proceed through considerable developmental stages during the first weeks of life, which result in physiologic responses normal only for the group of infants of the same age. These developmental changes occur in both the central nervous system and the middle and external auditory structures and thus affect the ERA results as well as the acoustic immittance results. However, given this consideration, these physiologic measures can be performed at birth and can provide a considerable amount of information about the auditory system.

Some centers routinely estimate hearing sensitivity with evoked response procedures in either well-baby or intensive-care neonatal units. However, the efficacy of such procedures has been plagued by the tendency of the measures to identify a high percentage of normal-hearing babies as having significant hearing loss. The problem has been so severe in some centers that the program has been dropped. As the infant's nervous system begins to mature during the first year of life, more definitive information concerning hearing can be obtained.

The Ewings in England pioneered behavioral hearing examination techniques for use with infants. Such procedures have come to be known as *behavioral observation audiometry,* or BOA. In 1958, they reported procedures they had developed and used over a period of twenty years.[159] The pioneer work in the United States in this area was done collaboratively by Johns Hopkins University School of Medicine and the Maryland State Department of Health—both located in Baltimore. In 1959, the Baltimore group reported test procedures based on the Ewing test battery and the results of a pilot study that utilized these procedures with 327 infants from three to fifty-two weeks of age, 111 infants from ten to twenty-nine weeks of age, and 107 newborn infants.[160]

Although the Ewings agree that deafness or profound hearing loss can be ruled out by observing the responses of babies of a few days of age to intense sound, they tend to dismiss the testing of the neonate as being too crude to yield significant information. They report cases of infants of very tender age who apparently did not respond to sound at all but who subsequently—say at age seven or eight months—demonstrated normal hearing. The Ewings prefer to concentrate their attention on infants of seven months of age and older. The Baltimore group reported reasonably good success in eliciting positive responses from newborn infants with a specially constructed wooden "clacker." This consists of two pieces of wood fastened together with a screen-door spring hinge. When the top piece is raised to a 90-degree angle with the lower piece and then released, a very brief sound of broad spectrum results (reported as a sound level of 64 dB with the "B" weighting network of a sound-level meter at a distance of 12 feet). The duration of the sound is estimated at 5 msec.

The response of a newborn infant to such a sound is a startle or Moro's reflex, which is a contraction of the limbs and the neck muscles. Sometimes an eye blink occurs simultaneously with the general muscular activity that characterizes Moro's reflex. The Baltimore group obtained "satisfactory" responses to the clacker in about 90 percent of the newborn infants with whom it was tried. Of course, a response to a stimulus of this intensity and spectrum does not rule out some hearing impairment, but it does indicate that the infant is not deaf. Failure of the newborn infant to respond to the clacker may or may not indicate a hearing impairment. In any event, the infant who does not respond should be studied closely as it matures over the next few weeks or months to discover whether hearing is impaired or there exists some neurological or other deficit that could have accounted for the failure to respond. Hardy, Dougherty, and Hardy suggest that pediatricians should be able to utilize this technique of hearing "evaluation" to advantage with newborn infants in the hospital nursery.[161]

[159] Irene R. Ewing and Alex W. G. Ewing, *New Opportunities for Deaf Children* (London: University of London Press Ltd., 1958).

[160] Janet B. Hardy, Anne Dougherty, and William G. Hardy, "Hearing Responses and Audiologic Screening in Infants," *Journal of Pediatrics* 55 (September 1959) :382–90.

[161] Ibid., p. 390.

Following the lead of Wedenberg in Sweden,[162] Downs and her colleagues at the University of Colorado Medical Center have focused attention on the auditory screening of newborn infants in the hospital nursery.[163] As a result of Downs's work, there are available on the market several electronic devices designed for auditory screening in the nursery. These are hand-held, battery-powered instruments that generate a warbling pure tone of 3000 Hz or a narrow-band noise centered at 3000 Hz and possibly also a wide-band noise. The output is variable from 70 to 100 dB SPL when delivered through a loudspeaker held a few inches from the infant's ear. Downs selected the frequency of 3000 Hz for screening so that infants with sloping hearing losses could be identified, whereas they might be missed by a test tone of lower frequency. She recommends 90 dB SPL as the criterion intensity for general use "because it is the lowest level that will consistently produce responses when presented to normal infants in the noise levels common to nursery situations."[164] A sound-pressure level of 90 dB at 3000 Hz is equal to a hearing level of 82.5 dB, according to the ANSI-1969 standard.

Downs originally proposed routinely screening every newborn infant in the nurseries of hospitals, utilizing trained and supervised volunteers, and following up the screening with audiological evaluations of all those infants who did not pass the screening criteria. She described and categorized various responses by awake and sleeping infants that indicated they were reacting to the acoustic stimuli. She reported that the incidence of "deafness" discovered in the Denver program was at least one in 2000 infants, or 0.05 percent. She stated that "false positive" results were found in 1.5 percent of the population tested, although among the false positives were infants later discovered to have nonauditory involvements of the central nervous system.[165] Silverman and Davis, quoting from the proceedings of a 1964 Canadian conference on the young deaf child, suggested that because of the low yield a widespread screening program of newborns may be economically indefensible. Also they questioned the validity and reliability of infant screening tests, saying, "The number of 'false positives' and the number of cases missed, which are both rather high, must be considered; the former will cause unfounded anxiety, and the latter will give a false sense of security and thus delay later recognition of

[162] Eric Wedenberg, "Auditory Tests on Newborn Infants," *Acta Oto-laryngologica* 46 (1956):446–61.

[163] Marion P. Downs and Graham M. Sterritt, "Identification Audiometry for Neonates: A Preliminary Report," *Journal of Auditory Research* 4 (April 1964):69–80; Marion P. Downs, "Testing Hearing in Infancy and Early Childhood," in *Deafness in Childhood*, eds. Freeman McConnell and Paul H. Ward (Nashville, Tenn.: Vanderbilt University Press, 1967), pp. 25–33; Marion P. Downs, "Organization and Procedures of a Newborn Infant Screening Program," *Hearing and Speech News* 35 (March 1967) :27–36.

[164] Ibid., p. 29.

[165] Downs, "Testing Hearing in Infancy and Early Childhood," p. 26.

an auditory impairment."[166] Ling et al. pointed out variables in testing that affect the validity of screening tests of newborn infants and concluded that without more definitive studies of "stimulus, response, and observer variables . . . newborn screening programs will continue to be assumption-ridden, time-consuming, and highly inefficient."[167] Goldstein and Tait criticized the rationale, method, and effectiveness of routine screening of newborn infants and proposed limiting testing of infants in the nursery to those in a "high risk" category—infants whose family history and prenatal and natal history are such that their hearing may be suspect.[168] A joint committee of the American Academy of Ophthalmology and Otolaryngology, the American Academy of Pediatrics, and the American Speech and Hearing Association refused to recommend the mass screening of newborn infants.

Taking cognizance of the criticisms of mass screening of neonates, Northern and Downs now advocate testing only those newborns who are on a high-risk register on the basis of meeting one or more criteria. The following criteria were proposed by the Joint Committee in a supplementary statement in 1982:[169]

1. Family history of hereditary hearing impairment
2. Maternal rubella or other intrauterine viral infection
3. Defects of the ear, nose, and throat of the infant
4. Birthweight of less than 1500 grams (3.3 pounds)
5. Bilirubin level in the blood greater than 20 mg/100 ml serum (associated with blood group incompatibility)
6. Bacterial meningitis, especially H. influenza
7. Severe asphyxia

The infant ideally should be in a "light" sleep state, although it is possible to test even when the subject is in a "deep" level of sleep. A test stimulus is presented for two seconds, and the infant is observed for three seconds after cessation of the signal. The only acceptable response is an awakening or arousal from sleep, indicated by opening of the eyes or by general bodily movement. After the infant has fallen asleep again, the stimulus is repeated. Two

[166] S. R. Silverman and H. Davis, "Hard-of-Hearing Children," in *Hearing and Deafness*, 3rd ed., eds. Hallowell Davis and S. Richard Silverman (New York: Holt, Rinehart and Winston, 1970), p. 428.

[167] Daniel Ling, Agnes H. Ling, and Donald C. Doehring, "Stimulus, Response, and Observer Variables in the Auditory Screening of Newborn Infants," *Journal of Speech and Hearing Research* 13 (March 1970):17.

[168] Robert Goldstein and Charles Tait, "Critique of Neonatal Hearing Evaluation," *Journal of Speech and Hearing Disorders* 36 (February 1971):3–18.

[169] "Joint Committee on Infant Hearing Position Statement," *Asha* 24 (1982):1017.

arousals must occur—and be agreed on by the volunteer observers—before the subject is passed.[170]

Simmons and Russ have described an automated system for testing the hearing of newborn infants in the nursery of a hospital. Their system, called the *Crib-o-gram*, utilizes motion-detecting transducers affixed to the cribs. Eight cribs can be monitored simultaneously by a multichannel strip chart recorder in another room. Twenty times a day, a test stimulus is introduced through loudspeakers in the ceiling. The stimulus is a band of noise from 2 to 4 kHz that reaches the crib at a sound-pressure level of 92 to 93 dB. The system is turned on automatically. The output of the transducers is recorded for ten seconds to establish a base line. The stimulus is turned on for one second, following which the output of the transducers is monitored for six seconds. Once a day the Crib-o-gram charts are scored. The scorer must decide whether or not there was a change in crib activity associated with the sound stimulus. Each infant's scores are totaled for the hospital stay. The infant passes the screening if responses are observed to at least 20 percent of the stimuli or if "two definite startle or arousal responses are present within two seconds after the test sound." Control events, or "silent" tests, are included periodically as a check on the validity of the scoring. Infants who fail the Crib-o-gram test are scheduled for screening tests at six months of age.[171]

With infants from three to fourteen weeks of age, the Baltimore group uses some of the articles and procedures suggested by the Ewings for older infants, plus some items of their own selection. In addition to the clacker used with newborns, these include a doorbell, a tonette, a xylophone, a squeaker, three rattles (low, middle, and high frequency), voiceless consonants *sss* and *kkk*, voice, crumpling tissue paper, and a spoon being stirred in a cup. As checked with a sound-level meter, these stimuli all produce sound levels of around 40 dB, with the exception of the squeaker (50 dB) and the bell and clacker (60 dB). These sound levels cannot be translated into *hearing* levels on the basis of the information reported. We can only say that the hearing levels of these sounds would probably be less than their sound levels.

The testing is performed by two examiners while the infant's parent, seated in a chair, holds the baby in the lap. The room in which the testing is performed should be reasonably quiet. One examiner sits in a low chair or kneels in front of the parent and baby, holding toys, puppets, dolls, and so forth, to attract the visual attention of the infant, while the other examiner introduces auditory stimuli behind the chair in which the parent is seated. The examiner in back holds a noisemaker to either side of the infant, well outside its peripheral vision. The infant should be supported under the arms and held

[170] Jerry L. Northern and Marion P. Downs, *Hearing in Children*, 3rd ed. (Baltimore: Williams & Wilkins, 1984), pp. 238–40.

[171] F. Blair Simmons and Frederica N. Russ, "Automated Newborn Hearing Screening, the Crib-o-gram," *Archives of Otolaryngology* 100 (July 1974):1–7.

away from the parent's body, so it is free to move its head or its body from side to side. The examiner in front serves as an observer to evaluate the infant's responses to the auditory stimuli produced by the examiner in back. Following a response, the infant's visual attention must be regained.

Infants in the three- to fourteen-weeks age group may respond by turning the head to seek the source of the sound (the response that is characteristic of older infants); they may exhibit "eye responses," such as turning the eyes, widening the eyes, and making searching movements with the eyes; they may exhibit Moro's reflex, with or without an accompanying eye blink, or a body "jump" or general muscular activity; or they may indicate by cessation of muscular activity, cessation of crying, or waking from a dozing or sleeping state that they are aware of the auditory stimulus. The most common response, especially to the stimuli of greater intensity, is Moro's reflex or a partial Moro's reflex. A surprising number of infants in this age group respond by head turning or eye responses, however. A "streamlined" version of the test, consisting of the voiceless consonants, the "middle" rattle, and voice, representing high-, middle-, and low-frequency ranges, respectively, can be given in about two minutes. If the infant does not respond, additional items should be introduced. If the infant still does not respond, a retest should be scheduled, and the infant should be periodically reexamined.

The same test procedures are followed with infants between fifteen and thirty weeks of age and between thirty-one and fifty-two weeks of age. In the former group, the predominant responses are turning the head toward the source of the sound and eye responses. Moro's reflex occurs infrequently except in response to the more intense stimuli. Because infants in the latter age group should all be sufficiently mature to turn the head toward the sound, they are required to respond in this fashion in order to pass the test. Furthermore, the head must be turned at least 45 degrees before the response is accepted.

As was mentioned earlier, the Ewings concentrate their efforts on infants beyond the age of seven months. The physical arrangements for the test are the same as described by the Baltimore group. The Ewings insist on obtaining the head-turning response, requiring that the infant look directly at the source of the sound before accepting the response. If the infant merely looks up and appears to be listening, or if the eyes and head are turned toward the sound but not directly at the sound source, the test is not considered passed because infants of seven months should demonstrate the ability to localize sound "automatically." The Ewings stress the importance of using "quiet" sound stimuli for the test. For infants from seven to nine months of age, they employ two "high-pitched" sounds (opening a small ball of crumpled tissue paper and "gently" shaking a high-pitched rattle) and two "low-pitched" sounds (metal teaspoon stirred quietly in the bottom of a china cup and low-pitched rattle). The child must localize all these sounds on both left and right sides in order to pass the screening test. According to the Ewings, the spoon and cup item is a sound of special interest to the infants, because it should suggest feeding time. It is interesting to note that the Baltimore group found the tissue crumpling and the spoon and cup sounds to be their least effective test stimuli. Murphy has reported the successful use of pure tones with infants in this age range. He checks the infant's localizing ability first with rattles and then substitutes a "telephone" connected to an oscillator for the rattles. He reports that localizing responses may be obtained at hearing levels as low as 40 dB for the frequencies from 400 to 6000 Hz.[172]

With infants from ten to fifteen months of age, the Ewings depend primarily on speech sounds to attract the baby's attention. The examiner calls the infant's name quietly and sings quietly at a distance of five to six feet, and the examiner utters the voiceless consonants *sss, ppp, ttt, kkk* "naturally and rhythmically" at three feet from either ear. If the infant does not respond to these speech stimuli, the test items used with younger infants are introduced.

Both the Ewings and the Baltimore group stress that their tests are screening tests—not diagnostic tests or tests designed to yield threshold information. The purpose of the testing is to detect infants whose responses to sound are not typical for their age, so that they may be more carefully tested in the audiology clinic or observed for signs of neurological or intellectual deficits. The younger the infant, the more gross the screening procedure. Failure of an infant to respond to any but intense stimuli—for example, the clacker—may indicate the presence of a hearing impairment or it may mean only that the child is not yet sufficiently mature to be interested in less intense sounds. On the other hand, the infant who does respond appropriately to the various "quiet" stimuli is demonstrating that there is no serious impairment.

Although the techniques of screening infants described here may appear to be simple, the success of these methods depends on the skill of both examiners and their experience in working together. Hardy, Dougherty, and Hardy believe that with some special training, nurses in "a clinic setting," for example, a well-baby clinic, will be able to perform these screening tests adequately with infants from thirty to fifty-two weeks of age. The screening of infants from three to thirty weeks of age, however, requires much more skill in evaluating the subtle responses they make to quiet sounds. About the testing of this younger age group, these investigators say, "It [the test] appears to be a useful diagnostic and research tool but because of the complexity of the responses obtained probably not applicable as a screening device on a general pediatric and public health level."[173] Ling et al. go a step further, saying,

> Many programs using localization responses, derived from the original work of Ewing, have proved to have levels of reliability and validity with children from about five months of age. These programs have the advantage of detecting

[172] K. P. Murphy, "Ascertainment of Deafness in Children," *Audecibel* 15 (Summer 1966) :89–93.

[173] Hardy et al., "Hearing Responses."

deafness arising postnatally. There appears to be no advantage to the infant from detection of deafness in the first few months. Parents are often quite unable to accept a diagnosis of sensory defect before they have time to develop a relationship with their child. They are, therefore, likely to frustrate very early efforts at training through hostility both to the baby and to the clinicians who press the immediate use of hearing aids.[174]

The Young Child

Children between the ages of twelve and twenty-four months will probably need to be evaluated on the basis of the tests described for the infant, although some of the children in this age group will cooperate adequately in at least a portion of the tests now to be described. Because the Ewing-type test gives only a general indication of the child's hearing abilities, it is desirable as soon as possible to administer a more formal hearing test in order to determine the child's thresholds with greater accuracy. This means that calibrated audiometric equipment must be employed. If suitable modifications of audiometric procedures are utilized, including in most instances the help of a trained observer or assistant, the examiner can often obtain valid and reliable threshold measurements on children as young as six months. Not infrequently, however, more than a single testing period will be required before satisfactory measurements can be achieved. The difficult task is in winning the child's confidence so that cooperation in the test will occur. For example, the child must be willing to accept earphones before the examiner can obtain threshold information on the ears individually. Many very young children refuse to permit the earphones to be placed on their heads. The examiner should be firm with the child and simply take for granted that the child will wear the earphones. In many cases, such a positive attitude on the part of the examiner is sufficient to convince the child that there is no choice but to accept the earphones. If the child believes it can get its own way by putting up a protest, then of course the child will refuse to accept the earphones. The examiner who approaches the young child with obvious trepidation will likely meet the anticipated resistance, much like the salesperson who asks the customer, "You wouldn't like to subscribe to this magazine, would you?" Sometimes it is helpful if the examiner, or someone else in the room, wears earphones for a short time before placing them on the child's head.

There will be occasions, however, when no amount of firmness or cajolery will induce the child to wear earphones. The examiner must exercise fine judgment in such cases, because to persist in forcing the earphones on the child may destroy completely any chance for establishing rapport at that time or in future sessions. The examiner, therefore, must know when to compromise. An acceptable compromise for both patient and examiner may be to hold one earphone to the ear instead of having the child wear the headset. It may be necessary, however, for the examiner to forego completely the use of

[174]Ling et al., "Stimulus, Response and Observer Variables," p. 16.

earphones and be content—at that time—to secure information through the use of sound-field procedures. Eventually, however, the answer to the question as to whether or not an impairment exists in either ear will require testing with earphones and perhaps also with a bone-conduction vibrator. If the examiner can keep from alienating the child, sooner or later, success in obtaining the measurement will follow.

In many cases, the examiner is more likely to succeed if the child's parent is not in the room, but frequently the parent's presence is a help rather than a hindrance. If the examiner has made the decision to invite the parent into the test room and this decision turns out to have been a mistake, it will be difficult to ask the parent to leave without upsetting the child and perhaps also the parent. When the child is scheduled for a reexamination, it can be suggested to the parent that it is time to try working with the child alone.

If the parent is to be present during the examination, it is perhaps best that he or she sit slightly to the side and behind the child. Care should be taken that no one is sitting between the child and any loudspeakers that are to be used in the hearing evaluation. The child should be given no reason to look toward loudspeakers unless there is an awareness of a sound originating from them. Usually, it is good practice to inform the parent before entering the room that he or she is not to speak or take part in the procedure unless requested to do so. The aim usually is to keep the parent out of the situation as much as possible but still make use of the parent's presence in the room as a comfort to the child.

A skilled assistant can be a great help to the examiner in working with a small child. Some of the testing procedure will require the examiner to be outside the room. The assistant stays in the room with the child and, it is hoped, keeps the child interested and happy while the examiner is operating the test equipment in the control room. The assistant serves also to supplement the examiner's observations of the child's reactions to the stimuli presented. Ideally, there should be communication from the examiner to the assistant by means of an amplifying system, so that the assistant can receive instructions through an earphone and be kept informed about what the examiner is doing and plans to do. The assistant can signal with a nod or shake of the head whether or not a response was observed, and because the examiner will be monitoring the talk-back system, the assistant can speak to the examiner whenever necessary.

The examiner will usually wish to begin the test by observing the child's reaction to speech and various noises introduced by sound-field through the microphone circuit of the speech audiometer. The child's responses to such signals are perhaps facilitated if, before any stimuli are presented, quiet play is allowed for a period of five to ten minutes, during which time no one speaks in the room and care is taken to present only toys that do not make any significant amount of noise. In this situation, the child is more likely to respond when low-intensity signals are presented through the loudspeaker than if these signals are introduced into an already noisy environment. The examiner may also attempt to observe the child's responses to pure-tone signals presented through a loudspeaker, but a more complex signal, such as speech or noise, is more likely to evoke an observable response.

For whatever group of signals is presented, an ascending intensity technique is usually most appropriate. The examiner should note each stimulus presented and rate the child's responses in some systematic fashion. For instance, a scale ranging from zero to 3 might be used to indicate the examiner's confidence in the child's response to a particular stimulus. A score of zero indicates "no observable response," and a score of 3 indicates "a definite response," such as a startle reaction or pointing toward the loudspeaker. Scores of 1 and 2 indicate less definite responses. This system of recording results is valuable when the examiner is reexamining a child and trying to recall what results were obtained on previous examinations.

After the possibilities of observing the child's response to stimuli presented through loudspeakers have been exhausted, the examiner may enter the test room and, working with the child directly, attempt to make more precise measurements. We shall now discuss more specifically the modifications of conventional speech and pure-tone audiometric procedures that may be found useful in evaluating a child's hearing.

Modifications of speech audiometry.   Initially, the examiner is interested in noting the child's reactions to speech stimuli—words, sentences, individual speech sounds, and noises made with the speech mechanism—when these are presented by sound-field through the microphone circuit. The assistant and the child will usually be seated at a child's table across from each other. The assistant will be showing the child some toys, trying to develop interest in a game or puzzle, or otherwise keeping the child reasonably quiet and occupied. The examiner can watch through the window between the control and test rooms, and the assistant will also be in a good position to evaluate the child's reactions whenever a stimulus is presented. Any indication that the child is aware of the stimulus should be noted and rated concerning confidence as previously suggested. Responses may consist of interruption of a task, head movements while trying to locate the sound, attempts to imitate the stimulus, interruption of vocal play, or eye responses—widening of the eyes, searching movements, or when an intense sound occurs, an eye blink. If two loudspeakers are available, the examiner can alternate the signal between them to see if the child appears to be aware of the differing sources of the sound within the test room.

One of the first stimuli the examiner should employ is whispered speech—saying the child's name, for example. Starting with zero hearing level, the examiner gradually increases the intensity of the whispered signal until a response is noted. Whispered speech emphasizes high frequencies. If the child responds to whispering at relatively low hearing levels, the examiner knows that the child's hearing for speech is adequate, or that at least there is no serious impairment of hearing. In such a case, the examiner may wish to proceed immediately to the pure-tone evaluation of the child's hearing or observation of the child's responses to other stimuli.

If the child does not respond to whispered speech at any hearing level, the examiner may next try saying the child's name aloud, starting at zero hearing level and gradually increasing the intensity until a response is noted or maximum intensity is reached. Other words than the child's name may, of course, be used. If no response is noted when the intensity is gradually increased, the examiner may elect to attempt to elicit a startle response by suddenly introducing a word at a high hearing level. The examiner should warn the assistant, so that the assistant does not give a startle response that attracts the child's attention.

In place of words or sentences, the examiner may use individual speech sounds in order to determine, for example, whether there is any difference in the child's responses to voiced and voiceless sounds. The examiner may make noises such as tongue clicks or perhaps animal noises. Various noise-makers—rattles, whistles, drum, and so forth may also be employed, including pulses of masking noise. Also, music may be introduced by using the phonograph or tape circuit of the speech audiometer.

A useful technique is to pair the auditory signal with a rewarding visual stimulus. Reddell and Calvert have described such a procedure, in which a hollow plastic toy animal is illuminated by a bulb mounted inside it whenever the examiner presses a button. The toy is mounted to the side of the child, so a head turn is required to look at it. In preliminary trials, the child is taught by the assistant to look at the animal when an intense sound stimulus is presented. When the child's head turns to look, the examiner presses the button that illuminates the animal. When the child is conditioned, the examiner presents another stimulus at a low level, gives the child time to respond, and then presents the stimulus at a 10-dB greater intensity. Each time the child responds appropriately by turning to look at the animal, the examiner reinforces the response activity by illuminating the animal. Reddell and Calvert call their procedure *CA-VR* for *Conditioned Audio-Visual Response Audiometry*.[175] Their technique was suggested by one developed in Japan called *COR* for *Conditioned Orientation Reflex*.[176] The basic difference between the two techniques is that with COR the examiner is evaluating the child's localizing behavior because two hollow plastic toys are used—one on each of a pair of speakers. With CA-VR, there is no attempt to assess localizing ability. The technique is designed only to assist the examiner by giving the

[175] Rayford C. Reddell and Donald R. Calvert, "Conditioned Audio-Visual Response Audiometry," *The Voice* (Journal of the California Speech and Hearing Association) 16 (May 1967) :52–57.

[176] Tokuro Suzuki and Yoshio Ogiba, "Conditioned Orientation Reflex Audiometry," A.M.A. *Archives of Otolaryngology* 74 (1961) :84–90.

child an interesting way to respond. CA-VR may be utilized while testing through earphones or with a bone-conduction vibrator as well as in a sound-field. Others have applied the term *visual reinforcement audiometry* (VRA) to the pairing of auditory and visual events.[177]

With children who are old enough or mature enough to respond to directions, and who have sufficient understanding of language, more refined techniques of speech audiometry may be employed. Special methods have been described by Keaster,[178] by Sortini and Flake,[179] and by Siegenthaler, Pearson, and Lezak.[180] These methods require that the child point to an object or picture of an object when directed to do so by the examiner. Before the test, the objects or pictures are shown to the child to make sure that they are recognized. Then the examiner, using the microphone circuit of the speech audiometer, asks the child to hold up an object or to point to a picture. An assistant may or may not be needed in this situation, depending on the maturity and cooperation of the child.

By starting the procedure at a hearing level at which the child can respond and then gradually decreasing the intensity until the child fails to respond, the examiner can ascertain the child's threshold for speech. Initially, the presentations would probably be made by sound-field. Monaural speech threshold can be determined in a similar fashion by having the child use earphones. If some of the objects or pictures have similar names that are easily confused, such as *bus* and *gun,* or *knife* and *light,* it is possible to gain some information about whether the child has speech-discrimination problems.

Ross and Lerman have standardized a picture-identification test for obtaining speech-discrimination scores with young hearing-impaired children who have limited vocabularies. Their final evaluation of the test was made with sixty-one children ranging in age from four years and seven months to thirteen years and nine months. Twenty-four of the subjects were enrolled in a school for the deaf. Ross and Lerman call their test WIPI for *Word Intelligibility by Picture Identification.*[181]

Children with greater language sophistication can be tested with the speech audiometer in a similar manner to adults. Special lists of spondees and

[177] G. Liden and A. Kankkonen, "Visual Reinforcement Audiometry," *Acta Otolaryngologica* 67 (1961) :281–92.

[178] Jacqueline Keaster, "A Quantitative Method of Testing the Hearing of Young Children," *Journal of Speech Disorders* 12 (June 1947):159–60.

[179] A. J. Sortini and C. G. Flake, "Speech Audiometry Testing for Preschool Children," *Laryngoscope* 63 (October 1953):991–97.

[180] Bruce M. Siegenthaler, Jack Pearson, and Raymond J. Lezak, "A Speech Reception Threshold Test for Children," *Journal of Speech and Hearing Disorders* 19 (September 1954):360–66.

[181] Mark Ross and Jay Lerman, "A Picture Identification Test for Hearing-Impaired Children," *Journal of Speech and Hearing Research* 13 (March 1970):44–53. (This test may be obtained from Stanwix House Inc., 3020 Chartiers Avenue, Pittsburgh, Pennsylvania 15204.)

phonetically balanced words have been compiled specifically for children, using a more restricted vocabulary than the adult lists. The appendix to this book contains word lists suitable for speech audiometric testing of young children.

Modifications of pure-tone audiometry. Special techniques are required to achieve pure-tone threshold measurements on very young children, and as has been mentioned previously, it frequently is necessary to spend more than one testing session with a child before satisfactory results can be achieved. If the purpose of the examination is to determine whether or not a significant hearing impairment exists, the sound-field procedures previously described should be sufficient. But if the purpose is to rule out the possibility of even a slight impairment in either ear, the examiner must try to obtain monaural thresholds at least by air conduction and probably also by bone conduction.

Very young children have to be trained to respond in some positive manner when they hear pure tones. This requires the presence of the examiner in the room with the child. The examiner sits at a small table opposite the child and operates the audiometer. It is advisable to use a portable audiometer that can be placed at the end of the table or on a chair next to the table, so it does not intrude between the examiner and the child.

Initially, the examiner may place the earphones on the table. Turning the frequency selector to 4000 Hz a brief burst of tone is presented that is clearly audible, while the child is observed for any reaction. If the child does respond, the intensity is lowered and the tone is presented again, continuing in this way until the child no longer gives evidence that the tone is perceived. If the child does not respond to the initial presentation of the 4000 Hz tone, the examiner increases the intensity and presents it again, continuing until the child responds or until the maximum output of the audiometer is reached. If the child responds to any of these presentations, the examiner knows the approximate level of the binaural hearing. Because the earphones are placed between the child and the examiner, the sound pressure at the child's ears should be about the same as it is at the examiner's ears. The tone selected for this initial screening is 4000 Hz because if the child responds at this frequency, the chances are good that there is no significant hearing impairment at any frequency. If the child does not give any evidence of hearing the 4000 Hz tone at any level, it may or may not indicate a hearing loss. The initial screening procedure is meaningful only if the child does respond.

Next, the child must be trained to make a positive, unequivocal response when a tone is heard. Usually, the response that is easiest for the young child to make is to place a block in a box, a smaller cup in a larger cup, a smaller wooden circle on a larger wooden circle in building a "Christmas tree" toy, or some similar definite motor act. The examiner's problem is to teach the child to wait for a tone to be heard before performing the required motor act. The child will usually want to complete the "game" without waiting for an auditory event to occur at each step.

A convenient and clinically useful method of teaching the child to wait for an auditory event before responding is to condition with tactile sensations from a bone-conductor vibrator that the child holds. The examiner sets the audiometer frequency selector at 500 Hz and the hearing-level control at maximum for bone conduction. Then, supposing that a nest of plastic cups is used for the objects the child is to manipulate, the examiner hands the first cup to the child and presents a brief signal from the audiometer so that the child feels it through the vibrator. The examiner then guides the child to a response, helping the child to place the cup on the table. The examiner hands the child the next cup, initially preventing placement of this cup in the first one, and then presents another signal through the vibrator and guides the child to a "response." After three or four such guided responses, the examiner tries handing a cup to the child and seeing if the child will voluntarily wait until the tactile signal is perceived before responding. If necessary, the examiner will continue guiding the child's hand until the child has learned to perform the task correctly. When an appropriate response occurs, the examiner compliments the child by gesture, expression, and words of praise, so the correct response is reinforced by reward in the form of approval from the examiner. There are distinct advantages in using a nonauditory stimulus for this training procedure, particularly when the examiner has no idea of the child's hearing levels. Otherwise, the examiner might be attempting to develop a response to a tone of a frequency outside the child's hearing range, or if earphones are in place, in a "dead" ear. In addition, with a nonauditory stimulus, the examiner has the opportunity to correct the child's mistakes before audition is tested as well as to see whether or not the child possesses the maturity and inclination to respond to this type of testing technique. A similar tactile conditioning procedure with a bone-conduction vibrator was described by Thorne.[182]

When the child has learned to respond appropriately to tactile stimuli, the examiner places earphones on the child and indicates to the child by word and gesture to listen through the earphones for a signal and to repeat the activity of building the nest of cups that has just been successfully accomplished. If necessary, the examiner will help the child to make responses when tones are presented, until the child is able to handle the task alone. Care must be taken to alter the intervals between tonal presentations so the child does not learn to respond to a rhythm pattern. The first tone to present in the test is usually 500 Hz because even deaf children will probably have some sensitivity at this frequency. The hearing level at which this tone is presented will depend on the information regarding the child's hearing the examiner has

---

[182] Bert Thorne, "Conditioning Children for Pure-tone Testing," *Journal of Speech and Hearing Disorders* 27 (February 1962) :84–85.

already obtained through the sound-field procedures described earlier. Or if no information has been obtained, the examiner will have to experiment with levels, seeking a level that is high enough to obtain a sensation of hearing but not so high that the child will be startled or perhaps frightened. Once the child has responded appropriately, the examiner will decrease intensity in successive presentations, seeking the minimum hearing level at which a response is observed.

When threshold in each ear has been established by this procedure at 500 Hz, the frequency is changed to 2000 Hz, and threshold in each ear is determined in similar fashion. Then threshold measurements are made at 1000 Hz, and if time permits and the child's cooperation continues at a satisfactory level, other frequencies can be tested as the examiner desires. The reason for testing at 2000 Hz after obtaining thresholds at 500 Hz is to get information on the highest of the speech frequencies while the child is still cooperating. In case the test must be discontinued before responses to all the speech frequencies have been obtained, the examiner will have a better notion of the child's hearing abilities for speech from the frequencies of 500 and 2000 Hz than from 500 and 1000 Hz.

If the air-conduction testing reveals some hearing loss, the examiner will wish to obtain information on the child's hearing by bone conduction. The same procedures can be followed for bone-conduction testing. It must be remembered that regardless of the vibrator placement, it is the response of the better ear by bone conduction that is being assessed. With a very young child, it is obviously not possible in most cases to utilize masking procedures. The examiner must be prepared to switch tasks for the child to perform whenever the child's interest seems to be waning. As was mentioned previously, the test of a very young child may frequently require several sessions, particularly if there is a problem in gaining cooperation or acceptance of the earphones. If the child can be taught to respond to auditory stimuli by performing a positive motor act when the tone is heard and to hold off performing the act if the tone is not heard, the examiner can use the same technique to obtain speech-detection thresholds with the speech audiometer. These speech-detection thresholds can be compared with pure-tone thresholds as a check on test reliability. It is even possible to use this type of response to observe improvement of the speech-detection threshold with a hearing aid.

Adaptations of pure-tone testing technique may be required also with somewhat older children. Because pure tones are not inherently interesting to children, their attention may have to be maintained by means that make the testing situation a game. Various play-audiometry procedures and "gadgets" to make the test enjoyable have been described in the literature.[183] Some pa-

[183] M. R. Dix and C. S. Hallpike, "The Peep Show: A New Technique for Pure Tone Audiometry in Young Children," *British Medical Journal* 2 (1947):719–23; F. R. Guilford and C. O. Haug, "Diagnosis of Deafness in the Very Young Child," *A.M.A. Archives of Otolaryngology* 55 (February 1952):101–106; Edgar L. Lowell, Georgina

tients who are difficult to test may respond well to an operant conditioning procedure developed originally for use with mentally retarded children. Called *TROCA* for *tangible reinforcement operant conditioning audiometry*, this procedure employs rewards for correct responses in the form of candy, cereal, or trinkets, and a mild punishment for false responses.[184] The important thing to remember in testing children, however, is that no ingenious procedure or fascinating gadget will substitute for a skillful examiner who "has a way" with children.

In summary, here are some guiding principles that the examiner of young children should keep in mind:

1. Obtain first information that is easiest to obtain. Getting the child to accept earphones may be a major hurdle. The following observations in a sound-field can be made before earphones are introduced and may be sufficient to establish a tentative diagnosis:

    a. Gross response to complex stimuli
    b. Gross response to pure tones
    c. Thresholds for pure tones
    d. Threshold of speech detection
    e. Estimates of speech discrimination

2. Obtain first that information which is most meaningful. It is short-sighted to spend time trying to obtain thresholds at 8000 Hz, for example, when it may be much more important to sample the child's bone-conduction hearing.

3. Perform tests as rapidly as possible without sacrificing accuracy. A child of two and a half years of age cannot be expected to yield accurate responses to pure tones for long periods. An experienced examiner, using 10-dB steps on the audiometer, can obtain approximations of thresholds at 500, 1000, and 2000 Hz in each ear by both air and bone conduction in ten to fifteen minutes, once the child has been trained to respond consistently to auditory stimuli. A more accurate audiogram can be obtained in later testing sessions.

4. Avoid asking the child to perform difficult motor acts. For example,

---

Rushford, Gloria Holversten, and Marguerite Stoner, "Evaluation of Pure Tone Audiometry with Preschool Age Children," *Journal of Speech and Hearing Disorders* 21 (September 1956):292–302; David S. Green, "The Pup-Show: A Simple, Inexpensive Modification of the Peep-Show," *Journal of Speech and Hearing Disorders* 23 (February 1958):118–20; John J. O'Neill, Herbert J. Oyer, and James W. Hillis, "Audiometric Procedures Used with Children," *Journal of Speech and Hearing Disorders* 26 (February 1961):61–66.

[184]L. L. Lloyd, J. E. Spradlin, and M. J. Reid, "An Operant Audiometric Procedure for Difficult-to-Test Patients," *Journal of Speech and Hearing Disorders* 33 (1968):236–45.

do not insist on placement of a block on a peg if this is a frustrating task. Switch to a simpler type of response, such as dropping the block on the floor when the tone is heard. Also do not inject irrelevant mental tasks into the testing situation, such as sorting sizes, colors, and so forth.

5. Always obtain complete history, including a description from the parent of the child's speech and hearing abilities. Such information may help to validate your hearing measurements or perhaps may shed a completely different light on your estimations of the problem.

6. Whenever possible, make your own observations of the child's "speech" and vocal characteristics. With some children who are unresponsive to you, observations of the child and parent alone in the test room might be made through the window while you monitor the talk-back system.

7. Be on the lookout for indications of other communicative problems, such as mental retardation, emotional disturbances, central auditory problems, and so forth. Remember, these may exist in combination and with or without peripheral hearing impairment.

Immittance testing.   Because it is an objective procedure requiring a minimum of patient cooperation and can be performed quickly, immittance testing is well suited for children and infants. According to Northern, "Impedance audiometry can provide substantial information about the hearing mechanism in very young children even when audiologic or otologic examinations prove to be difficult or impossible."[185] Some authorities feel that immittance tests should be performed first in evaluating the hearing of small children, and that the choice of what other tests to perform depends on these results.[186] As we pointed out earlier, techniques have been developed for predicting audiometric hearing threshold level and slope from the comparison of acoustic reflex thresholds for pure tones and for broad-band noise. Although such predictions might have to suffice for children who are too young or too uncooperative to test audiometrically, immittance testing is most useful to the audiologist and the otologist when viewed in conjunction with audiometric data.

Tympanometry and acoustic reflex testing can detect the presence of otitis media when audiometric testing cannot because of the mildness of the loss. The course of acute otitis media can be followed through observation of the changes in middle-ear pressure and of the absence or presence of reflexes. Normal tympanograms with absent reflexes suggest a severe sensori-neural impairment. On occasion, the finding of normal tympanograms and the

[185] Jerry L. Northern, "Clinical Measurement Procedures," in *Handbook of Clinical Impedance Audiometry,* ed. Jerger, p. 42.

[186] Lloyd E. Lamb and D. Craig Dunckel, "Acoustic Impedance Measurement with Children," in *Acoustic Impedance & Admittance,* eds. Feldman and Wilber, chap. 8, p. 192.

presence of acoustic reflexes at normal hearing levels, pointing to normal hearing or a sensori-neural impairment of mild to moderate degree, can obviate the necessity for further testing at that time with an infant or child who, for example, was suspected of being deaf.

Although, as we have said, immittance testing is objective and requires a minimum of cooperation, it is necessary for the child to be quiet—not talking or crying—for the brief time required for the test. If the child resists all efforts to be kept quiet, it may be necessary that sedation under the immediate supervision of a physician be considered. A recommended sedative is chloral hydrate in a dosage of 25 mg/kg body weight. The effect of this sedative is to make the child drowsy and initiate sleep, and the only effect on the immittance test battery is to depress acoustic reflex activity slightly but not enough that testing cannot be accomplished.[187]

DIFFERENTIATING DEAFNESS FROM OTHER AUDITORY DISORDERS

The audiologist is frequently confronted with the problem of making a differential diagnosis for children who apparently are not hearing but who may actually prove to have a normal peripheral hearing mechanism. There are other conditions that produce the behavioral symptom of apparent deafness. Myklebust has described the problem of differentiating the other disorders from genuine deafness and has suggested some techniques and procedures for making the differential diagnosis.[188] The child who is brain-injured, or aphasic, will frequently fail to attend to sound, so that the child may be suspected of being deaf or hard-of-hearing. Other conditions that are confused with deafness are severe mental retardation and psychological disturbances, which may vary from emotional maladjustment resulting in a psychogenic hearing loss to a full-blown psychosis. Every person concerned with diagnosing language difficulties in children should be aware of the differentiating characteristics of the various disorders. A diagnosis of deafness in a particular child must be approached with caution because the fact that a patient does not respond to sound in a testing situation is not incontrovertible evidence of an impairment of the hearing mechanism. The importance of a valid diagnosis is self-evident. A child who is mentally retarded and who has normal hearing does not belong in a school for the deaf. Likewise, a child who is severely emotionally disturbed requires entirely different handling from the child whose primary difficulty is an inability to hear normally. Differential diagnosis of auditory disorders is a subject in itself and is outside the scope of this book.

[187] Northern, "Clinical Measurement Procedures," p. 43.
[188] Helmer R. Myklebust, *Auditory Disorders in Children* (New York: Grune & Stratton, 1964).

REFERENCES

Barber, Hugh O., and Stockwell, Charles W. *Manual of Electronystagmography*, 2nd ed. St. Louis: C. V. Mosby, 1980.
Bess, Fred H., ed. *Childhood Deafness: Causation, Assessment and Management.* New York: Grune & Stratton, 1977.
Bradford, Larry J., ed. *Physiological Measures of the Audio-Vestibular System.* New York: Academic Press, 1975.
Coats, Alfred C. *Electronystagmography: A Compendium.* Houston: Baylor College of Medicine, 1972.
Feldman, Alan S., and Wilber, Laura Ann, eds. *Acoustic Impedance & Admittance—The Measurement of Middle Ear Function.* Baltimore: Williams & Wilkins, 1976.
Glattke, Theodore J. *Short-Latency Auditory Evoked Potentials: Fundamental Bases and Clinical Applications.* Baltimore: University Park Press, 1983.
Jerger, James, ed. *Modern Developments in Audiology*, 2nd. ed. New York: Academic Press, 1973.
———, ed. *Handbook of Clinical Impedance Audiometry.* Dobbs Ferry, N.Y.: American Electromedics Corporation, 1975.
———, ed. *Pediatric Audiology.* San Diego: College Hill Press, 1984.
———, ed. *Hearing Disorders in Adults.* San Diego: College Hill Press, 1984.
Jerger, Susan and Jerger, James, eds. *Auditory Disorders: A Manual for Clinical Evaluation.* Boston: Little, Brown, 1981.
Kaplan, Harriet, Gladstone, Vic S., and Katz, Jack, eds. *Site of Lesion Testing: Audiometric Interpretation*, Vol. II. Baltimore: University Park Press, 1984.
Katz, Jack, ed. *Handbook of Clinical Audiology*, 2nd ed. Baltimore: Williams & Wilkins, 1978.
Keith, Robert W., ed. *Central Auditory Dysfunction.* New York: Grune & Stratton, 1977.
Konkle, Dan F., and Rintelmann, William F. eds. *Principles of Speech Audiometry.* Baltimore: University Park Press, 1983.
Martin, Frederick N. *Introduction to Audiology*, 2nd ed. Englewood Cliffs, N.J.: Prentice-Hall, 1981.
———, ed. *Medical Audiology: Disorders of Hearing.* Englewood Cliffs, N.J.: Prentice-Hall, 1981.
———, ed. *Pediatric Audiology*, Englewood Cliffs, N.J.: Prentice-Hall, 1978.
Northern, Jerry L., ed. *Hearing Disorders*, 2nd ed. Boston: Little, Brown, 1984.
———, and Downs, Marion P. *Hearing in Children*, 3rd ed. Baltimore: Williams & Wilkins, 1984.
Reneau, John P., and Hnatiow, Gail Z. *Evoked Response Audiometry.* Baltimore: University Park Press, 1975.
Rintelmann, William F., ed. *Hearing Assessment.* Baltimore: University Park Press, 1979.
Ruben, Robert J., Elberling, Claus, and Salomon, Gerhard, eds. *Electrocochleography.* Baltimore: University Park Press, 1976.
Rupp, Ralph R., and Stockdell, Kenneth G., Sr., eds. *Speech Protocols in Audiology.* New York: Grune & Stratton, 1980.

CHAPTER EIGHT
PUBLIC SCHOOL
HEARING CONSERVATION
PROGRAMS

For many years, the public schools have assumed responsibility for discovering cases of hearing impairment in schoolchildren. Hearing conservation programs are now as much a part of school health examinations as measurements of height and weight and tests of visual acuity. Many states have passed legislation requiring all school districts to test the hearing of all their pupils, although generally the laws do not specify how frequently this should be done. Ideally, every pupil should be tested every year, but few districts can afford the personnel and equipment required to do so. Some school systems plan to test each child every three years, scheduling tests each year, for example, for the first, fourth, seventh, and tenth grades. In addition, provision is made for testing children from any grade referred by teachers, school psychologists, or school speech specialists. Children transferring into the district would be tested at the time of their transfer.

Larger school districts operate their own hearing conservation programs. Smaller schools may contract for hearing-testing services through the county superintendent's office. Some hearing conservation programs have audiometrists whose sole responsibility is to conduct hearing tests throughout the year. Other programs make use of school nurses, who of course have other responsibilities as well. Some larger school districts employ an audiologist, whose responsibility is to supervise the hearing conservation program, including the medical and educational follow-up of all children discovered to have impaired hearing.

The purposes of a school hearing conservation program are to reduce to the absolute minimum the number of children with permanently impaired hearing and to provide for the special educational needs of children whose hearing cannot be restored to normal limits through medical or surgical treatment. Because the discovery of children with hearing losses is prerequisite to providing for their needs, the testing program, which often includes both hearing and acoustic immittance measures, is at the heart of hearing conservation. The success of a hearing conservation program can be measured by the statistics developed in yearly testing. It is usually true that in the first two or three years of a hearing conservation program, testing may lead to the classification of as many as 10 percent of a school population as having "medically significant" hearing losses, whereas after the program has been in effect for a few years, this number may be reduced to a level of 3 to 5 percent. In any school system, the greatest number of medically significant hearing losses will be discovered in the primary grades, for the simple reason that very young children have a higher incidence of upper respiratory infections and of tonsil and adenoid problems. Because these conditions usually respond to proper medical treatment, it is important that they be discovered as soon as they become evident. In its early years, therefore, a hearing conservation program should concentrate on the primary grades. The discovery and treatment of conditions producing hearing loss then will reduce the number of hearing losses in the higher elementary grades and in junior and senior high school.

It is useless to discover cases of hearing impairment unless something is done to assist children who have hearing problems. Therefore, the medical and educational follow-up aspects of the program are extremely important. This chapter will be concerned primarily with the various methods of discovering hearing impairments in school populations but also, to some extent, with the requirements of medical and educational follow-up.

TESTING ENVIRONMENT

It is often a problem to find a satisfactory room in which to give school audiometric examinations. In the past, it has not been thought necessary to perform school tests in specially constructed rooms. Instead, it was felt that any room that was reasonably quiet would do. As a matter of fact, the screening level for individual sweep tests was traditionally set at 15 or 20 dB (re ASA-1951 calibration standards) because of the masking effect of room and outside noise in even "quiet" rooms. In 1960, a national conference on the subject of "identification audiometry" was held in Baltimore, and its major findings have been reported in monograph form.[1] One of the strong recom-

[1] Frederic L. Darley, ed., "Identification Audiometry," *Journal of Speech and Hearing Disorders,* Monograph supp. no. 9 (September 1961).

mendations that evolved from this conference was that school testing must be performed in an adequate environment, so that a more stringent criterion for passing the screening test can be employed.

> A good acoustic environment is necessary. It can safely be said that millions of dollars and thousands of man hours are now being spent on worthless programs simply because space has been utilized because of its convenience rather than because of its suitability for the purpose. If an examiner is screening at 15 dB above audiometric zero while the environment induces 20 dB of masking, spuriously large numbers of subjects will be identified as having hearing problems and will be referred on to successive stages of the program. Initial expenditure of money for a suitable testing environment results in substantial savings of money spent for the referral of children erroneously thought to have hearing impairment.[2]

It is to be hoped that school boards and school architects will plan for the inclusion of properly sound-isolated space for hearing testing in the construction of new school buildings. Because it is not economically feasible to remodel existing buildings to provide proper testing space, authorities should consider the purchase of prefabricated booths. Even though these booths are specially constructed to attenuate outside noise, care must be exercised to locate them in a quiet part of the building.

Assuming that specially constructed test rooms are not available, the school tests will have to be performed in the quietest space that can be found. Frequently, the nurse's office will be the most adequate space available. Regardless of which room is selected for the hearing tests, it is important that the ambient noise in and around the room be kept to a minimum. Because hearing testing involves only a few children of the total school population at a time, the rest are going about their regular activities. If there is much activity in the halls, or recess is in progress, the noise in the testing room may become intolerable. Most principals will cooperate with the audiometrist by selecting a room for the testing that is on the opposite side of the building from the playground, and by restricting traffic in the hallway outside the testing room. Also, it is helpful if during the days of testing, the bell system in the school is not operated. Rooms that are near lavatories should be avoided, if possible, because the noise of the plumbing may interfere with the testing.

Some school districts have solved the space problem by providing mobile testing units. These are buses or trailers that are specially sound-treated and fitted out for the sole purpose of providing a suitable environment for hearing testing. Although most mobile units are designed specifically for individual testing, some are equipped for testing groups of twenty to thirty children. Of course, individual testing may also be done in these units. The advantages of mobile units are self-evident. Most important, they provide uniform testing conditions at every school. They can be driven to the quiet side of any school and plugged into the nearest electric outlet. When group equipment is de-

[2] Ibid., p. 27.

cided on, it can be permanently installed. An advantage not to be overlooked is that the fully equipped mobile unit is unquestionably a laboratory on wheels in which scientific work is accomplished, and impressionable children may be more inclined to cooperate with the audiometrist in such a setting than in the more familiar surroundings of a classroom.

GROUP TESTS VERSUS INDIVIDUAL TESTS

The first school hearing surveys were conducted in 1927 with a group test devised by Dr. Harvey Fletcher of the Bell Telephone Laboratories and produced commercially by the Western Electric Company.[3] This test, designated the Western Electric 4A test, consisted of a phonograph record of spoken numbers which "faded" from 30 to − 3 dB. Popularly known as the "fading-numbers" or "group phonograph speech" test, it was used extensively for over twenty years and was succeeded by group forms of pure-tone tests. The primary advantage of a group test is that many more pupils can be tested by a single audiometrist. Also, the administration of a group test sometimes is simplified so that an audiometrist with a minimum of training can successfully operate it. The disadvantage of a group test is that it may sacrifice accuracy of testing in order to cover a wider population. The primary purpose of any hearing test is to identify individuals with hearing impairments. If a group test does not perform this function satisfactorily, it is a poor instrument.

The advantage of an individual test is that it is the most accurate means known of assessing the hearing of each individual. The disadvantage is that it is time-consuming, in comparison with the group test, and it requires an audiometrist who has skill in conducting individual tests of children. At the present time, almost all school testing is performed on an individual basis. Descriptions of the various group tests of the past were given in the previous editions of this book.

THE INDIVIDUAL SCREENING TEST

Most school districts prefer the individual type of screening examination because of its admittedly greater accuracy in discovering cases of hearing impairment. As was pointed out, the disadvantage of the individual method is the time it consumes; however, some people have speculated that because of the inadequacies of certain group tests in discovering cases of hearing impairment, the expense to the school district in the long run is greater with the group test than it would be to hire additional audiometrists to screen everyone individually.

[3] Aram Glorig and Marion Downs, "Introduction to Audiometry," in *Audiometry: Principles and Practices*, ed. Aram Glorig (Baltimore: Williams & Wilkins, 1965), p. 11.

A technique referred to as the "sweep" test has been devised to enable individual screening at a rapid rate. In the sweep test, the audiometrist sets the hearing-level dial of the audiometer at a fixed level, usually 20 or 25 dB (re ANSI-1969 calibration standards), and then "sweeps" from low through high frequencies, checking to see if the subject is responding at each frequency.

The 1960 conference on identification audiometry recommended that screening be performed at 1000, 2000, 4000, and 6000 Hz—and also at 500 Hz provided the test environment was sufficiently quiet. The conference recommended that a hearing level of 10 dB be employed for all frequencies except 4000 Hz. The recommended screening level for 4000 Hz was 20 dB, in recognition of the common occurrence of 4000-Hz "dips" considered to be insignificant.[4] Of course, these hearing levels were in reference to the ASA-1951 calibration standards. The corresponding hearing levels in reference to the ANSI-1969 calibration standards (for the Western Electric 705-A earphone) would be 20 dB at 1000, 2000, and 6000 Hz; and 25 dB at 500 and 4000 Hz. In other words, the new standard shifted audiometric zero by 10 dB at 1000, 2000, and 6000 Hz; by 15 dB at 500 Hz; but only by 5 dB at 4000 Hz. All these differences are approximations of the actual values, rounded to the nearest 5-dB step. The actual values are given in Table 5-2 in Chapter 5. The choice of a 20-dB screening level for the speech frequencies was rationalized on the basis that in some situations, individuals with hearing levels of 25 dB have difficulty understanding speech. If screening is performed at a hearing level of 25 dB, a child with a 25-dB hearing level is passed. A 20-dB passing criterion would screen out children with 25-dB hearing levels for additional testing.

In 1974 the Legislative Council of ASHA approved a set of guidelines— published in 1975[5]—for identification audiometry that had been proposed by the ASHA Committee on Audiometric Evaluation. They recommend that screening be done on an individual basis rather than by a group test. The committee's reasons for rejecting group tests are that those requiring written responses are nonusable with younger children, group tests pose problems of calibration and maintenance of multiple earphones, and they require excessive time for setting up and for retesting "false positive" failures. The committee maintains that group testing does not necessarily save time.

The ASHA guidelines specify that only three frequencies be used in screening: 1000, 2000, and 4000 Hz. The assumption is that the test environment will not be quiet enough to prevent masking of low frequencies, and so 500 Hz is not included. The committee eliminated 6000 Hz as a test frequency because of research evidence that this frequency produces too many failures,[6]

---

[4] Darley, ed., "Identification Audiometry," p. 31.

[5] "Guidelines for Identification Audiometry," *Asha* 17 (February 1975):94–99.

[6] William Melnick, Eldon L. Eagles, and Herbert S. Levine, "Evaluation of a Recommended Program of Identification Audiometry with School-Age Children," *Journal of Speech and Hearing Disorders* 29 (February 1964):3–13.

often because of "variable interactions between earphones and ears."[7] The guidelines recommend levels of 20 dB at 1000 and 2000 Hz and 25 dB at 4000 Hz (re ANSI-1969). When the differences in the 1951 and 1969 standards for audiometer calibration are taken into account, these screening levels are the same as those recommended by the 1960 conference on identification audiometry.

The audiometrist should take precautions to see that the subject is responding accurately. If the interrupter switch is used at each frequency, the validity of the subject's responses can be checked. The audiometrist should instruct the child to raise a finger when a tone is heard and lower it when the tone goes away. Although the prescribed hearing level for 4000 Hz is 25 dB, the audiometrist can save time by checking all three frequencies at the 20-dB hearing level. Then, only if the child does not respond at 20 dB at 4000 Hz will it be necessary to check at 25 dB. In beginning the test, the frequency control is set at 1000 Hz and the hearing-level control at 30 dB (so that the initial stimulus will be more clearly audible). The ear-selector switch is on "right ear." A tone is presented and left on until the child responds. If there is no immediate response, the interrupter is released, the hearing level is increased to 40 dB, and the tone is presented again. As soon as the child responds, the examiner releases the interrupter switch. The hearing-level control is then set at 20 dB, and the tone is presented again. The child's finger should be raised. Leaving the tone on, the examiner switches to 2000 Hz. The child's finger should remain raised. Now the interrupter is released, and the finger should lower. The examiner switches to 4000 Hz and depresses the interrupter. The finger should be raised. Leaving the tone on, the examiner switches to the left ear, with the frequency control still at 4000 Hz and the hearing-level control at 20 dB. The finger should remain up. The examiner then follows the same sequence of events for all three test frequencies in descending order in the left ear. The test ends with the frequency control back at 1000 Hz, and the examiner is ready for the next child.

Using this technique, a competent examiner should be able to screen at least thirty children an hour. In the interest of most efficient use of time, three children should be watching the testing procedure. Besides providing a steady flow of testees, this step minimizes the instructions required, because each child observes the tests of three children before his or her turn arrives.

In the sweep test, the audiometrist is interested in knowing whether or not a given pupil can hear at the screening level. If the pupil does not respond at the appropriate hearing level at any one of the frequencies screened, the child fails the sweep test and must be retested later with an individual threshold test, as described in Chapter 5. The ASHA guidelines specify that a child who fails the screening test must be rescreened, preferably on the same

---

[7] "Guidelines for Identification Audiometry," p. 96; E. Villchur, "Audiometer-Earphone Mounting to Improve Intersubject and Cushion-Fit Reliability," *Journal of the Acoustical Society of America* 48 (1970):1387–96.

day but at least within a week of the original test, before being referred for a threshold audiogram.[8] Wilson and Walton reported that rescreening reduced the number of failures by more than half, presumably because during the first test the earphones were not fitted properly or the child did not understand the examiner's instructions.[9] Other reasons why a child might pass the second screening after failing the first are apprehension during the first test; a cold or other respiratory condition that reduced hearing sensitivity on the initial screening (assuming that several days elapsed between the two screening tests); or the fact that hearing sensitivity actually might be on the borderline of normal, so that a very slight shift of threshold for whatever reason—perhaps just a matter of concentration or attention—could move the child from the "fail" to the "pass" group. Some audiometrists prefer to do the threshold test immediately upon discovering a pupil who fails the second sweep test. This step interrupts the steady flow of subjects to the test room, however, and thus decreases the efficiency of the procedure. Incidentally, although we have talked about "passing" and "failing" the screening test—and there are no good substitutes for these words—it is unwise to use the word "fail" in reporting the results of hearing tests to children or their parents because of the stigma attached to failure in any form.

FOLLOW-UP OF THE SCHOOL TESTS

The success of a hearing conservation program depends on the adequacy of medical and educational follow-up of pupils discovered to have "medically significant" hearing impairments. What is meant by this term? It was used in a classic monograph by Newhart and Reger that for many years was the "Bible" of school hearing conservation programs. Newhart and Reger said that a "hearing loss probably is of medical significance" if the impairment in either ear is at least 20 dB (re ASA-1951) for two or more frequencies. If the testing was performed in "an exceedingly quiet location," an impairment of 15 dB at two frequencies would constitute a medically significant loss.[10]

The 1960 conference on identification audiometry recommended that the same criteria that constitute failure of a screening test should be applied for referring a child for an otological examination. In terms of the ASHA guidelines, inability of either ear to hear 1000 or 2000 Hz at a hearing level of

[8] "Guidelines for Identification Audiometry," p. 96.

[9] W. Wilson and W. Walton, "Identification Audiometry Accuracy: Evaluation of a Recommended Program for School-Age Children," *Language, Speech, and Hearing Services in the Schools* 5 (1974):132–42.

[10] Horace Newhart and Scott N. Reger, "Syllabus of Audiometric Procedures in the Administration of a Program for the Conservation of Hearing of School Children," Supplement to the *Transactions of the American Academy of Ophthalmology and Otolaryngology* (April 1945):17, 18.

20 dB, or 4000 Hz at 25 dB, constitutes a failure of the screening test. A child who fails two screening tests is referred for a threshold audiogram. If the threshold audiogram confirms the validity of the screening test, the child should be referred for an otological examination. In other words, a "medically significant" impairment consists of hearing threshold levels of 25 dB or more at 1000 or 2000 Hz, or 30 dB or more at 4000 Hz. Because a threshold test includes frequencies other than those specified by the ASHA guidelines for screening, it is possible—though highly unlikely—that 1000, 2000, and 4000 Hz could be within the limits of passing and that some other frequency would have a threshold of 25 dB or greater. In this event, we can refer to the definition of the conference on identification audiometry of medically significant hearing impairment as HTLs of 25 dB or more at 1000, 2000, and 6000 Hz, or 30 dB or more at 500 or 4000 Hz (recommendations of the conference corrected to ANSI-1969 calibration standards for the Western Electric 705-A earphone). The conference's suggested levels have been generally well accepted over the years,[11] although Melnick, Eagles, and Levine recommended on the basis of their analysis of the frequencies most often failed that the same level be used for 6000 Hz as for 500 and 4000 Hz.[12]

If possible, bone-conduction tests with masking when appropriate should be given to all those pupils who have medically significant losses by air conduction. The comparison of air- and bone-conduction hearing levels on the school audiogram will assist the otologist to a diagnosis of a given pupil's hearing impairment. It is recognized that not all school districts will be equipped or have adequately trained personnel available to perform bone-conduction testing, in which case the audiogram will contain air-conduction HTLs only.

Experience has demonstrated that many schoolchildren have losses of 30 dB or more at only 4000 or 6000 Hz. Almost invariably, an otologist who examines children with this type of high-frequency loss finds no demonstrable pathology and nothing in the child's history of significance. Many otologists feel that such high-frequency losses are congenital and static (not progressive). The success of a hearing conservation program depends on securing the cooperation of the examining otologist. It may be advisable, therefore, for the school audiometrist to assign priorities to the pupils identified as having "significant" hearing impairments. Those with losses only at 4000 *or* 6000 Hz would be given the lowest priority. Thus, the otologist can decide whether or not individual examinations should be given to each of the pupils in the low-

---

[11] Marion P. Downs, Mildred E. Doster, and Marlin Weaver, "Dilemmas in Identification Audiometry," *Journal of Speech and Hearing Disorders* 30 (November 1965):360–64; Harold J. Weber, Frank J. McGovern, and David Zink, "An Evaluation of 1000 Children with Hearing Loss," *Journal of Speech and Hearing Disorders* 32 (November 1967):343–54.

[12] Melnick, Eagles, and Levine, "Evaluation of a Recommended Program of Audiometry," pp. 3–13.

priority group. Highest priority would be assigned to those who have a significant loss at any of the speech frequencies (500, 1000, or 2000 Hz). The next priority would include those children who have losses at *both* 4000 and 6000 Hz. Regardless of priority, all children who are found to have a medically significant loss should be retested in the schools at intervals of no greater than a year. Only by comparing the results of successive tests can it be determined whether a given loss is static or changing.

The purpose of identification audiometry is to discover cases of medically significant hearing impairment so that appropriate medical and/or educational follow-up procedures can be instituted. It would be nice if all those children who have otologically abnormal ears could also be identified, but unfortunately that is not the case. School hearing tests alone identify very few of the otologically abnormal ears in a school population, as has been demonstrated by Eagles and by Eagles and Wishik, reporting on a study in Pittsburgh under the sponsorship of the American Academy of Ophthalmology and Otolaryngology and the Graduate School of Public Health at the University of Pittsburgh. All children in the study were given an otological examination in addition to a hearing test. It was found that the median hearing levels of the otologically abnormal group varied by only 2 to 4 dB from the median hearing levels of the normal group. If only the speech frequencies are considered, 90 percent of the children in the otologically abnormal group could pass a screening test at the 15 dB level (re ASA-1951)—about 25 dB (re ANSI-1969).[13] Because so many of the otologically abnormal children have hearing levels within the range of normal, they could not be screened out by any hearing test, although many of them could be identified by immittance screening. The popularity of immittance testing in clinical audiological procedures, particularly in the identification of conductive pathologies, led to experimentation with the technique as a screening procedure. Several investigators reported on the comparative efficiency of immittance and audiometric screening in identifying ears that are otoscopically abnormal, with the not-surprising conclusion that the agreement between immittance screening and otoscopic examination results was much greater. Cooper et al., for example, reported 75 percent agreement between immittance screening and otoscopy, compared with 47 percent agreement between audiometric screening and otoscopy.[14] Some audiologists are so enthusiastic about immittance screening that they advocate its use in place of audiometric screening, but

[13] Eldon L. Eagles, "Hearing Levels in Children and Implications for Identification Audiometry," in "Identification Audiometry," ed. Darley, Appendix B, pp. 52–62; Eldon L. Eagles and Samuel M. Wishik, "A Study of Hearing in Children. I. Objectives and Preliminary Findings," *Transactions of the American Academy of Ophthalmology and Otolaryngology* (May-June 1961), pp. 261–82.

[14] J. C. Cooper, Jr., George A. Gates, Jeffrey H. Owen, and Harold D. Dickson, "An Abbreviated Impedance Bridge Technique for School Screening," *Journal of Speech and Hearing Disorders* 40 (May 1975):264.

most believe in a combined immittance and audiometric approach. Lamb and Dunckel suggest audiometric screening at 4000 Hz combined with tympanometry and acoustic reflex testing at 1000 Hz. They say, "Screening with pure tones at 4000 Hz usually will serve to identify meaningful sensori-neural problems while the combination of tympanometry and acoustic reflex tests will identify most middle ear problems, even those that may elude detection by otoscopic examination."[15] Much of the disagreement that occurs between immittance screening and otoscopic examination results occurs because tympanometry is sensitive to the beginning stages of otitis media before changes in the ear can be detected by otoscopy. Generally, failure of the immittance screen test is defined as a negative pressure in excess of -100 mmH$_2$O or absence of a reflex at 1000 Hz at 100 or 110 dB hearing level. Manufacturers are now producing equipment for combined immittance and pure-tone screening, and we can anticipate increasing interest in immittance testing in hearing conservation screening programs.

Medical Follow-up

All pupils found to have medically significant losses on the basis of the threshold test following the screening procedure should be referred for a medical follow-up. Many school systems, in cooperation with the crippled children services of the state department of health, conduct periodic otological clinics for children who have failed the school hearing test. As was stated, maximum otological cooperation can be achieved by grouping pupils who have failed the hearing test in terms of the priority of their hearing losses. The otologist can thus give attention first to pupils who have losses that might interfere with their ability to communicate. The duty of the examining otologist is to determine whether there is any condition of the ear or any significant information in the medical history of the child that could account for a hearing loss. The examining otologist thus makes a diagnosis and recommends treatment if the hearing loss is one that could be helped through medical or surgical care.

In one follow-up of 1000 pupils who were found to have medically significant hearing losses, 43 percent were diagnosed as conductive losses, 23 percent as sensori-neural losses exclusive of 4000 Hz "drop-off," and 34 percent were individuals whose only significant loss was at 4000 Hz. Through age eleven, the greatest number of impairments were conductive, with the highest incidence in the age group of six to seven. Beginning at age twelve, the 4000 Hz drop-off constituted the greatest number of cases, with the highest incidence at the oldest age group—sixteen and older. In the group of medi-

[15] Lloyd E. Lamb and D. Craig Dunckel, "Acoustic Impedance Measurement with Children," in *Acoustic Impedance & Admittance—the Measurement of Middle Ear Function,* eds. Alan S. Feldman and Laura Ann Wilber (Baltimore: Williams & Wilkins, 1976), chap. 8, p. 190.

cally significant losses as a whole, 62 percent were male and 38 percent were female.[16]

The findings of the examining otologist are recorded on the pupil's health record. These findings and recommendations are transmitted by the school to the pupil's parents. The parents are urged to take their child to their own family physician. If the parents are financially unable to provide the medical or surgical care that has been recommended, the crippled children services can assume this responsibility also.

The medical follow-up of a child discovered to have hearing impairment should include examinations by the examining otologist after the child has received medical or surgical care, so that the otologist can determine the effectiveness of the treatment. Audiometric tests should be administered before reexamination by the otologist, as the effectiveness of the treatment may be demonstrated by an improvement in the child's hearing. The value of the medical follow-up of children discovered to have significant hearing losses is demonstrated in a report indicating that 34 percent of the children who received treatment after their failure of the school tests demonstrated on subsequent tests a return to normal levels of hearing.[17] "Treatment" was defined as having included at least one known visit to a physician. Many children taken to a physician by their parents were found to have permanent and irreversible hearing losses. If these children are not considered in the statistics, 57 percent of those who received medical "treatment" demonstrated a return to normal levels of hearing. By contrast, only 18 percent of the children who did not receive medical "treatment" showed an improvement in hearing to normal levels on subsequent tests.

Educational Follow-up

As stated, the effectiveness of a school hearing conservation program is directly related to the thoroughness with which the follow-up program is conducted. In the otological examination, pupils whose hearing might be improved through medical or surgical care are identified, and provision is made to give them appropriate treatment. Many children with discovered hearing impairment have a loss that is irreversible even with medical care. In other words, these children will have congenital losses of a sensori-neural type, sensori-neural losses through adventitious causes, or static impairments due to previous middle-ear pathology. The otologist can make no medical recommendations, since the child has a permanent and irremediable type of impairment. This pupil then becomes the concern of the schools, which must provide

[16] Weber, McGovern, and Zink, "Evaluation of 1000 Children," pp. 344–46.

[17] Robert M. Cameron, "Summary of Hearing Conservation Program for 1955–1956 School Year," unpublished report submitted to the Palo Alto, California, Unified School District, 1956.

whatever education is required to help overcome or minimize the hearing handicap.

Naturally, the type of educational program planned will depend on the nature and degree of hearing impairment that an individual child demonstrates. The need for amplification should be considered. It may be that the child would benefit from having a wearable hearing aid. Or even though amplification may not be required, the child may benefit from some instruction in speechreading. Children with permanent hearing impairments may also have speech problems, and so they may need to be enrolled in a speech-therapy program. Even though a particular child may not have a speech problem at the time the hearing loss is discovered, it is possible that with the passage of time speech will deteriorate unless "preventive speech therapy" is given.

It is doubtful that children will be discovered in the public school system with such profound hearing impairments as would necessitate placement in a class for the deaf. Such children would be so obviously handicapped that they would be known without a hearing conservation program. It is possible, however, that a child may be discovered to have a mild hearing impairment of a progressive nature, and in a few years' time become so profoundly impaired that placement in a special class for the deaf would be necessary. The educational follow-up program in the schools, therefore, should include periodic audiometric examinations for all pupils who have a hearing loss. It is only through the follow-up tests that the progressive type of hearing impairment can be discovered.

In addition to providing special educational services for the child who is hard of hearing, the schools have the responsibility of informing parents of the extent of the handicap that their child has and helping them to assist their child. Some parents are completely upset at the discovery that they have a child with a hearing impairment. The schools and the physician must interpret the meaning of a specific hearing loss and counsel the parents on what can and cannot be done to help the child. The subject of parental counseling, as well as other aspects of the training of hearing-impaired children, will be discussed further in Chapter 11.

FUNCTIONAL HEARING PROBLEMS IN CHILDREN

Considerable attention has been focused on a very interesting clinical finding: the child who manifests a functional or nonorganic hearing problem. Juers was one of the first clinicians to refer to the existence of this problem.[18] Articles on the subject have appeared by audiologists working in clinical settings to which

[18] Arthur L. Juers, "Pure Tone Threshold and Hearing for Speech—Diagnostic Significance of Inconsistencies," *Laryngoscope* 66 (April 1956):402–409.

many children who fail school audiometric tests are referred for further evaluation.[19]

In a typical case of a functional hearing problem, the child will not have been suspected by parents or teachers of having a hearing impairment until a school hearing test is failed. Usually, an examination will be performed by a physician after the parents have been notified by the school that their child has a hearing impairment. If a hearing test is performed in the physician's office, generally the child will exhibit a bilateral hearing "loss" with air- and bone-conduction hearing levels of from 40 to 60 dB. The physician may or may not suspect the authenticity of the audiogram. In any event, the otological examination is negative in its findings, although there may be a history suggesting previous disease of the middle ear, and the physician refers the child to a hearing center or clinic for a complete hearing evaluation. Not infrequently, the referral will be for the purpose of selecting a hearing aid.

When interviewed by the examining audiologist, it will usually be noted that the child follows normal conversation. This observation is, of course, inconsistent with the degree of loss the child has shown on previous tests and should immediately alert the examiner to the possibility of a functional hearing problem. If the examiner were to start the evaluation with a pure-tone test, in all probability that audiogram would agree substantially with the ones obtained at school and in the physician's office. When the presence of a functional hearing problem is suspected, the examiner would be well-advised to commence the evaluation with the speech audiometer, monaurally with live voice. Best results will ordinarily be obtained with an ascending technique, that is, starting with the hearing-level control at minimum intensity and increasing intensity until the child responds.

The examiner may start the evaluation by asking the child casual questions or conversing on a subject that will be of interest to the child, for example, pets, sports, or television programs. If the child responds to the examiner's

---

[19] Robert L. Berk and Alan S. Feldman, "Functional Hearing Loss in Children," *New England Journal of Medicine* 259 (July 1958):214–16; Richard F. Dixon and Hayes A. Newby, "Children with Nonorganic Hearing Problems," A.M.A. *Archives of Otolaryngology* 70 (November 1959):619–23; Bengt Barr, "Nonorganic Hearing Problems in School-Children," *Acta Otolaryngologica* 52 (1960):337–46; Seymour J. Brockman and Gloria H. Holversten, "Pseudo Neural Hypacusis in Children," *Laryngoscope* 70 (June 1960):825–39; George J. Leshin, "Childhood Nonorganic Hearing Loss," *Journal of Speech and Hearing Disorders* 25 (August 1960):290–92; Donald R. Calvert, John P. Moncur, D. Wayne Smith, and Jack Synder, "Nonorganic Hearing Loss in School-Age Children," *The Voice* (The Journal of the California Speech and Hearing Association) 10 (November 1961):6–11; William Rintelmann and Earl Harford, "The Detection and Assessment of Pseudohypoacusis Among School-Age Children," *Journal of Speech and Hearing Disorders* 28 (May 1963):141–52; John L. Peterson, "Nonorganic Hearing Loss in Children and Békésy Audiometry," *Journal of Speech and Hearing Disorders* 28 (May 1963):153–58; Peter A. Campanelli, "Simulated Hearing Losses in School Children Following Identification Audiometry," *Journal of Auditory Research* 3 (1963):91–108.

questions in each ear at zero or near zero-dB hearing level, a more formal speech-reception threshold can be obtained, using spondee words. If no response occurs to the spondee words immediately, the examiner should "coax" a response from the child. It may be necessary to urge the child to respond on almost every word. Usually, SRTs within the range of normal can be established by using a combination of informal conversation and spondee words. Once an SRT has been established in each ear, the examiner should perform speech discrimination tests with PB word lists in each ear. Typically, the child will exhibit excellent speech discrimination at suprathreshold levels with no urging from the examiner.

Once the examiner has established SRT and obtained a discrimination score in each ear, a pure-tone evaluation is begun. It is best for the examiner to remain outside the test room, assuming that the equipment permits remote pure-tone testing. Before commencing the pure-tone test, the examiner should make sure that the child understands what to listen for and how to respond. It is probably best to make no mention to the child of the results of earlier tests at school or elsewhere. The examiner then proceeds to establish pure-tone thresholds in the conventional way. If the child fails to respond at levels consistent with performance in speech audiometry, the examiner should stop the test, inform the child that apparently the directions were misunderstood, and emphasize the necessity of the child's responding just as soon as the child is aware of the presence of the tone. The examiner may decide to present the tone in pulses and have the child report the number of pulses in each presentation. Perhaps because this is a new kind of task, the child may respond at appropriate hearing levels. Ross cautions that the emphasis should be on the counting task rather than on hearing, and he suggests alternating intensities above and below the child's admitted thresholds. Of course, any responses "below" threshold establish new threshold hearing levels.[20] Incidentally, the technique of having the child report the number of pulses may be successful even if they are not reported correctly. Sometimes, the child will consistently respond with the incorrect number after a series of pulses has been presented but always at the appropriate time. Sometimes, a child will respond "no" or "none" each time a series of tones is present, and it is possible to obtain reliable threshold measurements based on negative responses.

In most cases, by utilizing unusual techniques when necessary, the examiner can obtain pure-tone threshold measurements that agree well with the previously established speech thresholds. Only rarely is it necessary to employ neurophysiological techniques to establish thresholds. It is important that the examiner always treat the child with dignity and respect and give the child an

[20] Mark Ross, "The Variable Intensity Pulse Count Method (VIPCM) for the Detection and Measurement of the Pure-Tone Thresholds of Children with Functional Hearing Losses," *Journal of Speech and Hearing Disorders* 29 (November 1964):477–82.

opportunity to perform in a manner consistent with actual hearing levels without suffering "loss of face." In other words, the examiner must avoid giving the impression that the child is being accused of attempting to deceive the examiner.

Although occasionally it is obvious that a particular child who manifests a functional hearing problem is emotionally disturbed, in most instances there is no apparent reason for the child to exhibit atypical auditory behavior, and indeed it is only in a test that there is any indication of abnormal hearing. Reporting on their experiences with forty children found to have functional hearing problems, Dixon and Newby said,

> Most of the children seemed to be performing well academically, to be intellectually normal, and were without noticeable emotional disturbances. Nine children displayed symptoms which might be related to their "hearing problem." These symptoms included functional articulatory speech disorders, and—according to parent reports—strong sibling rivalry, persistent enuresis, anxiety reactions, possible nonorganic visual difficulties, and lack of satisfactory academic progress. It should be reemphasized, however, that children with any symptoms or history of psychological significance were definitely in the minority—less than 25 per cent of the total group. On the basis of our own observations, we cannot state why these children performed as they did on hearing tests.[21]

As stated earlier, the first clue an examiner obtains that a child may be exhibiting a functional hearing problem is that the ability to follow ordinary conversation is inconsistent with the degree of impairment demonstrated in tests. School audiometrists should be aware of discrepancies between a child's auditory behavior and test results. Too frequently, however, there is a tendency for those associated with the child to assume the validity of an audiometric test and to ignore the evidence of their own observation. It is not unusual to find that educational decisions of considerable importance to a child's future may be based on erroneous audiometric results. In the group of forty children studied by Dixon and Newby, fourteen were receiving instruction in speechreading, were receiving auditory training, or had been given preferential seating in the classroom; two were in special classes for the hard of hearing; one was in a class for the deaf; and one had been furnished with a hearing aid. All these children were found to have normal hearing.[22] The lesson to be learned from such experiences is that audiometrists, and others concerned with planning a child's educational program, must not place blind dependence on the results of an audiometric test when a child's behavior belies the evidence of the audiogram.

[21] Dixon and Newby, "Children with Nonorganic Hearing Problems," p. 620.
[22] Ibid.

CHAPTER NINE
INDUSTRIAL AUDIOLOGY

As we saw in Chapter 3, one of the causes of sensori-neural hearing impairment is exposure to noise. In our modern industrialized civilization, hardly anyone can escape some exposure to noise. Even the farmer, who traditionally is associated with the quiet environment of the wide open spaces, employs mechanized labor-saving devices that are noise producing and thus potentially damaging to hearing. The term *presbycusis* refers to the gradually increasing loss of hearing sensitivity associated with increasing age. It is quite possible that our daily exposure to just ordinary environmental noises contributes substantially to the "aging" of our hearing mechanism. There is evidence to suggest that primitive tribesmen in Africa who are completely removed from the noises of our modern civilization do not show any appreciable decrease in hearing sensitivity with advancing age.[1] Glorig has suggested that a better word to describe the progressive loss of hearing associated with increasing age would be "sociocusis"—the loss of hearing sensitivity because of all the hazards of living in our modern society, disease, and noise exposure as well as

[1] Samuel Rosen, Moe Bergman, Dietrich Plester, Aly El-Mofty, and Mohamed Hamad Satti, "Presbycusis Study of a Relatively Noise-Free Population in the Sudan," *Annals of Otology, Rhinology, and Laryngology* 71 (September 1962):727–43.

aging.[2] As noise becomes an increasingly important problem in our modern civilization, the control of noise and protection of the individual from damage as the result of exposure to noise become increasingly important. A variety of professional skills is required to deal with all the facets of noise control and hearing conservation. Included among the specialists whose skills are brought to bear on these problems are the expert in acoustics, industrial engineer, architect, industrial hygienist, safety engineer, industrial physician, otologist, and audiologist. This chapter will deal with the complexities of the problems created by noise, particularly in the context of industry, and the means to control these problems.

NOISE-INDUCED HEARING LOSS

Noise may cause a sudden hearing loss, as in the case of a blast or explosion that may rupture the tympanic membrane and also "jar loose" some of the hair cells of the organ of Corti in the cochlea; or noise may exert an insidious long-term effect on the hair cells that produces a gradually increasing hearing loss. The sudden loss of hearing from noise is called *acoustic trauma*; the gradual diminution of hearing sensitivity associated with noise exposure is referred to as *noise-induced hearing loss*. The amount of hearing loss incurred from noise exposure is proportional to the intensity of the stimulus and the length of the exposure. Also, there is the matter of individual susceptibility to consider. People differ considerably in their ability to withstand noise.

From animal experiments, it has been determined that the sensorineural loss associated with noise exposure is cochlear in origin. Confirmation of this conclusion comes from recruitment studies of humans who have incurred noise-induced hearing impairment. Typically, such individuals will demonstrate recruitment at the affected frequencies in loudness-balance tests or will yield SISI scores that are characteristic of cochlear involvement. Usually, the individual exposed to noise will manifest initially a "dip" or "notch" centered around 4000 Hz on the pure-tone audiogram. In its beginning stages, noise-induced hearing loss is reversible; that is, if the individual is removed from the noisy environment, hearing sensitivity will gradually improve until it reaches the pre-exposure level. For example, a worker tested on Friday evening after five days of on-the-job exposure to industrial noise may evidence a notch of 10 dB at 3000 Hz, 20 dB at 4000 Hz, and 10 dB at 6000 Hz, with all other frequencies at the zero-dB hearing level. After a weekend away from the noisy environment, this same worker may yield an audiogram on Monday

[2] Aram Glorig, Jr., *Noise and Your Ear* (New York: Grune & Stratton, 1958), p. 141. See also Alexander Cohen, Joseph Anticaglia, and Herbert H. Jones, " 'Sociocusis'—Hearing Loss from Non-Occupational Noise Exposure," *Sound and Vibration* 4 (November 1970):12–20.

morning that shows zero-dB hearing level at all the audiometric frequencies. The presumed explanation for this finding is that certain of the hair cells responsible for the reception of the frequencies from 3000 through 6000 Hz have not been destroyed or irreparably damaged by the noise exposure but have been "fatigued," and with rest they can recover their normal function. The results of fatigue we refer to as *temporary threshold shift,* abbreviated *TTS.* TTS can be demonstrated in the laboratory by presenting an ear with a fatiguing stimulus for as short a period as ten to fifteen minutes.

Now let us return to the example of the worker who demonstrated TTS at the end of a week of exposure to industrial noise. On a Monday morning, hearing sensitivity is back to its normal level. But then after another week in noisy work, on Friday night the audiogram shows a notch. Perhaps by the following Monday morning hearing sensitivity will be back to its normal level. If, however, this procedure is repeated for many weeks and months, there will come a time when even after a weekend of rest the worker's hearing at the affected frequencies will not quite return to its former level. With succeeding months of continued noise exposure, the worker will demonstrate on Friday evening audiograms a deepening and widening notch. Perhaps the audiogram will show levels of 10 dB at 2000 Hz, 20 dB at 3000 Hz, 40 dB at 4000 Hz, 20 dB at 6000 Hz, and 10 dB at 8000 Hz. On Monday morning, it may be found that instead of returning to zero dB at all frequencies, hearing levels are 10 dB at 3000 Hz, 20 dB at 4000 Hz, and 10 dB at 6000 Hz. In other words, this worker is now demonstrating some "permanent" noise-induced hearing loss in addition to a TTS. The word "permanent" is enclosed in quotation marks because it is possible that if this worker were removed from the noisy work environment for a period of several weeks or months, hearing sensitivity might gradually return to its former levels. On the other hand, it might not. One thing is sure: If this hypothetical worker remains in a noisy job for a period of several years, the degree of permanent hearing loss will increase both in the depth and width of the notch until the speech frequencies are affected and the worker is in fact hard of hearing. Figure 9–1 demonstrates a typical progression in hearing loss due to noise exposure with the passage of time.

What is particularly insidious about noise-induced hearing loss is that it can occur without the affected individual's being aware of it. As we saw in Chapter 2, sound does not become uncomfortably loud for most people until it reaches a sound-pressure level of 120 dB, and it does not produce pain until the sound-pressure level reaches at least 140 dB. Unfortunately, sound-pressure levels of considerably less than 120 dB can produce permanent damage to the ear in time. No one would endure sound-pressure levels in excess of 120 dB for long because of the discomfort, but we might be willing to work indefinitely in noise levels of 95 to 100 dB without suspecting that the noise was damaging us in any way.

Another way in which noise-induced hearing loss is insidious is that

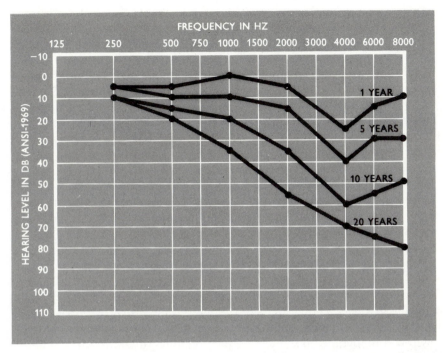

FIGURE 9-1.   Typical progression in hearing loss as a function of years of exposure to industrial noise of high intensity. Both ears would be affected similarly.

almost invariably the first evidence of damage to the ears is found in the frequencies above the speech range. Often, one can incur a substantial loss at frequencies above 2000 Hz without being aware of any difficulty in communication under good listening conditions. Only when the notch widens to include 2000 Hz is there usually any noticeable effect on our hearing for speech. Most people would not complain of being hard of hearing until there is some noticeable effect on their understanding of speech. By the time 2000 Hz is involved, there may be a considerable degree of permanent noise-induced hearing loss in the higher frequencies.

In advanced stages, noise-induced hearing loss may produce a sharply sloping audiogram curve for frequencies above 500 Hz. Although initially there is a notch effect, with the greatest loss somewhere between 3000 and 6000 Hz, in time the notch tends to become obliterated, so that the audiogram of the individual with noise-induced hearing loss becomes indistinguishable from other sensori-neural losses. Thus, the individual with noise-induced hearing loss that extends into the speech frequencies has problems in communication that are characteristic of those with typical sensori-neural impairment— primarily problems of speech discrimination.

THE MEDICOLEGAL PROBLEM

History

Following the lead of several European countries, the United States in 1908 enacted the first workmen's compensation law under which civilian employees of the federal government were protected against economic loss arising out of accidental injuries incurred on the job. By 1915, some thirty states had formulated workmen's compensation laws, and by 1949 all the states had done so.[3] Originally, compensation laws covered only accidental injuries, but subsequently the laws of most states were expanded to include occupational disease. In some states, these diseases were specified in "schedules"; in other states, the coverage was expanded to include any occupational disease that the claimant could prove was caused by employment. In order to qualify for awards under either the accidental injury or occupational disease provision of workmen's compensation, a claimant had to establish a loss of earnings.

When a loss of hearing is associated with a blast or single traumatic incident, it is clearly covered under the accidental injury provision of workmen's compensation. In cases involving the gradual onset of hearing impairment associated with one's occupation, the occupational disease provision would be applicable in those states where the definition of occupational disease is sufficiently broad to include noise-induced hearing impairment. In some states, a ruling has been made that a gradual hearing impairment associated with one's occupation is actually a series of separate "accidents," the effect of which is cumulative, so that such a noise-induced hearing impairment is held to be an accidental injury or "traumatic incident."

In 1948, a new principle in workmen's compensation was established through a ruling of the New York Court of Appeals by which compensation for a noise-induced hearing loss was awarded to a claimant who had not lost any time from a job and had thus demonstrated no loss of earnings. This decision resulted in the filing of many claims in New York State for noise-induced hearing impairment.[4] In the early 1950s a similar decision was rendered in Wisconsin. In both New York and Wisconsin, special legislation was enacted to establish a basis for compensating employees for occupational loss of hearing, rather than depending on the broad coverage provided by the laws relating to occupational diseases in general. In 1959, the State of Missouri followed the lead of New York and Wisconsin. Now in all but nine states there are legislative provisions for compensation for partial occupational hearing loss.[5] In general, the legislation that has been enacted by other states

[3] Harry A. Nelson, "Legal Liability for Loss of Hearing," in *Handbook of Noise Control,* ed. Cyril M. Harris (New York: McGraw-Hill, 1957), chap. 38, p. 4.

[4] Charles R. Williams, "Medicolegal Aspects," in *Industrial Deafness,* ed. Joseph Sataloff (New York: McGraw-Hill, 1957), chap. 5, p. 53.

[5] Jack Shampan and Richard Ginnold, "The Status of Workers' Compensation

recognizes the principles of compensation established in New York, Wisconsin, and Missouri. Let us, therefore, examine briefly the provisions of the laws of these three states.

Provisions of the Law in New York, Wisconsin, and Missouri[6]

In all three states, noise-induced hearing loss is considered to be an occupational disease, and a schedule of benefits is outlined. The principle that compensation is dependent on demonstrated wage loss is abandoned. In Wisconsin and Missouri, the new schedules reduce the amount of compensation payable for complete or partial loss of hearing in comparison to what the law provides in cases of traumatic hearing loss, but in New York no differentiation is made between the amount payable for occupational hearing loss and for traumatic hearing loss. In Wisconsin and Missouri, the "date of disablement" is considered to be the last day of a six-month period of separation from the noisy work that caused the hearing impairment; in New York, it is the last day of a six-month period following separation from the employment in which the noise exposure was received. In New York, in other words, there is no date of disability until the employee terminates the relationship with the employer. The purpose of the six-month waiting period is to allow for any recovery of hearing once the claimant has been removed from the noisy work environment. According to Symons, there is an additional advantage in the New York system because employers are encouraged to institute noise-control procedures without facing the danger that such procedures will focus workers' attention on noise problems and produce a flood of claims for noise-induced hearing loss.[7]

The laws hold the last employer liable for all of a claimant's noise-induced hearing impairment, unless that employer can present evidence that the employee had some hearing impairment at the time employment started. If it can be demonstrated that the claimant incurred some of the hearing impairment in previous jobs, those employers are held responsible for their "share" of the claimant's hearing impairment. This provision of the laws points up the importance of hearing testing as part of the physical examination procedure for all new employees. A given employer can then be held responsible for only that amount of hearing impairment an employee incurs after commencing work for that employer.

Programs for Occupational Hearing Impairment," in *Forensic Audiology*, eds. Marc Kramer and Joan Armbruster (Baltimore: University Park Press, 1982), chap. 14, pp. 286–89.

[6] *Background for Loss of Hearing Claims* (Chicago: American Mutual Insurance Alliance, 1964), pp. 1–7.

[7] Noel S. Symons, "Workmen's Compensation Benefits for Occupational Hearing Loss," *Noise Control* 4 (September 1958):29–30.

The states of New York, Wisconsin, and Missouri have all adopted the so-called AAOO method of computing percentage of hearing loss for purposes of determining degree of disability. It will be recalled from Chapter 5 that this method utilizes the average dB loss through the frequencies of 500, 1000, and 2000 Hz. As illustrated in Figure 5–13, the percentage loss in each ear is determined by subtracting 26 dB from the average dB loss through these three frequencies and then multiplying the remainder by 1½ percent. Binaural percentage hearing loss is computed by weighting the better ear five times the poorer ear.

A question that confronted the legislatures of the three states with which we are concerned was whether or not to make an allowance for presbycusis in determining an employer's liability for an employee's hearing impairment. In New York, no allowance is made for presbycusis. In Wisconsin, the practice for a number of years was to deduct from the percentage of compensable hearing loss ½ percent for each year of age over fifty. Wisconsin then changed its procedure and ceased to make any allowance for presbycusis. The Missouri law provides that before the percentage of hearing loss is determined, ½ dB for each year of age over forty shall be subtracted from the total average dB loss. The calculation is made on the basis of the employee's age at the time of the last exposure to industrial noise. In 1970, seventeen states made corrections for presbycusis, and in 1976 eleven states made corrections for presbycusis, based either on a formula, as in Missouri, or on medical evidence.[8]

Compensation for occupational hearing loss is usually expressed as so many weeks of a worker's salary as long as it does not exceed a statutory maximum. The stated number of weeks and maximum dollar amount of compensation is based on "total" loss of hearing. Compensation for less than a total hearing loss is computed on the actual percentage loss presented by a claimant. Thus, an employee found to have a 50 percent binaural loss of hearing would be entitled to half the compensation allowable for a total binaural loss. Among the states recognizing noise-induced hearing impairment, compensation for a total loss of hearing in both ears varies from two to six times the amount established for total loss of hearing in only one ear. For example, in Virginia in 1976, the compensation for total loss of hearing in both ears was 100 weeks, or a maximum of $16,200; the compensation for total loss in only one ear was 50 weeks, or a maximum of $8,100; in Wisconsin, the compensation for total loss of hearing in both ears was 216 weeks, or a maximum of $12,312, and the compensation for total loss in only one ear was 36 weeks, or a maximum of $2,052.[9]

The States of New York, Wisconsin, and Missouri led the way in legislation to provide compensation for occupational hearing loss. In all three, the

[8] Fox, "Hearing Loss Statutes."
[9] Ibid.

legislation enacted was the result of the cooperative efforts of labor, management, and medical and allied medical specialty groups, who joined to produce laws that were fair to both labor and industry and that were predicated on the best scientific information.

NOISE MEASUREMENTS

In order to determine whether or not an employer has a noise hazard, it is necessary to obtain accurate measurements of the noise levels at various locations within a factory. In addition to measurements of the overall sound level in a given location, it is necessary to have information concerning the spectral composition of the noise, because the danger of noise depends on both its intensity and frequency components. Noise measurements are made with an instrument called a *sound-level meter*, and spectral analyses are made with various kinds of analyzers.

The Sound-Level Meter

"A sound-level meter is an instrument including a microphone, an amplifier, an output meter, and frequency weighting networks for the measurement of noise and sound levels in a specified manner."[10] Measurements obtained with a sound-level meter are referred to as *sound levels*, which are weighted sound-pressure levels. The weighting networks provide three frequency-response characteristics, referred to as A, B, and C, the values of which are specified by the American National Standards Institute[11] (shown in Figure 9–2). The purpose of the weighting networks is to approximate the loudness function of the human ear at three different intensity levels. The A and B networks resemble equal loudness contours of the normal ear made at loudness levels of 40 and 70 phons, respectively. Network C provides a "flat" frequency response approximating the equal loudness contour at 100 phons. Readings obtained when the C network is employed and the meter is used with a flat response microphone are sound-pressure levels. Network A discriminates against low frequencies, and network B is intermediate in low-frequency weighting between A and C. Readings obtained with networks A and B are "sound levels" rather than sound-pressure levels. The weighting network employed in a particular sound-level measurement should always be specified. For example, if a reading of 50 dB were obtained when the A network was used, it should be reported as a sound level of 50 dB (A), or simply 50 dBA. Some manufacturers recommend that all three networks be

[10] "Psychoacoustical Terminology," *American National Standard,* ANSI S3.20-1973 (New York: American National Standards Institute), p. 49.

[11] "Specification for Sound Level Meters," *American National Standard,* ANSI S1.4-1971 (New York: American National Standards Institute).

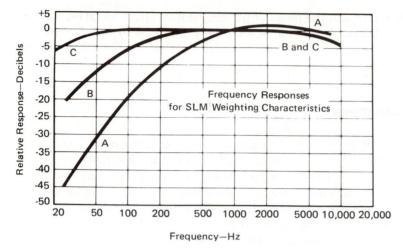

FIGURE 9-2. Frequency response of the weighting networks of sound-level meters. (From Arnold P. G. Peterson and Ervin E. Gross, Jr., *Handbook of Noise Measurement,* Concord, Mass.: General Radio, 1972, p. 8. Used by permission.)

used in measuring every noise. In the past, it was customary to use A weighting for levels below 55 dB, B weighting for levels between 55 and 85 dB, and C weighting for levels above 85 dB. Now, however, A weightings are most commonly used regardless of level.[12] Gross information about the frequency characteristics of the noise being measured may be secured by comparing the sound levels obtained by all three networks. If the readings are essentially the same, the noise is predominantly high frequency in spectrum; that is, its most prominent characteristics lie above 600 Hz. If lower sound-level readings are obtained with the A and B networks than with C, the noise is predominantly of low frequency. The greater the difference between the readings obtained with A and C networks, the more heavily weighted the noise is in the lower frequencies (below 600 Hz).[13] A typical sound-level meter is shown in Figure 9-3.

A sound-level meter is useful for measuring overall sound levels of continuing, or steady-state, noises. For measuring the levels of impulsive noises, such as a gunshot, it is necessary to use an impact-noise analyzer in conjunction with a sound-level meter. The meter response of the sound-level meter is too slow to give an accurate reading on an impulsive noise.

Noise Analyzers

The hazard of a particular noise usually cannot be determined without analyzing its frequency components. If a noise survey indicates that the

[12] Arnold P. G. Peterson and Ervin E. Gross, Jr., *Handbook of Noise Measurement* (Concord, Mass.: General Radio, 1972), p. 8.

[13] Charles R. Williams, "Principles of Noise Measurement," in *Industrial Deafness,* ed. Sataloff, chap. 7, p. 85.

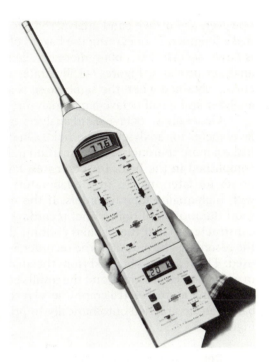

FIGURE 9-3.
A sound-level meter with attached filter set. (Courtesy of Bruel & Kjaer Instruments, Marlborough, Mass.)

overall sound levels obtained in a particular location are potentially hazardous, an analysis of the frequency components of the noise is in order. The most commonly used instrument for this purpose is an octave-band analyzer, which, as its name implies, measures the sound levels in various bands, each of which is one octave in width. When this instrument is used with the sound-level meter, the sound levels obtained in these bands are called octave-band levels. The "preferred" octave bands have center frequencies of 31.5, 63, 125, 250, 500, 1000, 2000, 4000, 8000, and 16000 Hz. Older octave-band analyzers included the following bands: 18.75–37.5, 37.5–75, 75–150, 150–300, 300–600, 600–1200, 1200–2400, 2400–4800, 4800–9600, and 9600–19200 Hz. Many test codes specify band levels in terms of the older bands, and considerable data have been reported based on the older series. Octave-band levels reported in the older series can be converted to octave-band levels based on the preferred center frequencies by referring to a table in the ANSI standard.[14] In Figure 9–3, the octave-band analyzer is attached to the sound-level meter.

In addition to the octave-band analyzer, other types of analyzers are available: half-octave and third-octave analyzers and continuously tunable narrow-band analyzers that accept a band of only $\frac{1}{30}$ octave in width. As the band width of an analyzer becomes narrower, the more precise is the information yielded about the frequency components of a noise. In general,

[14] "Specification for Octave, Half-Octave, and Third-Octave Band Filter Sets," ANSI S1.11-1966, R1971 (New York: American National Standards Institute).

however, the octave-band analyzer yields sufficiently precise information to make judgments concerning the hazard of a particular industrial noise, and it is rarely necessary to obtain more detailed information than the octave-band analyzer provides. Figure 9–4 illustrates the difference in the shape of the curves obtained when the same noise is analyzed with both an octave-band analyzer and a half-octave-band analyzer.

Generally an octave-band analyzer is used in conjunction with a sound-level meter for analyses in the field. On occasion, however, it is desirable to make a more thorough study of certain industrial noises than can easily be accomplished in the field. In such cases, tape recordings may be made of the noises for later analysis in the laboratory. Such recordings should be made with high-quality tape recorders. If the noise to be analyzed is of relatively short duration, or if only a brief recording has been made, a tape loop can be constructed so that the signal is continually passed over the playback head of the recorder. The output of the recorder is fed to the particular analyzer being used. The readings obtained from the analyzer can be recorded as the energy in each band is measured, and the results can then be plotted in the manner indicated in Figure 9–4. If a graphic level recorder is available, the energy in each band can be graphed automatically to produce the type of record shown in Figure 9–5.

Conducting a Noise Survey

Noise surveys are conducted usually for two basic reasons: to evaluate the hazard of noise for employees so that suitable protective measures may be taken to conserve hearing, and to obtain information concerning the noisiness of various pieces of machinery or manufacturing processes to improve design or the method of installation. In addition to constituting a hazard to hearing, noise may interfere with communication and have other annoying effects. Techniques have been evolved for translating the results of noise measurements into the subjective effects of the noise on exposed personnel, as we shall see later. In any event, a thorough study of the physical properties of noise is an essential first step to the development of a hearing conservation program or to noise-control procedures.

As Williams has said, noise measurement is an art, requiring not only technical proficiency in the handling of equipment but also a considerable amount of judgment in determining where measurements should be made and what kinds of analyses are indicated.[15] Noise measurements should be attempted only by individuals who are thoroughly acquainted with the uses and limitations of the equipment employed and who have an adequate background in the physical principles involved in noise measurement. The instructions contained in various technical manuals in regard to such matters as

[15] Charles R. Williams, "Principles of Noise Measurement," in *Industrial Deafness*, ed. Sataloff, chap. 7, p. 77.

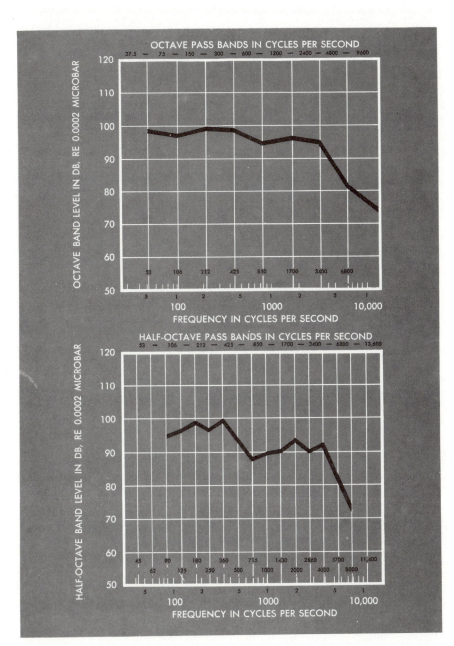

FIGURE 9-4.   Comparison of octave-band analysis and half-octave-band analysis of an industrial noise. (From Lewis S. Goodfriend, "Measurement of Noise," *Noise Control* 7, March-April 1961. Used by permission.)

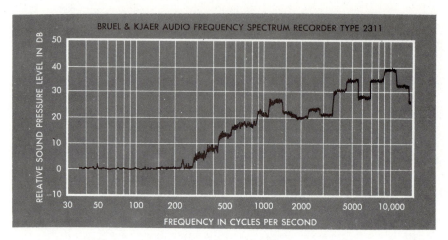

FIGURE 9-5.   Graphic record of one-third octave analysis of a stream of air. (Reproduced by permission of B & K Instruments, Inc., Marlborough, Mass.)

assessing the effect of background noise; choosing the right microphone and knowing what corrections must be made for it; and correcting measurements for cable length, the angle of incidence, and the effects of reflected sound are most bewildering to the novice. The validity of the measurements obtained is in direct proportion to the degree of knowledge on the part of the individual conducting a survey. It is not the purpose of this section to give detailed information concerning the use of measuring equipment, but rather to give the reader some appreciation of what is involved in conducting a noise survey.

The first step is to make sure that all equipment is calibrated and in proper working order. This determination in itself is no simple matter and requires an understanding not only of the particular instruments to be used but also of the physical principles involved in sound measurement. Once the equipment is found to be performing satisfactorily, the next step is to select the locations where measurements will be taken. This step is accomplished by obtaining rough measurements of the overall intensity at various positions around the noise to be evaluated. If the primary purpose of the survey is to assess the hazard to the hearing of the employees who work in the environment, the microphone placement should approximate the location of employees who work around the sound source. If the purpose of the survey is to derive the total acoustic power output and the directional characteristics of the noise, the measurements should be made in systematic geometric patterns around the source regardless of the location of the employees. In either event, the initial rough measurements of overall intensity may be made with the sound-level meter.

When the locations at which measurements are to be made have been selected, accurate readings of the overall levels at each location are taken with the sound-level meter. These locations should be plotted on a floor plan and clearly labeled, so that at some later time the measurements can be duplicated in the same locations. Once the overall sound levels have been recorded at each of the selected locations, the octave-band measurements should be made, or if the spectral analysis is to be accomplished later in the laboratory, tape recordings should be made at each location. The overall levels of the noise should be checked with the sound-level meter after the octave-band readings are obtained in order to make sure that the noise has not fluctuated appreciably since the time of the initial readings, and also as a check on the accuracy of the first readings. The accuracy of the octave-band analysis should be checked by adding the intensities in each band and comparing the total with the overall sound level obtained at a particular location. Octave-band levels may be added by using the chart of Figure 9–6, which enables one to determine the combined dB level of two or more sounds whose individual levels are known. For example, suppose there are two machines in a workspace, one of which produced a level of 84 dBA and the other a level of 82 dBA. To find their combined level, we enter the chart at 2 dB on the abscissa—the difference between the two levels we are combining. We then read 2.1 dB on the ordinate opposite the point where the 2 dB vertical line intersects with the curve, which means that the combined level is 84 plus 2.1, or 86.1 dBA. Note that the combination of two machines, each having the same level, will result in a level 3 dB greater than either machine alone. It will be remembered from Chapter 2 that doubling sound power results in an increase of 3 dB, whereas doubling sound pressure produces an increase of 6 dB. Why, then, when we combine the sound-pressure level readings on two machines of the same output do we not have a total that is 6 dB higher instead of 3 dB? The answer is that unless the sound sources to be combined are phase-coherent—and this is rarely the case—the power ratio applies.[16]

Now let us suppose that we have measured the following four octave-band levels and we want to combine them to check on the overall level:

Octave-band Center frequency	Band level
250	78
500	83
1000	79
2000	80

First, we arrange the band levels in a series from highest to lowest: 83, 80, 79, 78. Then we enter the chart in Figure 9–6 with 3 dB on the abscissa—the difference between the two highest levels to be combined. The combination of 83 and 80 yields a total of 84.8. Now, we enter the chart with the difference

[16] Frederick A. White, *Our Acoustic Environment* (New York: John Wiley, 1975), p. 41.

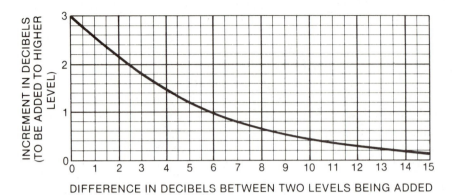

FIGURE 9-6.   Chart for combining noise levels. (From Arnold P. G. Peterson and Ervin E. Gross, Jr., *Handbook of Noise Measurement,* Concord, Mass.: General Radio, 1972, p. 9. Used by permission.)

between 84.8 and 79, or 5.8, which gives an increment of 1.0 dB, making the total for the first three octave-band levels of 85.8. Finally, the difference between 85.8 and 78 is 7.8, which yields an increment of 0.6, which when added to 85.8 gives 86.4 dB as the overall level from combining the four individual octave-band levels. The chart provides for differences in levels to be added of no more than 15 dB. If a difference exceeds 15 dB, the effect of the weaker intensity on the total is so minimal that it can be disregarded.

As stated earlier, overall sound levels measured on the A scale of a sound-level meter are the commonly used sound measurements, and most regulations for industrial or environmental noise are expressed in terms of dBA levels. If one wants to express a given spectrum of octave-band levels as a dBA value, the chart of Figure 9–7 can be used. Octave-band levels are plotted on the chart. The highest curve penetrated by the plotted octave-band levels is the approximate or "equivalent" dBA value of the overall sound. For example, assume a noise that has octave-band levels of 90 dB at every octave band from lowest to highest. The plot of octave-band levels (a straight horizontal line) would make its highest penetration into the dBA curves at 4000 Hz. Interpolating this penetration between the 95- and 100-dBA curves yields a value for this noise of about 97 dBA.

The recording of the data obtained is most important because it should be possible for someone else subsequently to duplicate the conditions of any noise survey from the information supplied on a report. The specific items of equipment utilized in the survey should be described by name, model, and even serial number. The settings of the equipment, for example, the weighting network employed and the meter speed utilized in making sound-level measurements, should be specified. The time of day and the duration of the measurements, and any corrections applied for microphone, cable, and so on, should be recorded. The environment in which the noise source is located

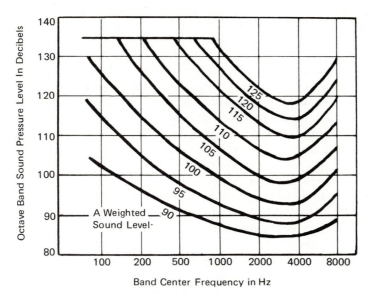

Band Center Frequency in Hz

FIGURE 9-7. Chart for converting octave-band levels into an approximate overall dBA value or "equivalent" A-weighted sound level. (From "Hearing Conservation Program," Bureau of Medicine and Surgery Instruction 6260.6B, Washington, D.C.: Department of the Navy, 1970. Used by permission.)

should be completely described, and the location of employees in relation to the source and the length of time of their daily exposure to the noise should be recorded. In other words, a complete description of the noise being measured, the way in which the measurements were obtained, and any extraneous factors that may have exerted any influence on the measurements should be included in any report.

DAMAGE-RISK CRITERIA

For many years, experts have sought an answer to the question concerning the levels of noise to which the average individual may be exposed during a working lifetime without incurring noise-induced hearing impairment. Many factors must be considered in evaluating the hazard of noise: the overall level of the noise, the frequency composition of the noise, the duration and distribution of exposure during the work day, and the number of years of exposure during one's lifetime. Another factor to be considered is the range of individual susceptibility to noise-induced hearing loss.[17]

In order to consider how best to specify noise exposures that are "safe"

[17] *Guide for Conservation of Hearing in Noise,* Supplement to *The Transactions of the American Academy of Ophthalmology and Otolaryngology,* 1973, p. 7.

for one's working lifetime, it will be helpful to review the principal efforts in this direction of the past three decades. Kryter, in 1950, suggested that an overall measurement of noise level was insufficient to yield information concerning the hazard to hearing presented by a given noise. He underlined the importance of making spectral analyses of noises in estimating their potential danger, and he suggested that the critical bands concept derived from masking experiments might profitably be employed in predicting the degree of hearing impairment from noise exposure. A "critical band" is the narrowest band that just masks out the pure tone that is the central frequency of the band when both the band and the central frequency contain equal sound power. In what he admitted might be a conservative "guess," Kryter suggested that the maximum safe sound-pressure level at any critical band for "long and intermittent exposures" was 85 dB.[18]

According to Yaffe and Jones,[19] Parrack introduced the concept of a "damage-risk criterion" about a year after the Kryter monograph appeared, and this concept was elaborated by Rosenblith and Stevens,[20] who proposed allowable safe limits for lifetime exposures for both wide-band and narrow-band noise in terms of octave-band levels. The Rosenblith and Stevens damage-risk criterion has been widely quoted and incorporated into various noise regulations and safety orders. It is reproduced in Figure 9–8.

Rosenblith and Stevens admit that their damage-risk criterion is based on incomplete data, and they anticipate that new curves will be derived from additional laboratory and field data. They do not hold any brief for the exact values plotted in the two curves of Figure 9–8 but feel that they are accurate within ± 10 dB. In the Rosenblith and Stevens criterion, the assumption is made that the risk of damage is greater for pure-tone stimuli, or noise in which the major portion of the energy is concentrated in a very narrow band of frequencies, than for wide-band noise.

In 1954, a report by a subcommittee of the American Standards Association attempted to relate hearing loss to noise exposure based on an analysis of data obtained from workers in industry.[21] "Trend" curves provided a way to estimate the degree of hearing loss at 1000, 2000, and 4000 Hz to be expected on the average for certain specified years of exposure to steady noise. The

[18] Karl D. Kryter, "The Effects of Noise on Man," *Journal of Speech and Hearing Disorders*, Monograph supp. 1 (September 1950):36–37.

[19] Charles D. Yaffe and Herbert H. Jones, *Noise and Hearing*, Public Health Service Publication No. 850 (Washington, D.C.: U.S. Government Printing Office, 1961), p. 43.

[20] Walter A. Rosenblith and Kenneth N. Stevens, *Handbook of Acoustic Noise Control*, vol. 11, *Noise and Man*, Technical Report 52-204 (Wright-Patterson Air Force Base, Ohio: Wright Air Development Center, 1953).

[21] *The Relations of Hearing Loss to Noise Exposure*, Report of the Z24-X-2 Exploratory Subcommittee of the American Standards Association Z24 Sectional Committee on Acoustics, Vibration, and Mechanical Shock (New York: American Standards Association—now American National Standards Institute—1954).

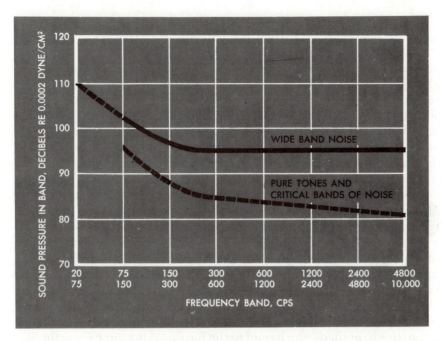

FIGURE 9-8. Damage-risk criterion for steady noise and for lifetime exposures. (From Walter A. Rosenblith and Kenneth M. Stevens, *Handbook of Acoustic Noise Control*, vol. II, Technical Report 52-204, Wright Air Development Center, June 1953. Used by permission.)

hearing levels at 1000 and 2000 Hz were shown to be more closely related to the octave-band level at 300–600 Hz than to any other octave-band level, whereas the hearing level at 4000 Hz was most closely related to the octave-band level at 1200–2400 Hz. The authors reported that they did not attempt to set damage-risk criteria or even to imply that it was possible to specify the limit of safe exposure at that time. Among other questions the authors of this report raised was the following: "What percentage of the people exposed to industrial noise should a standard be designed to protect? In view of the large individual differences in susceptibility to noise exposure, should a noise standard be aimed at preventing hearing losses in 50 percent, 90 percent, or even 99 percent of the population?"[22] An answer to this question must, of course, be forthcoming before allowable limits of noise exposure can be defined.

In 1956, the Air Force issued a regulation defining the limits of allowable noise exposure for Air Force personnel.[23] The allowable lifetime (twenty-five years) limit for an eight-hour day exposure to broad-band noise with ears unprotected was defined as a maximum band-pressure level of 85 dB at each of

[22] Ibid., p. 55.

[23] *Hazardous Noise Exposure*, Air Force Regulation No. 160–3 (Washington, D.C.: Department of the Air Force, October 29, 1956).

four octave bands: 300–600, 600–1200, 1200–2400, and 2400–4800 Hz. The Air Force recommends that when the band-pressure level in any of these bands exceeds 85 dB, personnel should wear ear protectors. When the band-pressure level in any of these bands reaches 95 dB, the use of ear protectors is mandatory. Based on the assumption that a short exposure to a noise of high intensity is equal in its injurious effect to a long exposure to a noise of lesser intensity, the Air Force regulation presents a method for calculating the allowable exposure time limits without ear protection for various band-pressure levels in excess of 85 dB by converting them to values equivalent to an eight-hour day of exposure to band-pressure levels of 85 dB. The same thing is done for allowable exposure time limits with ear protection for various band-pressure levels in excess of 95 dB. By using a nomogram reproduced in the Air Force Regulation, one can determine the allowable or "safe" time limit with or without ear protection for exposure to any given noise whose spectrum is known. The time limits are expressed in terms of the number of minutes a day to which personnel can be exposed to given noise intensities. Different allowances are made for different kinds of ear protectors, and an allowance is made also when the noise is found to be of the narrow-band type. The Air Force regulation employed the "equal energy hypothesis" that trades duration of exposure with intensity level of the stimulus. In other words, according to this hypothesis, the hazard to the hearing is the same for a stimulus of I intensity and D duration as it would be for a stimulus of 2I intensity and D/2 duration. By referring to Table 2–2 in Chapter 2, it can be seen that doubling intensity (power ratio) produces an increase of 3 dB. Thus, if a damage-risk criterion specifies that an exposure to an octave-band level of 85 dB for eight hours a day is allowable, the following exposures would also be allowable: 88 dB for four hours, 91 dB for two hours, 94 dB for one hour, 97 dB for thirty minutes, 100 dB for fifteen minutes, and so on.

The Subcommittee on Noise in Industry in 1957 stated that because of the limited information regarding the relation between noise exposure and hearing impairment, it was not possible to specify "safe" levels of exposure. The subcommittee took cognizance of the findings that workers exposed to noise tended to develop hearing impairments at frequencies higher than the dominant frequency of the noise stimulus. On the premise that it was most important to protect workers' hearing at the speech frequencies (500, 1000, and 2000 Hz), the subcommittee suggested that the octave-band levels at the two bands of 300–600 and 600–1200 Hz were the most important to consider in the development of damage-risk criteria. The subcommittee then proposed the following "tentative hearing conservation level," to be applied only in the case of long-term exposure to broad-band steady noises that have comparatively flat spectra:

> If the sound energy of the noise is distributed more or less evenly throughout the eight octave bands, and if a person is to be exposed to this noise regularly for many hours a day, five days a week for many years, then: if the noise level in

either the 300–600 cycle band or the 600–1200 cycle band is 85 dB, the initiation of noise-exposure control and tests of hearing is advisable. The more the octave band levels exceed 85 dB the more urgent is the need for hearing conservation.[24]

The subcommittee pointed out that the 85 dB level it specified applied only to the octave-band levels in two bands and that the overall sound pressure level of a noise may be as much as 20 dB higher than the level in a particular octave band.

Rudmose, in 1957, reviewed the report of the Z24-X-2 Exploratory Sub-committee of the American Standards Association (now the American National Standards Association), referred to previously in this section, and suggested a method for determining "safe" exposure limits.[25] His method is based on the "trend curves" for estimating hearing loss developed by the ASA Subcommittee, on data derived from hearing studies conducted at the Wisconsin State Fair, and on the principles of relating hearing impairment to compensation that were established by the Advisory Medical Committee to the State of Wisconsin when that state was developing regulations for adjudicating claims for noise-induced hearing impairment. Rudmose assumes that industry should aim to protect 80 percent of the workers, or in other words, that efforts should be made to control noise to the point where no more than 20 percent of the workers would incur compensable hearing impairment. Because the Wisconsin regulations related compensation to hearing loss only through the frequencies of 500, 1000, and 2000 Hz, the Rudmose method concentrates on the 300–600-Hz octave band, which Subcommittee Z24-X-2 had found to be most closely related to hearing loss for frequencies below 4000 Hz. Based on a number of assumptions, some of which would be untenable in certain circumstances, Rudmose developed a series of charts showing the percentage of compensable hearing loss (by the Wisconsin standards of that time) that would be equaled or exceeded by 20 percent of a group of workers as related to the band-pressure level in the 300–600-Hz octave band and the number of years of exposure. Separate charts were constructed for different age groups, thus reflecting the effect of presbycusis.[26] Although from these charts it is possible to derive damage-risk criteria (for the 300–600-Hz octave band only), Rudmose is more interested in proposing a method for industry, or actually society, to employ in arriving at damage-risk criteria than he is in suggesting a specific criterion. He says,

> It is hoped that [the charts previously referred to] will form the foundation for industry to set its own criteria for noise exposure. It is obvious that no single

[24] *Guide for Conservation of Hearing in Noise* (Los Angeles: Subcommittee on Noise in Industry of the Committee on Conservation of Hearing, and Research Center, Subcommittee on Noise in Industry, 1957), pp. 14–15.

[25] Wayne Rudmose, "Hearing Loss Resulting from Noise Exposure," in *Handbook of Noise Control*, ed. Harris, chap. 7.

[26] Ibid., p. 12.

number can be chosen as an undeniable criterion. Whether the matter is one of fully protecting 80 or 90 per cent of the workers or just 50 per cent is a policy decision industry must make. Certainly it seems reasonable that industry will try to protect as high a percentage of its employees as possible.[27]

Rosenwinkel and Stewart conducted a study of some 270 workers in a large machine shop, relating their audiograms to the length of time on the job and using a group of 290 office workers with the same distribution of ages as controls. The spectrum of the noise to which the experimental group was exposed was relatively flat through eight octave bands, with the highest octave-band level at 80 dB (300–600-Hz octave band). The authors asked the question, "Does a continuous occupational exposure to a steady-state noise of 80 dB per octave band cause a measurable change in pure-tone hearing sensitivity during man's normal working life span?" Their data showed that although the differences between the experimental and control groups were minimal up to a mean exposure time of sixteen years, comparisons between the groups indicate increasingly greater differences as the time of exposure increases. The groups differ significantly, however, only for the frequencies higher than 2000 Hz. The group that had a mean exposure time of thirty-four years demonstrated hearing levels at 4000 Hz that exceeded the control group's hearing levels at that frequency by an average of 25 dB. The authors concluded that although the experimental group's average hearing loss did not fall within the compensable range even for the longest exposure times, the difference between the hearing levels of the experimental and control groups at 4000 Hz demonstrated that exposure to steady-state noise that does not exceed a level of 80 dB in any octave band can produce measurable reduction in hearing sensitivity over a normal working life-span.[28]

In 1961, Yaffe and Jones reported on a study of the hearing sensitivity of prisoners who were exposed to various kinds of noisy work environments in federal prisons. The study was conducted over a period of seven years. The authors relate their data on shift in hearing level in various working environments to various published damage-risk criteria and reach the conclusion that their data lend considerable support to the criterion for exposure to wide-band noise that had been proposed in 1953 by Rosenblith and Stevens (see Figure 9–8). Their findings did not justify a lowering of the criterion for narrow-band noise, however, as Rosenblith and Stevens had proposed. Yaffe and Jones also agree with the recommendations of the Subcommittee on Noise in Industry that hearing conservation measures should be instituted when steady-state broad-band noise is characterized by octave-band levels as high as 85 dB.[29]

[27] Ibid., p. 13.

[28] N. E. Rosenwinkel and K. C. Stewart, "The Relationship of Hearing Loss to Steady State Noise Exposure," *American Industrial Hygiene Association Quarterly* 18 (September 1957):227–30.

[29] Yaffe and Jones, *Noise and Hearing.*

As can be seen by a comparison of the sources cited in this section, there is no agreement on the levels of noise to which workers may be exposed over long periods of time without incurring hearing impairment. If one is concerned only with compensable hearing impairment, then it would appear from the Rosenwinkel and Stewart study that octave-band levels of 80 dB and less are "safe," at least for the average worker over a lifetime of work exposure. One can only speculate as to what Rosenwinkel and Stewart would have concluded if they had applied Rudmose's principle of protecting 80 percent of the workers. It is possible that 20 percent of their experimental group might have incurred sufficient hearing impairment to warrant compensation from noise exposure that did not exceed 80 dB in any octave band. The Rosenblith and Stevens criterion has been widely quoted, and as we have just seen, the Yaffe and Jones study lends it considerable support. Yet even Yaffe and Jones favor the adoption of the more conservative practice advocated by the Subcommittee on Noise in Industry of becoming concerned when octave-band levels reach 85 dB. Air Force Regulation 160-3 represents a reasonable compromise between the Rosenblith and Stevens criterion and the recommendations of the Subcommittee on Noise in Industry in recommending the use of ear protectors when octave-band levels exceed 85 dB, and requiring their use when octave-band levels reach 95 dB.

In 1961, Glorig, Ward, and Nixon proposed damage-risk criteria for continuous steady-noise exposures for five hours a day, five days a week, for many years; continuous steady-noise exposures for less than five hours a day, five days a week, for many years; and steady-noise that is intermittently on during the day, five days a week, for many years.[30] Their recommendations are based on extensive research relating TTS to PTS (permanent threshold shift) and set the pattern for later thinking in regard to industrial hearing conservation.

Glorig, Ward, and Nixon's damage-risk criteria are based on research findings that if a worker demonstrates no "significant" TTS at the end of a day's exposure to noise, PTS will not develop for "habitual" exposure to that noise over a period of years. Whereas most TTS studies have been concerned with 4000 Hz, the frequency that generally shows the greatest loss from noise exposure, Glorig, Ward, and Nixon propose using the TTS at 2000 Hz for predicting PTS at 2000 Hz, and their criteria are based on avoiding PTS at 2000 Hz resulting from a lifetime noise exposure for 85 to 90 percent of the exposed population. Their reasoning for employing 2000 Hz instead of 4000 Hz for TTS and PTS studies is twofold: (1) PTS for 4000 Hz reaches a maximum after ten to twelve years, regardless of the level of the exposure noise; beyond this time, further increases in hearing level at 4000 Hz seem to be a function of aging; (2) 2000 Hz is the highest of the "speech frequencies," and hearing conservation measures should be aimed at protecting the worker's ability to hear and

---

[30] Aram Glorig, W. Dixon Ward, and James Nixon, "Damage Risk Criteria and Noise-Induced Hearing Loss," *A.M.A. Archives of Otolaryngology* 74 (October 1961): 413–23.

understand speech; generally, the frequencies above 2000 Hz are "expendable," in the sense that they are not important in communication by speech.

The criterion for steady (not impulsive) noise that is on for more than five hours a day is the International Organization for Standardization Noise Rating Number 85 (N-85). This refers to curves of octave-band levels covering a range from N-0 to N-130 in steps of five numbers. The numbers coincide with the sound-pressure level in dB re 0.0002 dyne/cm^2 for the octave band centered on the frequency of 1000 Hz. The curves of noise rating, which bear a resemblance to the sound-pressure level graphs of phon curves, were based on various studies and "educated opinions" of acoustical consultants from several countries and unanimously accepted by the group of consultants meeting in Stuttgart in 1959 under the aegis of the International Organization for Standardization. A noise having a rating of N-85 would have the following maximum levels at each octave band:[31]

Octave mid-frequency, Hz	Sound pressure level, dB	Octave mid-frequency, Hz	Sound pressure level, dB
63	102	1000	85
125	95	2000	82
250	91	4000	80
500	87	8000	79

The noise exposure criterion applicable to steady noise that is on less than five hours a day is determined from data relating noise-rating numbers and exposure time in minutes (up to 300 minutes) with the amount of TTS at 2000 Hz. After the "acceptable" amount of TTS at 2000 Hz has been decided, one can determine from the data how many minutes' exposure to a noise of a given rating is allowable to avoid PTS at 2000 Hz over a period of years. Glorig, Ward, and Nixon suggest that 12 dB should be the maximum allowable TTS at 2000 Hz as measured at the end of a working day. According to studies relating TTS and PTS, this criterion of allowable TTS will not result in any significant PTS at 2000 Hz for habitual exposure.

Additional data enable one to determine the relations among the "on-time," "off-time," and number of exposure cycles (combinations of on-time and off-time) allowable for exposure to intermittent steady noise of particular noise ratings. Glorig, Ward, and Nixon's criteria are based on recommendations of the International Organization for Standardization, which has also proposed methods of utilizing the noise-rating numbers for determining the effect of noise on communication and the annoyance effect of noise.

In 1966, Kryter et al. published the recommendations of a working group of the National Academy of Science–National Research Council Committee on Hearing, Bioacoustics and Biomechanics (NAS–NRC CHABA, usually

[31] Ibid., p. 421.

identified simply as CHABA).[32] The working group was established as the result of a request to CHABA by the Office of the Surgeon General of the U.S. Army to "reevaluate, on the basis of new knowledge in this field, the question of damage-risk criteria for exposure to sound." The working group adopted as its basic criterion the acceptability of noise exposures that would result in noise-induced permanent threshold shifts (NIPTS) after ten years of near-daily exposure of no more than 10 dB at 1000 Hz or lower frequencies, 15 dB at 2000 Hz, or 20 dB at 3000 Hz or higher frequencies. The working group believed that if the median NIPTS could be held at these levels, only 20 percent of workers exposed to them would incur compensable hearing impairments in a lifetime of work. The assumption was made that NIPTS from a particular noise environment over a period of years would be no greater than TTS measured two minutes after a full working day's exposure to that environment. In other words, it was assumed that essentially $TTS_2 = NIPTS_{10yr}$, so that a given noise environment would be "safe"—at least for 80 percent of the exposed workers—if it resulted in median TTS_2s of no more than 10 dB at 1000 Hz and lower, 15 dB at 2000 Hz, and 20 dB at 3000 Hz and higher. Based on field studies of NIPTS of workers in industries and laboratory studies of TTS, the working group then developed a series of damage-risk contours for various conditions of steady-state and intermittent noise exposures. With spectral information on the noise, one can determine from the contours the maximum allowable time per day for exposure to steady-state or intermittent noise, the maximum allowable level for short bursts of noise (two minutes or less in duration), or the amount of intervening quiet required between long bursts of noise (more than two minutes).

Botsford combined and consolidated the CHABA contours into fewer graphs. As a further simplification he suggested the use of A-weighted sound levels, instead of octave- or third-octave-band levels, which makes possible the combining of the CHABA contours into a single graph specifying the total allowable on-time per day and the allowable number of exposure cycles per day for manufacturing noises of various dBA levels.[33] Although casting some doubt on the usefulness of TTS_2 as a predictor of NIPTS, Eldredge and Miller support the notion of utilizing equinoxious contours based on TTS data that "allow us to chart our way through the complexities introduced by brief exposures, rest periods away from noise, etc., and provide the best guides to safety that we have."[34]

[32] K. D. Kryter, W. Dixon Ward, James D. Miller, and Donald H. Eldredge, "Hazardous Exposure to Intermittent and Steady-State Noise," *Journal of the Acoustical Society of America* 39 (March 1966):451–64.

[33] James H. Botsford, "Simple Method for Identifying Acceptable Noise Exposures," *Journal of the Acoustical Society of America* 42 (October 1967):810–19.

[34] Donald H. Eldredge and James D. Miller, "Acceptable Noise Exposures— Damage Risk Criteria," in *Noise as a Public Health Hazard, ASHA Reports 4*, eds. W. Dixon Ward and James E. Fricke (Washington, D.C.: The American Speech and Hearing Association, 1969), pp. 110–20.

Ward reported on a series of experiments in which TTS and recovery time were studied with a group of twelve normal-hearing young adults. The purpose of the experiments was to validate the damage-risk contours for steady and intermittent noise exposures that had been developed by the CHABA working group.[35] Specifically, Ward wished to see if the various CHABA contours were in fact accurate in predicting median TTS_2s of 10 dB at 1000 Hz and below, 15 dB at 2000 Hz, or 20 dB at 3000 Hz and above. He found that the CHABA contours are appropriate for eight hours of steady, continuous noise. The contours for eight-hour exposures to intermittent noise consisting of short bursts are apparently accurate in terms of predicted TTS_2s; but when the stimulus is a band of high frequencies (1400–2000 Hz) and the band level exceeds 100 dB, the recovery time to pre-exposure hearing levels may exceed sixteen hours, meaning that workers would begin a workday with some residual TTS. It was for intermittent noise consisting of longer bursts that the CHABA contours were most in error because even for exposures of relatively low intensity the recovery time for TTS_2 was significantly longer than had been assumed in the formulation of the contours. Ward suggests that the CHABA contours for longer bursts—and Botsford's derived single set of curves[36]—should be revised because Ward's findings indicate that the longer the duration of the bursts, the shorter should be the allowable cumulative daily exposure time. Ward concluded that TTS_2 was not a satisfactory measure to employ in evaluating the hazard of noise exposure. Because of the delayed recovery time from longer noise bursts and from shorter bursts of high frequency and high intensity, he suggests that TTS measured at some longer interval than two minutes following a day's exposure should be employed. Although ideally TTS_{1000}—that is, TTS measured approximately sixteen hours after exposure—should be the measure used to assure that workers would not begin a day with some residual TTS, Ward reports that TTS_{30} would have been adequate to rank order the TTSs of the subjects in his experiment. From inspecting the recovery curves of his subjects, Ward concluded that the CHABA contours should be constructed so that a particular allowable exposure would produce no more than median TTS_{30}s of 5 dB at 1000 Hz and lower, 7.5 dB at 2000 Hz, or 10 dB at 3000 Hz and higher. Ward believes that the CHABA method of presenting damage-risk criteria—with suitable modifications based on his and others' research—is superior to other methods that ignore the temporal distribution of energy, that is, the length of noise bursts and the intervals between noise bursts.[37]

In May 1969, the federal government put into effect an addition to the

[35] Kryter et al., "Hazardous Exposure to Noise."

[36] Botsford, "Simple Method."

[37] W. Dixon Ward, "Temporary Threshold Shift and Damage-Risk Criteria for Intermittent Noise Exposures," *Journal of the Acoustical Society of America* 48 (August 1970):561–74.

Walsh-Healey Public Contracts Act that places limitations on noise levels permissible in plants with federal contracts in excess of $10,000.[38] Noise exposures are expressed in dBA with meter on slow response. Contours are provided for translating octave-band levels into dBA values (see Figure 9–7). Table 9–1 gives the allowable noise exposures under the Walsh-Healey Act.

Note that the Walsh-Healey Act criteria depart from the equal energy principle, or what has come to be known as the 3-dB rule. The equal energy principle has been considered by many to be overly conservative because it does not take into account the recovery from fatigue that occurs during periods of relative quiet or harmless noise between bursts of intense noise. According to this theory, the hazard is the same from an eight-hour continuous exposure to 90 dBA of noise as it is for four one-hour exposures to 93 dBA of noise distributed over an eight-hour day. The Walsh-Healey Act adopts a 5-dB rule that presumably compensates for the decreased hazard of an intermittent noise. Thus, according to the act, 90 dBA of continuous exposure for eight hours is equivalent to four hours of 95 dBA exposure in an eight-hour day, whether that exposure is continuous or intermittent. In the 1973 revision of the *Guide for the Conservation of Hearing in Noise*, tables for determining acceptable noise exposures for less than eight hours a day based on dBA sound levels are given according to both the 3-dB rule and the 5-dB rule.[39]

The Walsh-Healey Act specifies a method for evaluating the cumulative effect of a series of exposures of different dBA levels and durations in terms of the criterion measure of a continuous eight-hour exposure to 90 dBA of noise. The method assumes continuous monitoring of plant noise with a sound-level meter and keeping a record of the duration of each exposure in excess of 90 dBA. The ratio of actual exposure time to allowable exposure time for each dBA level is computed. These ratios are then summed for the day. If the sum does not exceed unity (1.0), the Walsh-Healey criterion has been met.[40] For ex-

TABLE 9–1.   Permissible daily noise exposures according to the Walsh-Healey Act.

Duration per day, hours	Sound level, dBA
8	90
6	92
4	95
3	97
2	100
1½	102
1	105
½	110
¼ or less	115

[38] *Federal Register* 34, no. 96 (May 20, 1969): 7891–7954, Rules and Regulations 50-204.10.

[39] *Guide for the Conservation of Hearing in Noise*, 1973, pp. 16–19.

[40] *Federal Register*, 34:96.

ample, assume that during an eight-hour day, workers were exposed to the following dBA levels for the indicated times: 95 dBA for 1½ hours, 97 dBA for 1 hour, and 105 dBA for 15 minutes (¼ hour). The ratios of actual to allowable exposure times in hours would then be as follows (the allowable time taken from Table 9–1): 1.5/4, 1/3, and 0.25/1. These ratios reduce to .375, .333, and .250, respectively, and their sum is .958. Because this sum is less than 1.0, the Walsh-Healey criterion has not been exceeded. Although the kind of monitoring required to evaluate plant noise in terms of the Walsh-Healey provisions can be done with a sound-level meter and a watch, a much more convenient method is to use an automatic noise-exposure monitor that accumulates and integrates noise exposures throughout a workday. At any time during the day, the monitor will give a readout of the percentage of allowable exposure, based on the 5-dB tradeoff of exposure time and intensity. At the end of the day, the monitor will read less than 1.0, or 100 percent, if the noise levels in the area being monitored have not exceeded allowable limits. Individually worn noise dosimeters are now available. Dosimeters have been used for years to measure accumulated x-ray or atomic radiation, and they have now been developed for noise. They accumulate and integrate noise in a similar fashion to the automatic monitors just described. Some dosimeters give a direct readout when their cover is removed, and others must be connected with an external readout device. The Walsh-Healey Act states that where noise levels are found in excess of those permissible, "feasible administrative or engineering controls shall be utilized." If these fail to reduce the noise levels to acceptable values, then "personal protective equipment shall be provided and used."[41] Incidentally, the act specifies that exposure to impulsive noise should not exceed 140 dB peak sound-pressure level.

Following the lead of the federal government, the State of California in 1970 rewrote its standards for occupational noise exposure to specify the same allowable exposures to intermittent or continuous noise that were incorporated in the addition to the Walsh-Healey Act and reproduced in Table 9–1.[42] The 1970 revision replaced the standards for occupational noise exposure that had been in effect in California since November 1962. The exposure levels specified in the 1962 orders had been exactly those proposed in 1953 by Rosenblith and Stevens and reproduced in Figure 9–8. Also, the 1962 standards had incorporated the equal energy concept (halving exposure time increases the permissible exposure level by 3 dB). Thus, the 1970 revision lowers the allowable exposure level for an eight-hour day from band levels of 95 dB to sound levels of 90 dBA and substitutes the 5-dB rule for the 3-dB rule.

On December 29, 1970, the President of the United States signed into law the Occupational Safety and Health Act that extended to all manufactur-

[41] Ibid., 50-204.10(b).

[42] Revision of "Noise Control Safety Orders," Group 6.1, "General Industry Safety Orders" (Division of Industrial Safety, State of California Human Relations Agency, Department of Industrial Relations), effective September 19, 1970.

ing plants engaging in interstate commerce (about 55 million workers) the safety and health standards required of U.S. Government contractors through the Walsh-Healey Act.[43] The act authorized the Secretary of Labor to set mandatory occupational safety and health standards and adopted the Walsh-Healey standards until such time that they would be superseded by new standards promulgated by the Department of Labor. The act also created in the Department of Health, Education, and Welfare a new component of the National Institutes of Health—the National Institute for Occupational Safety and Health—for the purpose of conducting research, developing criteria to identify "toxic substances" (including noise), and recommending standards to the Department of Labor. Within the Department of Labor, an Occupational Safety and Health Administration, OSHA for short, was established to carry out the mandates of Public Law 91-596. The law became effective 120 days after its enactment, in late April 1971.

In August 1972, the National Institute for Occupational Safety and Health (NIOSH) provided the Department of Labor with a report recommending a noise standard to take the place of the Walsh-Healey regulation that had been incorporated into the Occupational Safety and Health Act. This report, known as the NIOSH Criteria Document, recommended a continuation of the 90-dBA standard for an eight-hour day that was already in effect but recommended that all new facilities be required to meet an 85-dBA standard.[44] Actually, in the Preface the director of NIOSH admitted that a majority of the review consultants recommended that an 85-dBA standard be applied to existing as well as to new factories, but somehow this majority recommendation did not get embodied in the report. Following receipt of the NIOSH Criteria Document, the Assistant Secretary of Labor for OSHA appointed a Standards Advisory Committee on Noise "to obtain and evaluate additional recommendations from labor, management, government, and independent experts."[45] This committee met for several months, received many written comments and oral presentations, and then made its report to OSHA. Finally, after studying the NIOSH Criteria Document and the Advisory Committee's report, OSHA published its proposed requirements and procedures in the *Federal Register* and invited written comments and requests for informal hearings.[46] Originally, OSHA expected to conclude the hearings within a few weeks, make whatever changes in the regulations seemed appropriate, and then issue them as official Department of Labor policy. The Environmental Protection Agency (EPA) raised such objections to the proposed OSHA

[43] Public Law 91-596, 91st Congress, S.2193, December 29, 1970.

[44] National Institute for Occupational Safety and Health, *Criteria for a Recommended Standard . . . Occupational Exposure to Noise* (Washington, D.C.: Department of Health, Education, and Welfare, Health Services and Mental Health Administration, 1972).

[45] *Federal Register* 39, no. 207 (October 24, 1974): 37,773.

[46] Ibid., pp. 37,773–78.

regulations, however, and so many professional people and labor representatives supported the EPA position, that OSHA scheduled additional hearings
and commissioned additional studies.

EPA became involved in industrial and environmental noise problems
through the Noise Control Act of 1972, which gave EPA the authority to
"coordinate the programs of all Federal agencies relating to noise research and
noise control."[47] All federal agencies were required to consult with the EPA
before prescribing noise standards or regulations. Any time the Administrator
of EPA "has reason to believe that a standard or regulation, or any proposed
standard or regulation, of any Federal agency respecting noise does not protect the public health and welfare to the extent he believes to be required and
feasible, he may request such agency to review and report to him on the ad-
visability of revising such standard or regulation to provide such protection."[48]
Within EPA, the responsibility for the noise program was vested in the Office
of Noise Abatement and Control, headed by a Deputy Assistant Administrator.

EPA challenged OSHA on two main components of the proposed
regulations: (1) OSHA proposed keeping the allowable level for an eight-hour
workday exposure to 90 dBA as specified in the Walsh-Healey amendments,
but EPA called for a reduction to 85 dBA within a three-year period and a com-
mitment to reduce the allowable limit further "when such a reduction is
shown to be feasible"; and (2) OSHA held to a 5-dB time-intensity tradeoff,
and EPA believed the tradeoff should be 3 dB, permitting only a 3-dB increase
in intensity for a halving of exposure time.[49] OSHA did accept EPA's recommendation regarding a standard for exposure to impulse noise that specifies a
10-dB decrease in the maximum level for each tenfold increase in the number
of impulses. OSHA allowed a daily exposure of up to 100 impulses at a maximum peak level of 140 dB. Thus, if the exposure is 1000 impulses a day, the
maximum peak level must be reduced to 130 dB.[50]

Although EPA would settle for an 85-dBA workday standard to be
achieved in three years (presumably from the time the OSHA regulations
become effective), its long-term objective is to achieve even a stricter standard
for an eight-hour exposure. One of the requirements of the Noise Control Act
of 1972 was that EPA shall "publish information on the levels of environmental noise the attainment and maintenance of which in defined areas under
various conditions are requisite to protect the public health and welfare with
an adequate margin of safety."[51] In July 1973, EPA and the Air Force jointly
published two monographs that sought to specify the risk to hearing of various

---

[47] Public Law 92-574, 92nd Congress, HR 11021, October 27, 1972.

[48] Ibid., sec. 4. (c) (2).

[49] *Federal Register* 39, no. 244 (December 18, 1974): 43,802.

[50] Ibid.

[51] Public Law 92-574, sec. 5. (a) (2).

A-weighted eight-hour workday exposures.[52] These monographs reviewed various studies that attempted to relate hearing loss to noise exposures. According to Johnson, studies that allowed calculation of NIPTS at various percentile points for the frequencies 500, 1000, 2000, and 4000 Hz were accepted for analysis.[53] The data of three researchers met this requirement: Passchier-Vermeer, Robinson, and Baughn.[54] Johnson averaged the data reported in these three studies and summarized the results in tabular form, as shown in Table 9–2. For each noise exposure are given (1) the "maximum" NIPTS, meaning the NIPTS occurring over forty years of exposure, that will not be exceeded by 90 percent of the population; (2) the NIPTS after ten years of exposure that will not be exceeded by 90 percent of the population; (3) the forty-year NIPTS averaged over all percentiles; and (4) maximum hearing risk, which means the difference in percentage of people whose hearing levels exceed the AAOO "low fence" in the noise-exposed population and in a non-noise-exposed (but otherwise equivalent) population. The maximum risk usually, but not always, occurs after forty years of exposure. The columns of Table 9–2 present threshold shifts in dB for the average of the three speech frequencies, for the average of four frequencies (the speech frequencies plus 4000 Hz), and for 4000 Hz alone.

In March 1974, EPA published what has come to be known as its "Levels Document," which states noise-exposure levels that will protect 96 percent of the population over a working lifetime from "significant" changes in hearing level at 4000 Hz, which is admittedly the most "noise-sensitive" frequency.[55] A significant change is defined as 5 dB or more. These levels are based on the data presented in Table 9–2, with certain corrections and roundings. In discussing these levels, EPA makes clear that it is concerned only with the health and welfare effects of noise and not with technical or economic prob-

---

[52] J. C. Guignard, *A Basis for Limiting Noise Exposure for Hearing Conservation,* Joint EPA/USAF Study Publication Nos. AMRL-TR-73-90 and EPA-550/9-73-001-A (Wright-Patterson Air Force Base, Ohio: Aerospace Medical Research Laboratory, 1973); Daniel L. Johnson, *Prediction of NIPTS Due to Continuous Noise Exposure,* Joint EPA/USAF Study, Publication Nos. AMRL-TR-73-91 and EPA-550/9-73-001-B (Wright-Patterson Air Force Base, Ohio: Aerospace Medical Research Laboratory, 1973).

[53] Ibid., p. 2.

[54] Wilhemina Passchier-Vermeer, *Hearing Loss Due to Exposure to Steady-State Broadband Noise,* Report No. 35 (The Netherlands: Institute for Public Health Engineering, 1968); D. W. Robinson, *The Relationships Between Hearing Loss and Noise Exposure,* NPL Aero Report Ac 32 (Teddington, Eng.: National Physical Laboratory, 1968); William L. Baughn, *Relation Between Daily Noise Exposure and Hearing Loss Based on the Evaluation of 6,835 Industrial Noise Exposure Cases,* Joint EPA/USAF Study, Publication No. AMRL-TR-73-53 (Wright-Patterson Air Force Base, Ohio: Aerospace Medical Research Laboratory, 1973).

[55] *Information on Levels of Environmental Noise Requisite to Protect Public Health and Welfare with an Adequate Margin of Safety,* Publication No. 550/9-74-004 (Washington, D.C.: Environmental Protection Agency, 1974).

TABLE 9–2. Summary of predicted effects from various A-weighted exposures to continuous noise.

	Speech (.5, 1, 2)	Speech (.5, 1, 2, 4)	4 kHz
75 dBA for 8 hours			
Max NIPTS (90%-ile)	1 dB	2 dB	6 dB
NIPTS at 10 yrs (90%-ile)	0	1	5
Average NIPTS	0	0	1
Max Hearing Risk	N/A	N/A	N/A
80 dBA for 8 hours			
Max NIPTS (90%-ile)	1 dB	4 dB	11 dB
NIPTS at 10 yrs (90%-ile)	1	3	9
Average NIPTS	0	1	4
Max Hearing Risk	5%	N/A	N/A
85 dBA for 8 hours			
Max NIPTS (90%-ile)	4 dB	7 dB	19 dB
NIPTS at 10 yrs (90%-ile)	2	6	16
Average NIPTS	1	3	9
Max Hearing Risk	12%	N/A	N/A
90 dBA for 8 hours			
Max NIPTS (90%-ile)	7 dB	12 dB	28 dB
NIPTS at 10 yrs (90%-ile)	4	9	24
Average NIPTS	3	6	15
Max Hearing Risk	22.3%	N/A	N/A

From Guignard, *A Basis for Limiting Noise Exposure for Hearing Conservation*, p. 12, based on data from Johnson, *Prediction of NIPTS Due to Continuous Noise Exposure*, p. 59.

lems of setting standards. EPA is thus tacitly admitting that its standards may not be economically feasible. EPA believes that in order to protect the public health and welfare, long-term average sound levels must be kept to a maximum of 70 dBA. By "long-term," EPA means sound levels averaged over a twenty-four-hour period on the "equal energy" principle or 3-dB tradeoff of time and intensity. Thus, two sounds of different intensity and length but of equal energy would have the same "equivalent" sound level, or L_{eq}. So, according to EPA, an $L_{eq(24)}$ of 70 dBA averaged over a year will be sufficiently protective to a worker over a forty-year work life. In evaluating the annoyance effect of noise in a community, EPA believes it is appropriate to give a greater weight to sounds that occur during the night. Such sounds are more intrusive because at night, background noise is less. L_{dn} is a twenty-four-hour equivalent level computed by giving a 10-dB weighting to nighttime sounds—those occurring between 10:00 P.M. and 7:00 A.M. The subscript *dn* stands for "day-night."

Occupational noise exposures are expressed as $L_{eq(8)}$ because the typical workday is eight hours. Assuming that for the other sixteen hours of a day noise exposures are negligible (60 dBA or less), an $L_{eq(8)}$ of 75 dBA is the maximum allowable workday exposure that will result in a $L_{eq(24)}$ of no more than 70 dBA. OSHA's mandate under the Occupational Safety and Health Act was to "set the standard which most adequately assures . . . that no employee will suffer material impairment of health or functional capacity" over a working lifetime,[56] whereas EPA was charged by the Noise Control Act with protecting "the public health and welfare with an adequate margin of safety."[57] OSHA argued that EPA's objective of protecting virtually the entire population from an NIPTS of more than 5 dB at 4000 Hz over a working lifetime may be appropriate for a "public health and welfare" goal, but it goes beyond the "material impairment" mandate of OSHA. OSHA pointed out that the AAOO-AMA low fence (an average hearing level of 26 dB for the frequencies 500, 1000, and 2000 Hz) has been "accepted by the medical profession as marking the beginning of impairment."[58] Obviously, the AAOO-AMA formula ignores the hearing level at 4000 Hz. OSHA maintained that its proposed standard of 90 dBA for an eight-hour workday provides "adequate protection" and pointed to evidence in the literature that "the risk of impairment is minimal under either an 85 dBA or 90 dBA standard, being limited to the most sensitive 2 percent of the population at risk."[59] By "impairment" in the preceding quotation, OSHA presumably meant hearing levels in excess of the AAOO-AMA low fence. After issuing the proposed regulations in 1974 and subsequently revising them, OSHA issued a final rule which became effective April 7, 1983.[60] The final rule included some significant points. First, it specified that a hearing conservation program must be implemented if a noise exposure equalled or exceeded a time-weighted average of 85 dBA over an 8-hour period. Second, it stated that hearing protectors must attenuate an employee exposure which exceeds this level, to at least an 8-hour time-weighted average of 90 dBA for all employees and to 85 dBA or lower for those employees who have experienced an average shift in threshold sensitivity of 10 dB or more from a baseline audiogram at the frequencies of 2000, 3000, and 4000 Hz.

Before concluding this section, mention should be made of a radical damage-risk criterion proposed in 1973 by Kryter, whose 1950 suggestion that the "safe" limit for any critical band was 85 dB began our discussion of damage-risk criteria. Although even EPA believes that an $L_{eq(8)}$ of 75 dBA over a working lifetime will prevent an NIPTS of more than 5 dB at 4000 Hz for 96 percent of the population, Kryter proposes a maximum level of 55 dBA for an eight-hour workday exposure, citing evidence that this criterion will protect 90 percent of the population from incurring noise-induced hearing impairment over a working lifetime of forty-five years.[61] Kryter defines *hearing impairment*

---

[56] Public Law 91-596, sec. 6.(b) (5).

[57] Public Law 92-574, sec. 5.(a) (2).

[58] *Federal Register* 40, no. 53 (March 18, 1975):12,336–37.

[59] Ibid., p. 12,337.

[60] *Federal Register* 48, no. 46 (March 8, 1983):9738–9785.

[61] Karl D. Kryter, "Impairment to Hearing from Exposure to Noise," *Journal of the Acoustical Society of America* 53 (May 1973):1211–34.

as an average hearing level at 500, 1000, and 2000 Hz in excess of 16 dB, or an average hearing level at 1000, 2000, and 3000 Hz in excess of 26 dB. In a world that is arguing the efficacy of an 85-dBA versus a 90-dBA criterion for an eight-hour workday, nobody can give serious consideration to the 55 dBA criterion proposed by Kryter. Most people would tend to agree with Ward, who said at the 1968 Conference on Noise as a Public Health Hazard, ". . . when the worker's noise environment is below 80 dBA, the probability is zero that the noise caused his hearing loss; when the level has been at 95 dBA, the probability is about 50 percent. At 105 dBA, steady, continuous exposure produces losses in nearly all men who are habitually exposed."[62]

INTERFERENCE OF NOISE WITH COMMUNICATION

Quite apart from the potentially damaging effects of noise exposure to hearing, noise can create problems that require noise-control procedures. One of these problems concerns interference with speech communication. Because of the obvious importance of maintaining adequate communication in military activities, a great deal of research on the interference effects of noise on speech has been sponsored by the Army, Navy, and Air Force. Naturally, the importance of maintaining speech communication in the presence of various kinds of noise has been recognized by industries also, and particularly by the American Telephone and Telegraph Company, whose Bell Laboratories have contributed a great deal of our present knowledge of the characteristics of speech and the effects of distortion and masking on speech intelligibility.

In order to make an accurate assessment of the effect of noise on speech communication, it is necessary to conduct speech-intelligibility tests with actual talkers and listeners in the presence of the interfering noise. The test materials utilized may be sentences, digits, bisyllabic words, monosyllabic words, or nonsense syllables. The listeners are scored according to the percentage of the speech materials heard correctly, in the manner of scoring discrimination tests in speech audiometry as explained in Chapter 6. Because it is not practical to conduct this kind of testing in the presence of the actual noise with which one is concerned, in practice the noise is recorded and the speech-intelligibility testing is performed in the laboratory in the presence of the recorded noise. From such experiments, it is known that speech intelligibility is affected by both the intensity and the frequency characteristics of an interfering noise. The relationship between the intensity of the speech and the intensity of the noise is known as the *signal-to-noise ratio*, abbreviated *S/N*. According to Licklider and Miller, "For most noises encountered in prac-

---

[62] W. Dixon Ward, "Effects of Noise on Hearing Thresholds," in *Noise as a Public Health Hazard*, eds. Ward and Fricke. p. 44.

tical situations S/N should exceed 6 dB for satisfactory communication, although the presence of speech is detectable for S/N as low as −18 dB."[63] If the signal (speech) is more intense than the noise, the S/N is plus; if the noise is more intense than the signal, the S/N is minus. Figure 9–9 from Licklider and Miller, adapted from Hawkins and Stevens,[64] shows the effect of white noise on the thresholds of detectability and intelligibility of running speech. It will be noted from Figure 9–9 that the threshold of intelligibility is not seriously affected until the sound-pressure level of the noise exceeds the sound-pressure level of the speech by about 6 dB (S/N of −6 dB). As the sound-pressure level of the noise is increased above 30 to 40 dB, the threshold of intelligibility is proportionally increased, so that the S/N of −6 dB remains constant over a wide range of intensities, in this experiment involving running speech and white noise. For other kinds of speech materials and different kinds of noise, the relationships between the threshold of intelligibility and

FIGURE 9-9.   The effect of white noise on thresholds of detectability and intelligibility of running speech. (Reproduced from *Handbook of Experimental Psychology* by permission of the publishers.)

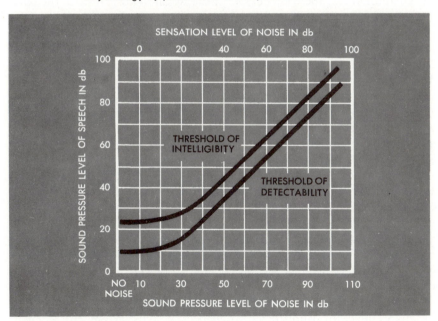

[63] J. C. R. Licklider and George A. Miller, "The Perception of Speech," in *Handbook of Experimental Psychology*, ed. S. S. Stevens (New York: John Wiley, 1951), chap. 26, p. 1049.

[64] J. E. Hawkins, Jr., and S. S. Stevens, "The Masking of Pure Tones and of Speech by White Noise," *Journal of the Acoustical Society of America* 22 (January 1950):12.

the level of the interfering noise would not necessarily be the same. Note that the running speech is detectable at an S/N of -18 dB.

Because of the expense and time involved in measuring the effects of noise on the intelligibility of speech in this manner, engineers have sought simpler ways of arriving at interference effects of noise on speech communication. A widely accepted method is to compute what has been termed the *articulation index* by analyzing the intensity and frequency components of both the speech signal and the noise and working out their interactions mathematically on the basis of data available from laboratory experiments in psychoacoustics. French and Steinberg[65] of the Bell Laboratories developed a method for arriving at the articulation index based on the following assumptions: (1) the range of important speech frequencies is from 200 to 6100 Hz; (2) this range can be divided into twenty frequency bands, each of which contributes equally to the intelligibility of speech provided the signal-to-noise ratios are equal in each band; (3) a 30-dB change in signal-to-noise ratio will span the entire range of word-intelligibility scores from 0 to almost 100 percent; (4) each of the twenty frequency bands will contribute 0.05 (5 percent) to the articulation index, and each decibel of the signal-to-noise ratio in the band will contribute $\frac{1}{30}$ of this 0.05 of the articulation index.[66] Thus, to calculate the articulation index in a given situation, one needs to determine the signal-to-noise ratio (at the ear of the listener) in each of twenty frequency bands of specified width to arrive at the proportion of the 0.05 that band contributes to the total articulation index. The sum of the contributions of each band, then, is the articulation index. Figure 9–10 from Hawley and Kryter plots typical intelligibility curves in relation to articulation index. According to Beranek, speech communication is probably satisfactory if the articulation index exceeds 0.6 (60 percent), unsatisfactory if it is less than 0.3 (30 percent), and in between these two values more study is required.[67]

Calculation of the articulation index is not a simple matter because it is necessary to determine the signal-to-noise ratio for twenty frequency bands, a process that requires special laboratory equipment. A simpler means of estimating the effect of noise on speech communication has been devised, making use of octave-band levels as measured in a typical noise survey. What is called the *speech-interference level*, abbreviated SIL, can be obtained by computing the arithmetic average of the octave-band levels in the three octave bands of 600–1200, 1200–2400, and 2400–4800 Hz. It has been determined that reliable speech communication can exist when the overall rms (root-mean-square) level of undistorted speech is 12 dB above the speech-interference level at the ear of the listener. This relationship between speech

[65] N. R. French and J. C. Steinberg, "Factors Governing the Intelligibility of Speech Sounds," *Journal of the Acoustical Society of America* 19 (January 1947):90–119.

[66] Mones E. Hawley and Karl D. Kryter, "Effects of Noise on Speech," in *Handbook of Noise Control*, ed. C. Harris, chap. 9, p. 6.

[67] Leo L. Beranek, *Acoustics* (New York: McGraw-Hill, 1954), p. 415.

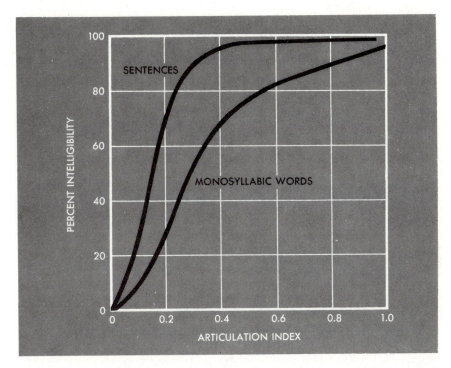

FIGURE 9–10.   The relation of intelligibility to articulation index. (From Mones E. Hawley and Karl D. Kryter, "Effects of Noise on Speech," in *Handbook of Noise Control,* ed. Cyril M. Harris. Copyright 1957. New York: McGraw-Hill Book Co., Inc. Used by permission.)

level and noise level is equivalent to an articulation index of 0.4.[68] Beranek suggests that if the band level in the 300–600-Hz band exceeds the band level in the 600–1200-Hz band, the speech-interference level should be computed by including the level in the 300–600-Hz band in the average.[69]

Beranek has worked out a table that represents the speech-interference levels that "barely permit reliable word intelligibility" at various distances between speaker and listener and at various voice levels, assuming that no reflecting surfaces are present. This information is presented in Table 9–3. If women's voices are involved, the speech-interference levels should be decreased by 5 dB from those values shown in Table 9–3.

Webster has related SILs based on the average of band levels in the three octaves with the preferred center frequencies of 500, 1000, and 2000 Hz to those shown in Table 9–3. The correction from the data reported in Table 9–3, which were based on the octave bands 600–1200, 1200–2400, and 2400–4800 Hz, to data based on octave bands with center frequencies of 500,

[68] Hawley and Kryter, "Effects of Noise on Speech," p. 10.
[69] Bernanek, *Acoustics,* p. 419.

TABLE 9–3.   Speech interference levels (in dB re 0.0002 dyne/cm²) that barely permit reliable word intelligibility at the distances and voice levels indicated.

Distance, feet	Normal	Voice Level (average male) Raised	Very loud	Shouting
0.5	71	77	83	89
1	65	71	77	83
2	59	65	71	77
3	55	61	67	73
4	53	59	65	71
5	51	57	63	69
6	49	55	61	67
12	43	49	55	61

After L. L. Beranek, "Airplane Quieting II—Specification of Acceptable Noise Levels," *Transactions American Society Mechanical Engineers* 67 (1947): 97–100, in Beranek's *Acoustics*, 1954, McGraw-Hill.

1000, and 2000 Hz involves simply adding 5 dB to each of the values in Table 9–3.[70] Later, Webster refers to this SIL based on the preferred center frequencies for octave-band analyzers as *PSIL*, the *P* standing for *preferred*.[71] In a 1977 ANSI standard, the Acoustical Society of America defined speech-interference level as "The arithmetic average of the sound pressure levels of the interfering noise in decibels *re* 20 μPa, in the four octave bands centered on the frequencies 500, 1000, 2000, and 4000 Hz." To avoid confusion with other speech-interference levels used in the past, the ANSI standard uses an abbreviation that specifies the center frequencies in kHz: SIL (0.5, 1, 2, 4).[72] The speech-interfering effects of various noises can also be rated by A-weighted sound-level meter readings, according to Webster, or by modifying dBA readings by the difference between C-weighted and A-weighted levels, as suggested by Botsford.[73]

In its "Levels Document," EPA identifies an L_{eq} of 45 dB in the home as necessary to provide for 100 percent intelligibility of sentences. On the assumption that there will be an attenuation of 15 dB of outside noise with partially open windows, the maximum outside L_{eq} that will ensure an inside L_{eq} of 45 dB is 60 dB. For communicating outdoors, EPA says that an L_{eq} of 60

[70] J. C. Webster, "Speech Communications as Limited by Ambient Noise," *Journal of the Acoustical Society of America* 37 (April 1965):694.

[71] John C. Webster, "Effects of Noise on Speech Intelligibility," in *Noise as a Health Hazard,* eds. Ward and Fricke, p. 68.

[72] "American National Standard for Rating Noise with Respect to Speech Interference," ANSI S3.14-1977 (New York: Acoustical Society of America).

[73] Webster, "Speech Communications," pp. 60–63: James A. Botsford, "Predicting Speech Interference and Annoyance from A-Weighted Sound Levels," *Journal of the Acoustical Society of America* 42 (November 1967):1151 (abstract).

dB will allow "normal conversation at distances up to 2 meters with 95% sentence intelligibility."[74]

OTHER EFFECTS OF NOISE

Physiological Effects

There is no question that exposure to very high levels of sound will produce temporary extra-auditory physiological effects. In his 1950 monograph, Kryter[75] cites a study performed by Parrack, Eldredge, and Koster for the Engineering Division of the Air Materiel Command in 1948 of the effects of exposure to noise from turbojet engines and from sirens at sound-pressure levels of around 150 dB. In addition to producing severe temporary threshold shifts, the noise was reported to produce some heating of the skin, a sensation of vibration in the bones of the cranium and movement of air in the sinuses and nasal passages, some blurring of the vision, and some difficulty in maintaining posture thought to be associated with the proprioceptive reflex mechanism.

Broadbent also refers to the Parrack, Eldredge, and Koster study, and in addition he mentions some biological effects noted in response to sudden, unexpected sound, such as a shot.[76] He notes that in such situations there will be a rise in blood pressure, an increase in pressure inside the head, increased perspiration, increase in heart rate, changes in breathing, and perhaps general muscular contractions. It would seem logical to conclude that if these reactions are repeated frequently, they might cause harmful effects to the health, for example, digestive disorders, because one of the by-products of such startle responses is a decrease in peristalsis and in the flow of saliva and gastric juices. Broadbent also mentions the possibility of harm resulting from increased activity of the adrenal glands in response to sudden, unexpected noise. Apparently, however, there are no long-term effects from repeated exposures to "unexpected" noises because with repetitions a noise no longer serves to produce a startle effect. Broadbent also refers to a study indicating that such biological effects as increased blood pressure, heart rate, and respiration rate tended to disappear or adapt over long periods of exposure to intense noise.

There is question about whether workers exposed to industrial noise incur any risks to their health other than NIPTS. Unfortunately, few studies have been reported and these tend to be inconclusive, because factors other

---

[74] *Information on Levels of Environmental Noise Requisite to Protect Public Health and Welfare with an Adequate Margin of Safety,* p. 21.

[75] Kryter, "Effects of Noise on Man," p. 21.

[76] Donald E. Broadbent, "Effects of Noise on Behavior," in *Handbook of Noise Control,* ed. C. Harris, chap. 10, pp. 8–10.

than noise may be influencing the results. One of the most widely quoted bits of information is a figure from a study reported in a 1961 German publication by Gerd Jansen.[77] The figure consists of bar graphs comparing the percentage of occurrence of peripheral circulation problems, heart problems, and equilibrium disturbance between workers in "very noisy" and "less noisy" industries. The figure shows a greater incidence for the workers in the very noisy industries in all cases, the differences between the two groups in regard to peripheral circulation problems and heart problems reaching statistical significance.

Summarizing the information presented by various authors, Cohen reports that the following "distinctive functional changes" can occur during noise exposure: vasoconstriction of small blood vessels and compensating increases in diastolic blood pressure, increase of corticosteroids in the blood and in the urine representing a marshalling of bodily defenses against a threat, reduction in rate of respiration and decrease in salivary and gastric secretions with a resulting slowing of digestive processes, and a generalized increase in muscular tension and in the activity of muscle reflexes. Cohen says, "Taken together, these physiological reactions to noise constitute a generalized response of the body to stress."[78]

In an earlier publication, Cohen cited some results from the 1972 report of a contract between the Raytheon Service Company and the National Institute for Occupational Safety and Health. As part of the contract research, the records for five years of workers exposed to noise of 95 dBA or higher were compared with the records of workers in noise of 80 dBA or lower in regard to number of accidents, number of diagnosed medical problems, number of discrete absences, and number of days of absence. In one industrial study (a boiler factory), there were statistically significant differences in favor of the noise-exposed workers on each of these four dimensions. Respiratory problems constituted the most commonly diagnosed disorder. Among the noise-exposed workers, many of the respiratory disturbances involved vocal problems—hoarseness and laryngitis—and sore throats, which probably resulted from the vocal strain required to communicate in high noise levels. Other disorders characterized by a much higher incidence among the noise-exposed workers were allergenic, musculoskeletal, cardiovascular, digestive, glandular, neurological, and urological. Cohen admits that the research he was reporting,

---

[77] Karl D. Kryter, *The Effects of Noise on Man* (New York: Academic Press, 1970), p. 509; James D. Miller, "Effects of Noise on People," *Journal of the Acoustical Society of America* 56 (September 1974):761; Alexander Cohen, "Extra-Auditory Effects of Noise," in *Industrial Noise and Hearing Conservation*, eds. Julian B. Olishifski and Earl R. Harford (Chicago: National Safety Council, 1975), chap. 10, p. 261; Frederick A. White, *Our Acoustic Environment* (New York: John Wiley, 1975), p. 462.

[78] Cohen, "Extra-Auditory Effects of Noise," p. 260.

as well as other research of a similar type, can be criticized for "the inability to control other adverse workplace or job factors, apart from noise, which may have influenced the results."[79]

Most of the research on the physiological effects of noise exposure has been performed with animals. Welch contends that "our whole framework of neuroendocrine knowledge about the human body is based upon information derived from . . . basic animal models." He points to animal research that indicates noise affects many aspects of physiology, such as the reproductive and cardiovascular systems, and argues that information gleaned from animal studies is "referable to and relevant to the human situation."[80] Miller is skeptical about the applicability of animal research to human beings. He points out that rodents have frequently been used in animal studies and comments that rodents "seem to have special susceptibility to the effects of certain sounds." In regard to the physiological effects of noise on humans, Miller says, "Perhaps the stress of continued exposure to high levels of noise can produce disease or make one more susceptible to disease, but the evidence is not conclusive. . . . The only conclusively established effect of noise on health is that of noise-induced hearing loss."[81] Essential agreement with Miller's position has been expressed by Ward, von Gierke, and Kryter.[82]

Davis dispels the notion that there are any mysterious biological effects from exposure to certain sounds or combinations of sounds or from exposure to ultrasonic frequencies. He says, "There is no magic in any strange disharmony or in any high-frequency 'ultrasonic death ray' at any practical intensity."[83]

In engineering contexts, noise and vibration are considered to be problems of equal concern to the acoustical engineer. "Vibration is an oscillation wherein the quantity is a parameter that defines the motion of a mechanical

[79] Alexander Cohen, "Industrial Noise and Medical, Absence, and Accident Record Data on Exposed Workers," in *Proceedings of the International Congress on Noise as a Public Health Problem, Dubrovnik, Yugoslavia, May 13–18, 1973*, ed. W. Dixon Ward, Publication No. 550/9-73-008 (Washington, D.C.: U.S. Environmental Protection Agency), pp. 441–53.

[80] Bruce L. Welch, *Public Hearings on Noise Abatement and Control, vol. VII, Physiological and Psychological Effects, Boston, October 28 and 29, 1971* (Washington, D.C.: Environmental Protection Agency), p. 240.

[81] Miller, "Effects of Noise on People," p. 761.

[82] W. Dixon Ward, *Public Hearings on Noise Abatement and Control*, pp. 270–77; Henning von Gierke, *Public Hearings on Noise Abatement and Control*, p. 277; Karl D. Kryter, "Extraauditory Effects of Noise," in *Effects of Noise on Hearing*, eds. Donald Henderson, Roger P. Hamernik, Darshan S. Dosanjh, and John H. Mills (New York: Raven Press, 1976), p. 543.

[83] Hallowell Davis, "Conservation of Hearing or Prevention of Hearing Loss," in *Hearing and Deafness*, 4th ed., eds. Hallowell Davis and S. Richard Silverman (New York: Holt, Rinehart and Winston, 1978), chap. 5, p. 152.

system."[84] A mechanical system is an aggregate of matter comprising a defined configuration of mass, mechanical stiffness, and mechanical resistance."[85] The human body comes under this definition of a mechanical system and is affected by vibration. The body as a whole is subject to vibration while in a rough-riding vehicle, and harmful effects may result from such abuse. One of the receptors for mechanical stimulation is the auditory system, and another is the vestibular system. Frequently, these interact, so that high-intensity sound stimulation can produce reflexive head motions and displacement of the visual field. It is not the purpose of this section to discuss the biological effects of vibration but only to mention that high-intensity noise stimulation sufficient to produce vibratory effects can cause other physiological effects than have been discussed.[86]

Psychological Effects

Many studies have been conducted on the psychological effects of exposure to noise, including studies on the ability of subjects to perform various kinds of tasks in the presence of noise and studies on the annoyance of noise. Cohen states that high-level noise (90 dB SPL) has adverse effects on tasks requiring vigilance, where a subject must monitor many dials, looking for slight needle deflections or variations of signal strength, and requiring some response from the subject. With noise, subjects detect fewer signal variations and their response time is slower. In studies of mental and psychomotor abilities, the results have been equivocal. Cohen says, "Studies of performance in noise on mental tasks involving arithmetic computations, mechanical and abstract reasoning, clerical sorting and coding, and on psychomotor tasks of reaction time and tracking sometimes show losses, sometimes improvement, and in most cases no significant change when compared to performance under non-noise conditions." One of the variables affecting the results of such studies is the level of the noise used. Studies that use levels of less than 90 dBA rarely show any decrement of performance.[87]

James Miller formulates several general conclusions regarding the effects of noise on the performance of mental or motor tasks: (1) steady, non-meaningful noise does not seem to affect performance at levels below 90 dBA; (2) random bursts of noise—even at levels below 90 dBA—are more disruptive than steady-state noise; (3) components of high frequency—above 1000 to

---

[84] "American Standard Acoustical Terminology (Including Mechanical Shock and Vibration)," *American National Standard*, ANSI S1.1-1960 (New York: American National Standards Institute), p. 9.

[85] Ibid. p. 16.

[86] David E. Goldman, "Effects of Vibration on Man," in *Handbook of Noise Control*, ed. C. Harris, chap. 11, p. 3.

[87] Alexander Cohen, "Effects of Noise on Psychological State," in *Noise as a Health Hazard*, eds. Ward and Fricke, pp. 74–88.

2000 Hz—are more disturbing than components of lower frequency; (4) although noise does not affect the overall rate of work, it may produce a variability in the rate of work—periods when little or nothing is accomplished followed by periods of increased activity—that does not affect the overall rate; (5) although not reducing the quantity of work produced, noise may reduce the accuracy of the work; (6) complex rather than simple tasks are more likely to be affected adversely by noise. Miller suggests that even when a person maintains a high level of performance in noise, there may be a price to pay in terms of fatigue and a reduced capacity to react to additional demands.[88]

Laymon Miller explains that sometimes the introduction of a noise into a work environment will result in a temporary improvement in performance, because the need to adjust to the presence of the noise represents a change in what otherwise was a monotonous environment. Miller states that exposure to high noise levels, whether or not it affects performance, is likely to produce annoyance and irritability. He points out that annoyance increases with increasing intensity of the noise; a noise having most of its energy in a narrow band, thus producing a whine or hum, is more annoying than a noise with a broad spectrum; an impact, or intermittent type of noise, is more annoying than a steady-state noise; and (excluding impact noises) longer noises are more disturbing than shorter ones.[89]

Broadbent observes that a high-pitched noise (above 1500 Hz) is more annoying than a low-pitched noise of the same loudness, and he suggests that the reduction of high-frequency components in a noise will yield greater benefits than reduction of low frequencies.[90] Another factor involved in assessing annoyance is the localization of the noise. Apparently, a noise that cannot be localized is more annoying than one that can. Other parameters contributing to annoyance are the degree to which a given noise is "necessary" or "unnecessary" and the degree to which a noise is inappropriate to one's own activities. The unnecessary noise evokes more complaints, and a noise that is manifestly inappropriate to a situation—such as a laugh at a funeral—is most annoying.[91]

THE CONTROL OF INDUSTRIAL NOISE

The control of noise may be desirable in order to reduce the hazard of noise-induced hearing impairment, to improve communication, or to reduce annoyance. The reduction of noise can be accomplished through improved

[88] Miller, "Effects of Noise on People," p. 757.

[89] Laymon N. Miller, "Does Noise Affect You and Your Work?" *Safety Maintenance* (June 1956):44.

[90] Broadbent, "Effects of Noise on Man," p. 5.

[91] Ibid., pp. 7–8.

engineering design of machinery, proper mounting of machinery, alterations in the path of sound emanating from the machinery, and finally the use of ear protectors that reduce the level of sound reaching the hearing mechanism.

Improved Engineering Design

If designers of machinery considered the desirability of minimizing noise, many of the noise-control measures now needed in factories would become unnecessary. Frequently, parts can be designed with materials that are relatively noiseless at no sacrifice of efficiency, durability, or expense. Sometimes, the design of machinery to minimize noise production may create additional expense, but when it is compared to the costs of instituting noise-control procedures in factories and the possible economic effects of workmen's compensation claims, the additional initial investment for "quiet" machines may appear to be well worthwhile. Manufacturers of machinery are responsive to consumers' demands, so if the consumers insist on quieter machinery and are willing to pay the price, the manufacturers of machinery will produce quieter products.

Peterson and Gross refer to some ways in which noise can be controlled at its source:[92]

1. Decrease the energy available for driving the vibrating system.
2. Change the coupling between this energy and the acoustical radiating system.
3. Change the structure that radiates the sound so that less is radiated.

Although these suggestions refer to the modification of existing machinery, they could apply as well to the original design. The energy that drives the vibrating system can be decreased by keeping the speed of moving parts as slow as possible, by keeping air streams at low velocity, and by using structural materials that inherently are less noisy. Noise resulting from the coupling system can be reduced by providing special mounts that absorb vibration and by installing mufflers on intake and exhaust systems. Changing the radiating structure may involve only reducing the external surface areas of vibrating parts, or it may involve special treatment of the radiating surfaces to reduce the efficiency of radiation.

Alterations in the Pathway of Sound

Peterson and Gross suggest three ways in which noise control can be achieved through altering the pathway of sound:[93]

[92] Peterson and Gross, *Handbook of Noise Measurement*, p. 217.
[93] Ibid., p. 218.

1. Change in relative position of source and listener
2. Change in acoustic environment
3. Introduction of attenuating structures between source and listener

If most of the noise is directly radiated from the source, rather than being bounced off reflecting surfaces, it may be sufficient simply to move employees further away from the source—at least those employees who do not have to be close to the source. If the source is directional, rotating it to achieve minimum exposure of the workers around the source may be helpful. The acoustic environment can be changed by adding acoustical absorbing material to the room in which the machinery is located. Acoustical tiles and other absorbing materials are useful primarily in reducing noise levels at some distance from the source and in reducing the sound energy reflected from walls and ceiling. Such treatment does not substantially reduce the noise that emanates directly from the source, and so it will not be very effective in protecting workers who are in that vicinity.

Usually, the most effective way of altering the pathway of sound to achieve noise control is through the use of attenuating structures of various types. These may consist of walls, standing or hanging barriers, or even total enclosures of the sound source. By using one or more enclosures around a machine, it is possible to reduce the noise level by almost any desired amount. It must be kept in mind, however, that the isolating integrity of an enclosure can be nullified if sound can be transmitted through ventilating ducts or doors and windows in the enclosure. Ducts should be lined with absorbing materials and built with interior baffles like a muffler, and doors and windows should be designed for maximum acoustical attenuating characteristics in the same manner that openings into audiometric "soundproof" rooms are designed. It goes without saying that as the complexity of the enclosure increases, the expense of the noise-control measure increases. Thus, as we stated earlier, it may be more economical in the long run to pay an increased price for a machine that is designed to minimize noise than to go to the expense of isolating the machine in an enclosure. Figure 9–11 from Peterson and Gross[94] shows a hypothetical example of what typically can be anticipated in the way of noise reduction by various noise-control measures. First, this figure shows the octave-band levels, measured at the position M, of the noise produced by a machine that is simply sitting on the floor of a factory. The machine produces a wide-band noise that is relatively flat through all the eight octave bands. The band levels range from about 83 to 92 dB. The next seven parts of the figure show the decrease in band levels that would typically occur with various kinds of noise-control measures, from the use of vibration mounts to the employment of a double enclosure of a rigid, sealed type and vibration mounts on

[94] Ibid., pp. 220–21.

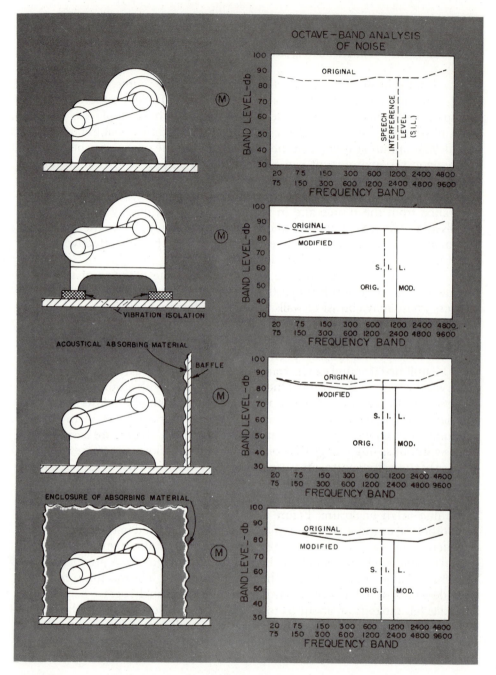

FIGURE 9-11.   Noise reduction by various noise-control measures. (Reproduced by permission of General Radio Company from Arnold P. G. Peterson and Ervin E. Gross, Jr., *Handbook of Noise Measurement,* 1972.)

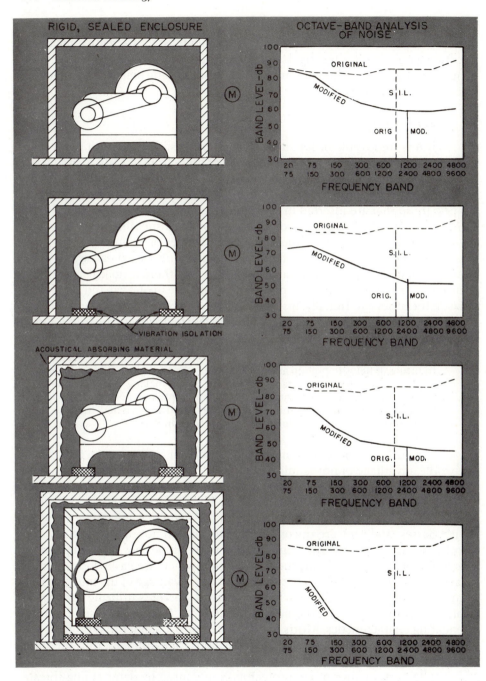

FIGURE 9-11. (Continued.)

both the machine and the inner enclosure. It should be noted that enclosing the machine with sound-absorbing material alone is an ineffective means of reducing noise; a massive, rigid, sealed enclosure is much more effective. Lining the interior of a rigid structure with sound-absorbing material, however, increases its effectiveness.

Ear Protectors

If it is impossible or for some reason not feasible to control noise at its source, or to create barriers to the radiation of noise from its source, so that the resulting sound level is potentially hazardous to hearing, the individuals exposed to the noise may be protected by "ear protectors." These are of two types: those that are inserted in the external canal and those that fit over the entire auricle. Insert-type protectors may be of the disposable variety, such as wax-impregnated cotton, or they may be of rubber or neoprene. The latter types are made in from three to five sizes for different size ear canals. To be effective, an insert must fit the canal snugly, so that there is no leakage around the insert. The same individual may require one size in one ear and a different size in the other ear. Initially, inserts should be fitted by a trained person to ensure that the proper size is selected. Maas gives the following instructions for fitting ear protectors:

> In fitting, it helps to pull up and back on the ear lobe slightly. This enlarges and tends to straighten the entrance to the ear canal, making it easier to insert a proper-sized device. When the lobe is released, the tissues of the canal will then hold the protector firmly in the ear. If properly fitted and inserted, the device will seem to *stay put* when an attempt is made to withdraw it.[95]

Earmuffs are becoming increasingly popular as ear protectors. They have the advantage of not requiring special fitting, as do the inserts, and they may be more comfortable for long-time wear. Also, they are somewhat more efficient in attenuating sound than inserts. The disadvantage to the earmuffs is that there may be a problem in getting an adequate seal when they are worn with glasses, and they are uncomfortable to wear in hot rooms. Initially, the cost of the earmuffs is higher, but over a period of time they may not prove to be any more expensive than the insert types, which are easily lost and may have to be replaced several times. An additional advantage of the muff is that a supervisor can see at a glance whether or not a worker is utilizing ear protectors. Earmuffs may have liquid-filled seals that further increase their attenuating characteristics. Muffs may be fitted into a helmet that protects the whole head. Muffs may also be used as cushions for earphones, thus serving a dual purpose. Insert protectors and muffs are shown in Figure 9–12.

The performance of ear protectors is measured by determining thresh-

[95] Roger Maas, "Ear Protection—Why . . . How?" *Supervision* (February 1960): 19.

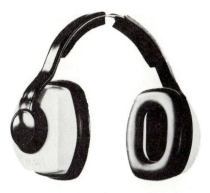

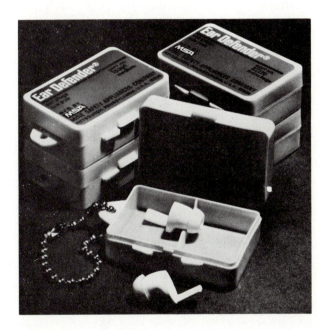

FIGURE 9–12. Muff-type ear protectors above and insert-type ear protectors below. (Courtesy of Mine Safety Appliance Company.)

old shifts of normal-hearing subjects when they are wearing the protectors. The testing is performed in a sound-field. A subject's thresholds for a wide range of frequencies are measured binaurally. Then thresholds are measured again while wearing the defenders to be tested. The difference between the thresholds at each frequency is the attenuation of the protector. Standard procedure calls for using a group of ten subjects and determining each subject's threshold with a given protector three times at each frequency. An average threshold shift at each frequency is then determined for each subject, and a mean for the ten subjects is computed to give a mean attenuation curve for that defender.[96] A 1957 ANSI standard specified the procedures for measuring the attenuation of ear protectors.[97] A 1975 NIOSH publication reported attenuation data on 175 protective devices from forty manufacturers. The attenuation data were furnished by the manufacturers.[98] The 1957 ANSI standard was revised and reissued in 1974.[99] The 1974 standard specifies the use of third-octave bands of noise instead of pure tones as the test stimuli and the use of a reverberant test room for the measurements of attenuation instead of a sound-absorbent test chamber. Also, an objective method for determining the attenuation of earmuffs is described.[100]

In conditions of extreme noise, it may be necessary to wear both the insert-type defenders and earmuffs. The two types of protectors used together result in more attenuation than that provided by either one alone. Table 9–4 compares the attenuation of a typical earplug and a typical earmuff and shows the attenuation resulting from the simultaneous use of both.

It is of concern to supervisory personnel that although good protective devices are available, it is not easy to persuade workers to use them. Maas reports a study by the Employers Mutual Liability Insurance Company of Wausau, Wisconsin, indicating that only 22.5 percent of 1148 plants polled reported having had much success with getting workers to accept ear protectors for a period of six months or more. Maas lists some of the following reasons given by workers for not utilizing ear protection: The protectors "hurt" and are uncomfortable; they are too much bother; they get lost; they cause headaches and nervousness; with the protectors in place one cannot hear wanted sounds; one gets used to the noise so it is not bothersome.[101] If ear protectors are properly selected and fitted, they need not be uncomfortable, and it is actually easier to carry on conversation in a noisy environment with ear protectors than without them. The hardest argument to overcome is that the noise really does not bother people when they get used to it. Many men seem to feel that they are being "sissy" if they use ear protectors. They like to

[96] Richard L. Swift, "Personal Hearing-Protective Devices," in *Industrial Noise and Hearing Conservation*, eds. Olishifsky and Harford, chap. 20, p. 545.

[97] "Method for the Measurement of the Real-Ear Attenuation of Ear Protectors at Threshold," ANSI Z24.22-1957 (New York: American National Standards Institute).

[98] Patricia Kroes, Roy Fleming, and Barry Lempert, *List of Personal Hearing Protectors and Attenuation Data*, HEW Publication No. (NIOSH) 76-120 (Washington, D.C.: U.S. Department of Health, Education, and Welfare, 1975).

[99] "Method for the Measurement of Real-Ear Protection of Hearing Protectors and Physical Attenuation of Earmuffs," ANSI S3.19-1974 (New York: American National Standards Institute).

[100] Kroes, Fleming, and Lempert, "List of Personal Hearing Protectors," p. 1.

[101] Roger A. Maas, "Hearing Protection in Industry," *Nursing Outlook* 9 (May 1961):281.

TABLE 9–4. Mean real-ear attenuation in dB of typical ear plug, typical ear muff, and combination of the plug and muff.

	Frequency in Hz								
	125	250	500	1000	2000	3000	4000	6000	8000
Ear plug	25	24	25	28	36	37	34	40	37
Ear muff	19	23	36	36	31	41	41	45	35
Combination plug and muff	37	35	40	40	39	48	51	48	40

Adapted from Andrew D. Hosey and Charles H. Powell, *Industrial Noise, a Guide to Its Evaluation and Control,* Public Health Service Publication No. 1572 (Washington, D.C.: U.S. Department of Health, Education, and Welfare, 1967), p. N-12-2.

think that their ears are "tougher" than other people's, and they believe it would be an admission of weakness to use ear protectors. As we said at the beginning of this chapter, noise is insidious in its effect on the hearing because noise levels below those required to produce the sensation of discomfort may cause permanent damage, and in the absence of regular audiometric tests a worker may incur a serious hearing loss in the higher frequencies without being aware of it. In the experience of insurance companies and factory management, it is necessary to carry on continuing employee education programs about the need for and advantage of ear protection, and even to insist on threat of discharge from employment that employees in certain very noisy operations wear ear protection at all times. At the same time, management has the responsibility for seeing that ear protection is available to every employee in noisy areas and that the protectors issued are of proper size and fit for maximum comfort.

Incidentally, a word should be said about the ineffectiveness of dry cotton as ear protection. Because for many years no specially designed ear protectors were manufactured, cotton was used by individuals who were exposed to gunfire in the armed services. In comparison with the attenuation provided by even a relatively inefficient earplug of rubber or neoprene, however, dry cotton is almost useless.

Fletcher has described an ingenious method for making use of the ear's own protective device, the intra-aural muscle reflex, for protection from impulsive sounds, such as bursts of gunfire. When the tensor tympani and stapedius muscles contract, the amount of sound transmitted to the inner ear is reduced. In a burst of machine-gun fire, the muscles will contract after the first shot, but that first shot may cause damage to the hair cells of the cochlea. It takes 10 msec or more for the ear reflex to occur, whereas the rise time of a gunshot is less than 2 msec. Fletcher devised a system for presenting a 1000-Hz tone through a loudspeaker at a sound-pressure level of 98 dB some 200 msec before a burst from a machine gun was fired. Thus, the ear reflex was activated prior to the initial shot of the burst. Fletcher then compared the amount of TTS obtained from two groups of subjects firing machine guns:

one in which the acoustic reflex was activated in the manner described, and the other (control group) in which there was no activation of the acoustic reflex prior to the first shot. His results indicated that the experimental group showed an average of 10 dB less TTS than the control group for frequencies of 1000 Hz and higher. He stated that for certain "highly sensitive" individuals, the protection afforded by the acoustic reflex may be as great as 50 dB at some frequencies. Fletcher then compared the protective effect of the ear reflex with that of an ear insert protector. He found that the ear reflex produced slightly better protection for frequencies of 1000 Hz and lower, but that the insert provided superior protection for frequencies higher than 1000 Hz.[102] Although Fletcher's work is interesting, it is doubtful if a method of activating the ear reflex will prove feasible for industrial use, especially because readily available ear protectors provide almost as good protection for the lower frequencies as does the ear reflex, and better protection for the higher frequencies.

As was already stated, although ear protectors may be used if it is impossible or unfeasible to control noise at its source, the use of defenders should not be considered an acceptable substitute for engineering or administrative controls. Ear protective devices should be used as interim measures until such time as engineering or administrative controls can reduce noise exposure to safe levels.

INDUSTRIAL HEARING CONSERVATION PROGRAMS

Since noise-induced hearing impairment has become a compensable disability, hearing conservation has assumed an economic importance to industry and to the companies that write industrial compensation insurance. The principle of apportionment of liability, referred to earlier in this chapter, holds an employer liable for only that portion of a claimant's hearing loss that was incurred during the period of work for that employer, provided the employer can prove that the claimant had some hearing loss at the initiation of employment. It follows, then, that to protect against being held liable for a claimant's entire hearing loss, an employer must perform a hearing test on each new employee. This initial audiogram then becomes a "reference" with which future audiograms will be compared to determine what changes, if any, have occurred in an employee's hearing levels during the period of employment. Because the decision about where to place a new employee may hinge to some extent on the degree of "toughness" or "tenderness" of the ears, the initial audiogram is frequently called a *preplacement audiogram*. If in the initial audiogram a new employee shows evidence that some noise-induced hearing

---

[102] John L. Fletcher, "Reflex Response of Middle-Ear Muscles: Protection of the Ear from Noise," *Sound* 1 (March-April 1962):17–23.

impairment has occurred, the employer is warned that placing this employee in a noisy work environment may be inviting a future claim, because the employee has already demonstrated a susceptibility to noise.

Another purpose of the reference audiogram is to identify individuals who have hearing problems whether or not they are related to noise exposure. Such individuals should have careful diagnostic audiometry performed to determine whether their hearing impairments are conductive, sensori-neural, or mixed in type, and insofar as it can be determined, the site of the lesion and its etiology. Naturally, an otological examination is required to establish the medical diagnosis of any hearing impairments identified by reference audiograms. Individuals who have hearing impairments that are treatable by medical or surgical means should be advised to seek treatment in the interest of conserving their hearing. The primary interest in discovering hearing impairments that are not related to noise exposure, however, as far as the employer is concerned, is protection from future claims that noise exposure on the job has been the primary agent in producing an employee's hearing impairment, when in fact there may have been an entirely different etiology.

Establishing a system through which the hearing of all new employees is routinely tested is certainly desirable, for the reasons that have been cited. It may not, however, be economically feasible for an employer to provide hearing tests for all new employees. If this is the case, there should be provision for obtaining reference audiograms for all new employees who will be working in environments that the employer considers to be at least potentially hazardous to the hearing. The OSHA regulations require employers to obtain a reference or "base-line" audiogram within six months of an employee's first exposure to noise levels of at least 85 dBA for eight hours a day.[103]

For those employees who are working in noisy environments, there should be provision for periodic retesting to determine whether or not there has been a change in hearing level. Because exposure to noise is known to produce a temporary threshold shift, the periodic retests, referred to frequently as *monitoring audiometry*, should be performed on Monday mornings after the employee has had the weekend to recover. After forty-eight hours, any change in hearing levels from the reference audiogram should be regarded as "persistent," if not permanent, threshold shift. The detection of a persistent threshold shift should alert management to the need to prevent further deterioration of an employee's hearing—by insisting that the employee use available ear protection, attempting to reduce excessive noise levels at their source through improved engineering, limiting the employee's exposure time if possible, or in extreme cases, removing the employee entirely from the noisy environment.

As in the case of reference audiograms, monitoring audiometry also serves the purpose of discovering changes in hearing levels that may be due to an etiology other than noise exposure. Whenever monitoring audiometry

[103] *Federal Register* 48, no. 46 (March 8, 1983):9777.

reveals significant differences from the reference audiogram, there should be an audiological and otological evaluation of the employee whose hearing has been affected to determine wherever possible the cause for the change in hearing levels. Glorig suggests that the first monitoring audiogram should be scheduled for a period of about ninety days after the reference audiogram, unless the employee complains of hearing impairment or tinnitus, in which case the first monitoring audiogram should be obtained earlier. If the first retest following the reference audiogram shows that there has been no change at any frequency of 10 dB or more, future monitoring audiograms can be scheduled annually.[104] The annual audiograms are compared with the base-line test results. Whenever this comparison reveals a threshold shift of 10 dB or more at any frequency, appropriate action should be taken to protect the employee's hearing from further loss: providing appropriate ear protection, reducing the amount of time spent in noise, or reducing noise exposure by job reassignment.[105]

The Reference Audiogram

The reference audiogram should be obtained under conditions of testing that assure validity. The room in which the testing is performed should be properly sound-treated for excluding outside interference. A normal-hearing listener wearing the usual binaural earphones with MX41/AR cushions should be able to hear all test tones from 500 through 6000 Hz at zero-dB hearing level re ANSI-1969 calibration standards provided the octave-band levels for the octave bands with preferred center frequencies do not exceed the following values within the test room:[106]

500 Hz	21.5 dB
1000 Hz	29.5 dB
2000 Hz	34.5 dB
3000 Hz	39.0 dB
4000 Hz	42.0 dB
6000 Hz	41.0 dB

Of course, the amount of attenuation required to achieve the necessary levels within the room will depend on the amount of noise in the environment in which the test room is placed.

The reference audiogram should include thresholds by air conduction for the following frequencies: 500, 1000, 2000, 3000, 4000, and 6000 Hz. The frequency of 3000 Hz is included because some states utilize this frequency in

---

[104] Glorig, *Noise and Your Ear*, p. 129.

[105] *Guide for Conservation of Hearing in Noise*, p. 29.

[106] "American National Standard Criteria for Permissible Ambient Noise during Audiometric Testing," ANSI S3.1-1977 (New York: Acoustical Society of America).

computing percentage of hearing loss for purposes of compensation, and also because a loss at 3000 Hz is known to affect discrimination of speech materials under conditions of difficult listening.[107] The highest frequency tested is 6000 Hz rather than 8000 Hz, because of the comparative unreliability of test results at 8000 Hz.[108] Some authorities prefer to include 250 Hz as a test frequency, but most favor its elimination. Whether or not it is included will depend on local preferences and legal requirements.

The reference audiogram is usually obtained by an audiologist, nurse, or audiometric technician operating a pure-tone audiometer in the standard method for individual threshold testing. Automatic audiometry, however, on either an individual or group basis, is becoming more popular, especially in those industries in which there is a large turnover of the labor force, so that it is not feasible to administer individual tests in the customary manner because of sheer numbers.

Some automatic audiometers have been designed with "programmers" that present single pulses of tone to a listener, who responds by pushing a button if the tone is heard. The machine then attenuates the tone by 10 dB and presents another stimulus. As long as the subject responds correctly, the tone is attenuated in 10-dB steps. When the subject does not respond, the next presentation is at a level 5 dB higher in intensity. When the subject again responds, the intensity of the tone is decreased in 5-dB steps. Several threshold crossings are provided, and the machine makes a "decision" about thresholds at that frequency, which is then printed out automatically. Such automatic audiometers are designed to determine threshold by following the logical pattern employed by a human tester. One such instrument that has had wide military use was described by Brogan, its designer.[109]

A Grason-Stadler automatic audiometer built on the Békésy principle is shown in Figure 9–13. This instrument tests at seven discrete frequencies: 500, 1000, 2000, 3000, 4000, 6000, and 8000 Hz. At the conclusion of the test on the second ear, it presents 1000 Hz again as a check on the test validity. At each frequency, the rate of intensity change is rapid until the subject first responds. Then the intensity changes more slowly as threshold is approached. Thus, the threshold region is reached quickly and more time is spent in defining the actual hearing threshold levels. These devices tend to be computer-based so the results can be sent easily to a main computer for storage and analysis.

[107] J. Donald Harris, H. L. Haines, and C. K. Myers, "The Importance of Hearing at 3 KC for Understanding Speeded Speech," *Laryngoscope* 70 (February 1960):131–46.

[108] Hallowell Davis, Gordon Hoople, and Horace O. Parrack, "The Medical Principles of Monitoring Audiometry," A.M.A. *Archives of Industrial Health* 17 (January 1958):18.

[109] F. A. Brogan, "An Automatic Audiometer for Air Force Classification Centers," *Noise Control* 2 (May 1956):58–59, 67.

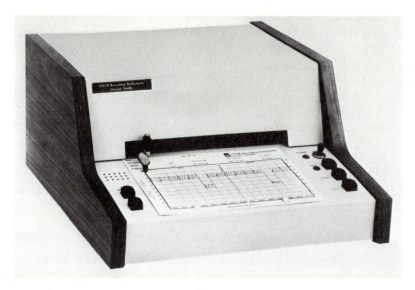

FIGURE 9-13.   The Grason-Stadler automatic audiometer. (Reproduced by permission of Grason-Stadler, Inc., Littleton, Mass.)

Monitoring Audiometry

The purpose of monitoring audiometry is to determine if there has been any significant change at any frequency since the preceding test. A significant change is one greater than the acceptable variation from test to retest, which, as stated in Chapter 5, is ± 5 dB. Of course, the kind of change the examiner is concerned about is an increased hearing impairment—an increase at any frequency of 10 dB or more. The OSHA regulations specify that audiometric tests shall include as a minimum the frequencies 500, 1000, 2000, 3000, 4000, and 6000 Hz.[110] Thus, any monitoring test—as well as the base-line test—must include these frequencies.

Personnel Requirements

The OSHA regulations specify that "audiometric tests shall be performed by a licensed or certified audiologist, otolaryngologist, or other physician, or by a technician who is certified by the Council of Accreditation in Occupational Hearing Conservation or by other technicians.[111] A Certified Audiometric Technician is a person who has successfully completed a two and a half day training period, consisting of both didactic material and practicum, under the direction of a person who has been certified as a faculty member by the Council for Accreditation in Occupational Hearing Conservation. The

[110] *Federal Register* 48, no. 46 (March 8, 1983): 9777.
[111] Ibid.

council awards certification to successful students and maintains a roster of the holders of certificates. Requirements for certification of faculty and audiometric technicians and the syllabus for the training program were established by the Board for Industrial Hearing Conservation Technicians. The council and the board were created by an intersociety committee consisting of representatives of the American Association of Industrial Nurses, the American Academy of Occupational Medicine, the American Council of Otolaryngology, the American Industrial Hygiene Association, the American Speech and Hearing Association, the Industrial Medical Association, and the National Safety Council.[112]

Audiometric technicians are trained to administer only air-conduction pure-tone tests. They must be responsible to a professional, preferably an audiologist. When the technician identifies a significant threshold shift, it is the supervisor's responsibility to perform whatever additional testing is required to help a physician establish a diagnosis of the hearing impairment. The supervisor needs to keep check on the procedures employed by the technicians to ensure comparability of test results. The supervisor is responsible also for checking on the calibration of audiometers and assuring proper acoustical environment within test rooms.

NOISE SUSCEPTIBILITY

It has been generally recognized that there are individual differences in the susceptibility of ears to damage from exposure to noise. Many references have been made in the literature to "tough" ears and "tender" ears, referring to differences in degree of susceptibility. Considerable attention has been focused on the problem of identifying those individuals who, when placed in a noisy working environment, would be most susceptible to noise-induced hearing loss. The assumption has been that if such individuals could be identified, they could be assigned to less noisy working environments, or at the least, could be provided with the best possible ear protection when they are working in noise. Attempts have been made, therefore, to devise tests for susceptibility that could be administered at the time the reference audiogram is obtained. Several such tests have been reviewed and evaluated by Summerfield, Glorig, and Wheeler[113] and by Rowland.[114]

By far, the most popular type of test is some measure of the temporary

[112] Olishifsky and Harford, eds., *Industrial Noise and Hearing Conservation,* pp. 1000–1010, app. D.

[113] Anne Summerfield, Aram Glorig, and D. E. Wheeler, "Is There a Suitable Industrial Test of Susceptibility to Noise-Induced Hearing Loss?" *Noise Control* 4 (January 1958):40–46, 54.

[114] Roy C. Rowland, Jr., "Tests for Identifying Noise-Susceptible Individuals" (unpublished M. A. thesis, Stanford University, 1960).

threshold shift (TTS). The method involves presenting a subject with a "fatiguing" stimulus that may be either a pure tone or a wide-band noise. After a prescribed period of exposure to the fatiguing stimulus, the degree of shift of the subject's threshold at some frequency—usually around 4000 Hz—is measured immediately or from one to five minutes (most commonly two minutes) following the cessation of the fatiguing stimulus. Predictions of susceptibility are then made on the basis of either the absolute amount of threshold shift observed or the time required for the subject's threshold at the criterion frequency to return to normal, that is, its prestimulation level. The individual who incurs the greatest amount of threshold shift, or who requires the longest time for the threshold to return to its "normal" level, is then presumed to be the most susceptible to permanent, irreversible hearing impairment if placed in a noisy environment.

Several investigators have found that individuals with high preexposure hearing levels will incur less TTS to a given exposure than individuals with good hearing to begin with. Kryter believes that the best index of susceptibility is a subject's postexposure hearing level two minutes after exposure (HL_2) plus the threshold shift two minutes after exposure (TTS_2). Thus predicted NIPTS = HL_2 + TTS_2. Kryter says that if both HL_2 and TTS_2 are low, the individual has successfully resisted NIPTS in the past and probably will continue to do so in the future. Further, Kryter says, "A high postexposure HL and low TTS would imply that the person probably had susceptibility to NIPTS for that noise equal to a person with a somewhat lower HL but a larger TTS."[115]

Another type of test that seems to have predictive value is the aural harmonics test of Lawrence and Blanchard.[116] This test attempts to determine the minimum intensity at which the response of the ear to a particular frequency becomes distorted or nonlinear and produces harmonics. The assumption of the test is that at some point as intensity is increased the ear will "overload," that is, be unable to respond without distorting. Distortion is manifested by the production of aural harmonics (multiples) of the stimulating frequency. The presence of an aural harmonic is detected by introducing to the ear of the listener a second tone that is almost exactly twice the frequency of the original stimulus. If a harmonic is being generated within the ear, the second tone, called the *probe* tone, will interact with the aural harmonic to produce the sensation of beats. (See Chapter 2 for a discussion of the phenomenon of beats.)

For example, suppose the stimulating tone was at a frequency of 1000

[115] Kryter, *Effects of Noise on Man*, p. 170.

[116] Merle Lawrence and Cyrus L. Blanchard, "Prediction of Susceptibility to Acoustic Trauma by Determination of Threshold of Distortion," *Industrial Medicine and Surgery* 23 (May 1954):193–200.

Hz. It is presented at some arbitrary level above the subject's threshold for that frequency, say 70 dB. A probe tone of 2004 Hz is introduced into the same earphone at a level of 60 dB above the subject's threshold for 2000 Hz. The subject is instructed to adjust the intensity of the stimulating tone and the probe tone up and down in relation to each other until "best" beats are heard, that is, until the beats appear to be most pronounced. Then beats will occur at the rate of four per second, representing the difference in cycles between the probe tone (2004 Hz) and the aural harmonic (2000 Hz—the second harmonic of the stimulus tone of 1000 Hz). The tester then gradually decreases the intensity of both tones until the subject reports that the beats have disappeared. The subject then adjusts the intensity of the probe tone alone to see if the beats recur. If they recur, the tester again reduces the intensity of both tones until once more the subject reports the beats are no longer heard. Again the subject attempts to restore the beats by adjusting the intensity of the probe tone. This procedure is repeated until the beats have finally disappeared regardless of the adjustment of the probe tone in relation to the stimulus tone. The hearing level of the 1000-Hz tone at which the beats finally disappear is considered to be the threshold of nonlinearity. The threshold of nonlinearity is usually determined for two frequencies, 1000 and 2000 Hz, which would require the use of probe tones of 2004 and 4004 Hz, respectively.

Lawrence and Blanchard believe that when an ear is driven into nonlinearity by high-intensity stimuli and this condition, which produces distortion in the ear, is allowed to persist for any considerable length of time, a breakdown in the auditory system will occur. The earlier nonlinearity occurs, the lower the intensity of the stimulus required to produce breakdown in the auditory system. Lawrence and Blanchard assume that subjects who have comparatively low thresholds of nonlinearity or overload are therefore susceptible to noise-induced hearing loss. Their assumptions were based on laboratory experiments with guinea pigs. The animals that showed the lowest thresholds of nonlinearity sustained the greatest losses after exposure to noise; those that showed the highest thresholds of overload sustained the least losses following noise exposure.

After reviewing all the tests thought useful in identifying those individuals who are noise-susceptible, Summerfield, Glorig, and Wheeler concluded that none of them was suitable in its present form for use in industry. They suggest certain criteria that any test for susceptibility should satisfy if it is to be acceptable for industry. The equipment to be employed must be "simple and rugged." It must be sufficiently uncomplicated so that subjects and relatively naive testers can perform the test without difficulty. The test must not consume more than a brief portion of the time available for medical examinations of new employees. It must be demonstrated to be both valid and reliable; that is, it must pick out those individuals who are truly noise-susceptible, and the results of the test must be repeatable within acceptable limits of variability. Also, the test results must be immediately classifiable into degrees of susceptibility that are meaningful to industrial personnel who have to assign employees to specific tasks.[117]

Although the search for a simple, valid, and reliable test of susceptibility will probably continue, the protection of workers' ears from NIPTS for the foreseeable future will depend primarily on the effectiveness of industrial hearing conservation programs. The early detection of significant threshold shifts and the adoption of appropriate measures to prevent further impairment are the first line of defense against NIPTS, rather than trying to predict in advance which individuals can safely work in a noisy environment.

NOISE POLLUTION

Recently, a great deal of attention has been focused on the preservation of our environment. Ecologists have increased our awareness of the danger of destroying our environment by polluting the air and the water with the waste products of our technological civilization. As our civilization has become more "advanced," it has also become noisier. In 1961, it was estimated that our urban noise levels were increasing by 1 dB a year,[118] which if true means that by 1976 the intensity (power) of urban noise had doubled five times. Obviously, without effective controls at various levels of government, our civilization will get noisier and noisier. As Vern O. Knudsen, a pioneer acoustic physicist, has said, "Noise, like smog, is a slow agent of death. If it continues to increase for the next 30 years as it has for the past 30, it could become lethal."[119]

In light of our present concern with pollution, it is natural to refer to the proliferation of unwanted sound as *noise pollution*. Although the consequences of uncontrolled noise pollution are not nearly as dire as the possible results of air and water pollution, they are quite properly of concern to an increasing segment of our population. Although life itself is not threatened by noise, certainly the quality of life can be affected by the environment in which we live. It is appropriate, therefore, to devote some attention to community noise problems and their control.

What are the principal sources of noise pollution within a community? Without any attempt to rank-order them either on the basis of frequency of occurrence or level of noise, we can identify the following chief offenders: traffic noise—from automobiles, motorcycles and scooters, trucks, and buses; construction noises—from bulldozers, pile drivers, jackhammers, compressors, chain saws, and so on; subway or surface trains; sirens of emergency vehicles;

[117] Summerfield, Glorig, and Wheeler, "Is There a Suitable Industrial Test?" pp. 44–45.

[118] *Noise Control* 7 (July-August 1961):39.

[119] Quoted by W. H. Ferry, "The Citizen's View," in *Noise as a Health Hazard*, eds. Ward and Fricke, p. 303.

power mowers; aircraft flyovers, including sonic booms; barking dogs; children's screaming; air-conditioning equipment or ventilating fans; garbage or trash collections. Such a list does not include industrial noises (assumed, not always correctly, to be confined within a factory or office) or noises within one's home or apartment from various kinds of equipment, such as dishwashers, blenders, laundry equipment, vacuum cleaners, and so on, and of course the ubiquitous television and stereo sets. In all these examples of noise pollution, we are concerned for the most part not about damage to the hearing (such as workers in a noisy industry might incur over a working lifetime), but about the invasion of our privacy and the threat to the tranquillity of our existence. And who is to say that the cumulative effects of all the daily environmental noises with which we are bombarded might not contribute substantially to the statistical curves of decreasing hearing sensitivity by decade of age that we term *presbycusis*, or more properly, *sociocusis?*

There is one possible exception to the statement just made that environmental noise is not a threat to one's hearing sensitivity, and that is the discotheque or the rock concert. For some unexplainable reason, our youths today demand that their music be loud. And with electric guitars hooked to powerful amplifiers and all instruments and voices boosted with public-address systems, the hundreds of hirsute rock groups give our youths what they demand. Newspapers and popular magazines have carried stories about the dangers of hearing damage in such environments, and sound-level meter readings in discotheques have confirmed that the audience is exposed to levels that greatly exceed industrial damage-risk criteria. Because the exposures are intermittent, however, with periods of days or weeks between them, there is probably little or no danger that members of the audience will incur any NIPTS, although it is quite likely that many will demonstrate TTSs after attending a concert. The situation may be different, however, for members of performing groups—at least those groups that are in such popular demand that they perform several times a week—although even here the evidence is contradictory. Jerger and Jerger found that all members of such a group incurred TTSs ranging from 15 to 50 dB for frequencies of 2000 Hz and higher after playing for four and a half hours. Measurements made in the center of the group revealed octave-band levels in the 300–600-Hz and 600–1200-Hz bands ranging from 104 to 124 dB, with occasional peaks as high as 130 dB. Three of the five musicians in this group had preexposure audiograms showing threshold hearing levels in at least one ear ranging from 30 to 70 dB for frequencies above 2000 Hz. Because the group had been playing about three nights a week for a two-year period, it is likely that at least some of their preexposure hearing levels represented NIPTS from their rehearsals and performances.[120]

[120] James Jerger and Susan Jerger, "Temporary Threshold Shift in Rock-and-Roll Musicians," *Journal of Speech and Hearing Research* 13 (March 1970):221–24.

On the other hand, Rintelmann and Borus studied six different rock groups, making some 165 overall sound-level measurements and octave-band analyses of forty-four musical selections. They then performed hearing tests on forty-two rock musicians. The mean SPL for the six groups was 105 dB with a range of 91 to 144 dB. The mean spectral distribution was relatively flat over the range 63 to 2000 Hz, with a dropoff of from 5 to 10 dB per octave for frequencies above 2000 Hz. The criteria for inclusion in the study for the musicians were (1) no history of hearing loss, (2) never served in armed forces, (3) never worked in a noisy industry, (4) infrequent gun shooting, and (5) no family history of hearing loss. The musicians had been associated with rock groups for a mean of 2.9 years. They averaged 3.7 hours per week in practice and 7.7 hours per week in performance, for an average total of 11.4 hours per week of exposure to rock music at high levels. Surprisingly, forty of the forty-two musicians had hearing within normal limits for all frequencies from 125 through 8000 Hz.[121]

Community noise control requires some means of measuring noise in terms of its nuisance or annoyance characteristics. Annoyance is a subjective judgment, and so a method must be used of equating judgments of annoyance with the physical characteristics of a noise because regulations must be based on physical measurements. Because the jet aircraft is one of the noisiest objects to which a wide segment of our population is exposed, much time, effort, and money have been expended in trying to reduce the annoyance of airport operations to surrounding communities. Some of the measures of control attempted have been changing of flight patterns for landings and takeoffs and even relocation of major airports. In studying the reactions of listeners to aircraft noises, Kryter and his associates in a large consulting firm found it helpful to develop a new subjective measure, *perceived noisiness*, expressed in units called *noys*.[122] A scaling method for noisiness was developed in a similar manner to the way in which Stevens developed his scaling of loudness in sones.[123] The loudness scale indicates how loud a sound appears to a listener. A value of 1 sone is assigned to the loudness of a 1000-Hz tone that has a sound-pressure level of 40 dB. Then a sound that is half as loud is assigned a value of 0.5 sone, and a sound that is twice as loud as the reference tone is assigned a value of 2 sones. Similarly, a value of 1 noy was assigned to the perceived noisiness by listeners of a band of frequencies from 910 to 1090 Hz presented at a sound-pressure level of 40 dB, and values of 0.5 noy and 2 noys were assigned to sounds of half the noisiness and twice the noisiness, respectively, of the reference sound.

[121] William F. Rintelmann and Judith F. Borus, "Noise-Induced Hearing Loss and Rock and Roll Music," *Archives of Otolaryngology* 88 (1968):57–65.

[122] Karl D. Kryter, "Scaling Human Reactions to the Sound from Aircraft," *Journal of the Acoustical Society of America* 31 (November 1959):1415–29.

[123] S. S. Stevens, "Calculating Loudness," *Noise Control* 3 (September 1957): 11–22.

In Chapter 2, reference was made to the *phon*, which is the unit for measuring loudness level. The phon and the decibel are equated at the frequency of 1000 Hz by definition. When we say a sound has a loudness level of 50 phons, we mean that according to listeners' judgments it is equal in loudness to a 1000-Hz tone that has a sound-pressure level of 50 dB. In audiometric work, phons and decibels are equated at 1000 Hz in terms of hearing level rather than sound-pressure level. *Perceived noise level,* measured in units called *PNdB*, was devised by Kryter as the analog of loudness level in phons. According to Kryter, the perceived noise level of a sound in PNdB is the sound-pressure level of the 910–1090-Hz band of random noise that a listener judges to be as acceptable or unacceptable as the sound in question.[124] In 1960, Kryter published noys curves for bands of sound as a function of sound-pressure level, tables for determining noisiness in noys for each of eight octave bands and each of twenty-two ⅓ octave bands once the band level in dB is known for each band, a formula for determining the total noisiness in noys for a given sound, and a table for converting noisiness in noys to perceived noise level in PNdB.[125] Kryter and his associates believe that these measures of noisiness and perceived noise level should contribute greatly to the development of quantitative methods of expressing the subjective effects of noise, and thus will lead to methods of control to keep noise within acceptable limits. One example of the usefulness of this method of evaluating noisiness is in airport operation. One community specified that jet aircraft must not be noisier than propeller-driven aircraft, and it was possible to compare the noisiness of the two types of aircraft by means of PNdB values at various points along their flight paths. As a result of this study, airlines were forced to specify altitudes and power cutbacks for various kinds of jet aircraft to keep them within the prescribed noise limits at certain points along their flight paths in proximity to the airport.[126]

In the years since Kryter first proposed that PNdB be used as a measure of annoyance or the "unwantedness" of a noise, dozens of articles have appeared refining the concept of perceived noise level and citing its usefulness in determining not only the acceptability of aircraft noise but also, applying appropriate corrections or modifications, the acceptability of various environmental noises. These studies have been reviewed by Kryter.[127] No attempt to describe the various uses of perceived noise level will be made here.

---

[124] Kryter, "Scaling Human Reactions to the Sound from Aircraft," p. 1425.

[125] K. D. Kryter, "The Meaning and Measurement of Perceived Noise Level," *Noise Control* 6 (September-October 1960):12–27.

[126] Laymon N. Miller, Leo L. Beranek, and Karl D. Kryter, "Airports and Jet Noise," *Noise Control* 5 (January 1959):24–31.

[127] Karl D. Kryter, "Psychological Reactions to Aircraft Noise," *Science* 151 (18 March 1966):1346–55; K. D. Kryter, "Concepts of Perceived Noisiness, Their Implementation and Application," *Journal of the Acoustical Society of America* 43 (February 1968):344–61.

At the present time the scaling of noises in PNdB offers probably the best method available of setting community noise criteria. As far as measuring perceived noise level from aircraft flyovers, takeoffs, and landings is concerned, a good approximation of PNdB can be made by adding 13 dB to A-weighted sound-level meter readings.[128]

Sonic booms, resulting from flyovers of aircraft whose speed exceeds the velocity of sound, represent a special kind of hazard to our environment. They have been known since the middle 1940s when high-performance fighter planes dived at supersonic speeds. Now, with military aircraft commonly exceeding the velocity of sound (Mach 1), sonic booms are heard frequently during military maneuvers or sometimes when a military plane accidentally exceeds the speed of sound. A boom is a shock wave generated by the "piling up" of air particles when a sound source moves at a greater speed than the velocity of propagation of the disturbance.[129] The shock wave can be likened to a bow wave from a speeding boat. When the shock wave hits the ground, a sudden increase in air pressure, called *overpressure*, occurs, causing a booming sound like a single clap of thunder. In addition to the startling noise that disturbs and jolts unsuspecting listeners, the sudden overpressure from a sonic boom may cause damage to buildings. Many studies of sonic booms—both actual and produced in the laboratory—have been conducted for the purpose of determining the acceptability of the noise. The results are not encouraging. There is little evidence that most people can learn to adapt to sonic booms as they do to a certain extent to various other noxious sounds. The French, British, and Russians now have operational supersonic transports (SSTs). Reacting to overwhelming public opinion, Congress eliminated funding for the development of an American SST. In 1976, the secretary of transportation in President Ford's cabinet gave permission for a limited time for the French and British SST—the Concorde—to schedule regular flights in and out of Washington's Dulles International Airport and New York's John F. Kennedy International Airport. The SSTs are forbidden to fly over U.S. land at supersonic speeds, however, thus preventing sonic booms. Although at present there is no known "cure" for the sonic boom, it is possible that supersonic aircraft in the future may be designed to minimize the intensity of the boom, if not eliminate it altogether.

REFERENCES

Baron, Robert Alex.   *The Tyranny of Noise*. New York: St. Mary's Press, 1970.
Berendt, Raymond D.; Corliss, Edith, L. R.; and Ojalvo, Morris S.   *Quieting: A Practical Guide to Noise Control*. Washington, D.C.: National Bureau of Standards, U.S. Department of Commerce, 1976.

[128] Leo L. Beranek, "General Aircraft Noise," in *Noise as a Public Health Hazard*, eds. Ward and Fricke, p. 257.

[129] Harvey H. Hubbard, "Sonic Booms," *Physics Today* 21 (February 1968):31–37.

BURNS, WILLIAM. *Noise and Man*, 2nd ed. Philadelphia: J. B. Lippincott, 1973.

CUNNIFF, PATRICK F. *Environmental Noise Pollution*. New York: John Wiley, 1977.

DAVIS, HALLOWELL, and SILVERMAN, S. RICHARD, eds. *Hearing and Deafness*, 4th ed. Chaps. 5 and 9. New York: Holt, Rinehart and Winston, 1978.

HENDERSON, DONALD; HAMERNIK, ROGER P.; DOSANJH, DARSHAN S.; and MILLS, JOHN H., eds. *Effects of Noise on Hearing*. New York: Raven Press, 1976.

KRAMER, MARC B., and ARMBRUSTER, JOAN M., eds. *Forensic Audiology*. Baltimore: University Park Press, 1982.

KRYTER, KARL D. *The Effects of Noise on Man*. New York: Academic Press, 1970.

LIPSCOMB, DAVID M., ed. *Noise and Audiology*. Baltimore: University Park Press, 1978.

OLISHIFSKY, JULIAN B., and HARFORD, EARL R., eds. *Industrial Noise and Hearing Conservation*. Chicago: National Safety Council, 1975.

PETERSON, ARNOLD P. G., and GROSS, ERVIN E., Jr. *Handbook of Noise Measurement*. Concord, Mass.: General Radio, 1972.

ROBINSON, D. W., ed. *Occupational Hearing Loss*. New York: Academic Press, 1971.

SALMON, VINCENT; MILLS, JAMES S.; and PETERSEN, ANDREW C. *Industrial Noise Control Manual*. HEW Publication No. (NIOSH) 75-183. Cincinnati, Ohio: National Institute for Occupational Safety and Health, U.S. Department of Health, Education, and Welfare, 1975.

WARD, W. DIXON, ed. *Proceedings of the International Congress on Noise as a Public Health Problem, Dubrovnik, Yugoslavia, May 13–18, 1973*. Publication No. 550/9-73-008. Washington, D.C.: U.S. Environmental Protection Agency, 1973.

WARD, W. DIXON, and FRICKE, JAMES E., eds. *Noise as a Public Health Hazard*. Washington, D.C.: The American Speech and Hearing Association, ASHA Reports 4, February 1969.

WELCH, BRUCE L., and WELCH, ANNEMARIE S., eds. *Physiological Effects of Noise*. New York: Plenum Press, 1970.

WHITE, FREDERICK A. *Our Acoustic Environment*. New York: John Wiley, 1975.

YERGES, LYLE F. *Sound, Noise and Vibration Control*. New York: Van Nostrand Reinhold, 1969.

CHAPTER TEN
THE HANDICAP
OF HEARING IMPAIRMENT

In the previous parts of this book, we have been concerned with the physiology and pathology of hearing and with the measurement of hearing loss. Problems of hearing impairments have been considered thus far impersonally and hypothetically. Actually, of course, a hearing impairment cannot be separated from the patient who possesses it and has to live with it. Hearing is perhaps our most important sense, and naturally any marked interference with its functioning will produce difficulties in communication and in adjustment to our environment. Almost invariably, a hearing impairment produces psychological problems that add to the handicap imposed by the purely sensory dysfunction. The difficulties experienced will be proportional to the severity of the hearing impairment and related to its time of onset, to cite two of the most important variables involved. It is the purpose of this part of the book to analyze the handicap produced by a hearing impairment and to discuss the general principles of rehabilitation.

It is difficult to discuss rehabilitative needs generally because of the infinite number of possible variations of hearing loss, both in the severity of loss and in the configuration of the audiogram curve. It is difficult for hard-of-hearing persons themselves to recognize that their hearing problem is different from that of another hearing-impaired individual. Frequently, the audiologist hears the complaint, "But Mr. Smith swears that Blank hearing aid makes it possible for him to attend lectures, and I can't understand why it won't do the same for me." What the complainer fails to realize, of course, is that the hearing loss may be entirely different from Smith's. Some patients will search for years for the "perfect" hearing aid, acquiring an imposing array of different makes and models in the process. They will be dissatisfied with each aid because it does not restore their hearing as they think it should, when the source of their difficulty is not the hearing aid but their own peculiar pattern of hearing loss, which may not be helped by *any* hearing aid. Thus, in discussing the rehabilitative needs of the hard of hearing, it is necessary to differentiate somewhat on the basis of the degree and type of hearing loss involved.

SEVERITY OF HEARING IMPAIRMENT

The term *deafness* is used loosely to refer to any amount of hearing loss, but in planning a rehabilitative program for adults, or an educational program for children, it is necessary to make a distinction between the "deaf" and the "hard of hearing." In the mind of the layman, *deaf* means "completely without hearing." Actually, there are very few individuals whose auditory mechanism is completely dead. Most persons educationally classified as deaf have some shreds of hearing remaining, that is, some level of hearing that is demonstrable on an audiometric test. It is the *usefulness* of this residual hearing that determines whether a person is deaf or hard of hearing.

Some audiologists prefer to use more scientific terms to describe the degree of hearing impairment. *Hypacusis* (sometimes *hypoacusis*) means "loss of hearing that is less than complete." *Anacusis* means "deafness"—literally, "without hearing." Another scientific term is *dysacusis*, which designates an auditory disorder that is other than just a loss of sensitivity. Most frequently the term is applied to a central auditory dysfunction—a disturbance in the processing of auditory stimuli—although it can also refer to such phenomena as a loss of tonality and diplacusis. In this book, we shall refer to hard-of-hearing and deaf individuals instead of to hypacusic and anacusic ones.

In 1937 the Committee on Nomenclature of the Conference of Executives of American Schools for the Deaf proposed the following definitions, which are still valid:

1. *The Deaf:* Those in whom the sense of hearing is nonfunctional for the ordinary purposes of life. This general group is made up of two distinct classes based entirely on the time of the loss of hearing:
   a. The congenitally deaf: Those who were born deaf.
   b. The adventitiously deaf: Those who were born with normal hearing but in whom the sense of hearing became nonfunctional later through illness or accident.

2. *The Hard of Hearing:* Those in whom the sense of hearing, although defective, is functional with or without a hearing aid.[1]

In 1975, the Conference of Executives of American Schools for the Deaf adopted the following definitions, which are intended to replace the 1937 ones:

> *Hearing Impairment.* A generic term indicating a hearing disability which may range in severity from mild to profound: it includes the subsets of *deaf* and *hard of hearing.*
>
> A *deaf* person is one whose hearing disability precludes successful processing of linguistic information through audition, with or without a hearing aid.
>
> A *hard-of-hearing* person is one who, generally with the use of a hearing aid, has residual hearing sufficient to enable successful processing of linguistic information through audition.[2]

Although it is not possible to draw firm boundaries between the deaf and the hard of hearing on the basis of the extent of loss shown on an audiogram, the following classification, based on the average of pure-tone hearing threshold levels at 500, 1000, and 2000 Hz, is a general guide to the degree of severity of hearing losses:

20–30 dB	slight
30–45 dB	mild
45–60 dB	moderate
60–75 dB	severe
75–90 dB	profound
90–110 dB	extreme

Conversational speech averages a sound-pressure level of about 70 dB or a hearing level for speech of about 50 dB. The difference between "weak" and "loud" conversational speech is about 30 dB, covering a range of average hearing levels for speech of 35 dB (weak) to 65 dB (loud).[3] Speech sounds of English range in power some 28 dB from the weakest sound (the voiceless *th* as in *thin*) to the strongest sound (the vowel *aw* is in *law*).[4] A person with an HTL for speech of 30 dB would just barely be able to hear average conversational

[1] S. R. Silverman and H. S. Lane, "Deaf Children in *Hearing and Deafness,* 3rd ed., eds. Hallowell Davis and S. Richard Silverman (New York: Holt, Rinehart and Winston, 1970): 386.

[2] S. Richard Silverman, Helen S. Lane, and Donald R. Calvert, "Early and Elementary Education," in *Hearing and Deafness,* 4th ed., eds. Hallowell Davis and S. Richard Silverman (New York: Holt, Rinehart and Winston, 1978), chap. 17, p. 434.

[3] Hallowell Davis, "The Articulation Area and the Social Adequacy Index for Hearing," *Laryngoscope* 58 (August 1948):766.

[4] Harvey Fletcher, *Speech and Hearing in Communication* (New York: D. Van Nostrand, 1953).

speech with the unaided ear; the weaker sounds would be at about threshold level. A great deal, if not most, of weak conversational speech would be inaudible. Such a person would probably benefit from a hearing aid.

For many years, it was a rule of thumb that unless a patient's loss for speech in the better ear was at least 30 dB, a hearing aid would not be recommended. The advent of head-worn aids and "all-in-the-ear" aids has caused us to revise our thinking. There are many patients with losses of less than 30 dB for speech, and some with unilateral losses, who are at least part-time users of hearing aids—and satisfied users. As yet, the upper limit of hearing loss that can be benefited by a hearing aid has not been accurately determined. As aids have become more powerful, their benefit has been extended to a greater proportion of the hearing-handicapped population. Some patients with HTLs for speech of as much as 100 dB obtain "usable" hearing from a hearing aid. Others, with less extreme losses, are unable to utilize aids successfully. The factor of recruitment of loudness, which is characteristic of many cases of sensori-neural loss, may militate against a hearing aid. As was stated in Chapter 5, the configuration of the audiogram curve, as well as the extent of loss through the speech frequencies, is important in determining whether or not a given patient can benefit from amplification.

TIME OF ONSET

The degree of handicap produced by a hearing loss depends to a considerable extent on its time of onset. This is true of the handicap of communication and of the problems of a psychological nature that accompany the hearing impairment. The effect of time of onset on the individual's ability to communicate is easy to understand. Language is learned through the auditory pathway. To learn to speak, the child must first understand or comprehend the speech that is heard. If a child is born with defective hearing, or incurs a hearing impairment in the first year to year and a half of life, language development will be affected—to what extent depends, of course, on the severity of the loss and other factors, such as intelligence. If, however, hearing is normal throughout the period when the child is acquiring basic language concepts, both receptive and expressive, the effect of an acquired hearing loss on ability to communicate will be considerably less, again depending on the severity of the loss. The child with a severe congenital hearing impairment will have to be taught to recognize speech through minimal auditory clues and visual clues and will have to learn to speak laboriously on a word-by-word basis. Without the help of skilled teachers of the deaf, such a child would go through life deprived of oral communication.

On the other hand, the child who loses hearing after learning to comprehend speech and to speak will in time lose the ability to communicate unless given special instruction. Nevertheless, the job of teaching such a child is relatively easy because the teacher does not have to begin with basic language concepts. The problem here is to keep the child from losing what has already been acquired in the way of language ability, while helping to develop a constantly increasing facility in language.

The problems of the adult who incurs a hearing impairment are usually quite different from those of children. In the first place, an adult seldom incurs a complete loss of hearing. Usually there is sufficient residual hearing present so that speech can be heard to some extent. In the second place, the adult has well-established language patterns. Although there may be a need for help in learning to understand speech with impaired hearing, the hearing-impaired adult should have a minimum of difficulty with speech production.

PSYCHOLOGICAL PROBLEMS

A hearing impairment almost always produces some maladjustment in the individual. Sometimes, the psychological difficulties arising from the hearing loss are a greater problem for the hard-of-hearing person than is the communicative disorder. Psychological difficulties are not always proportionate to the severity of the loss, but they are usually related to the time of onset. According to some points of view, those who are born with impaired hearing or who lose their hearing early in life do not have as severe adjustment problems as those who suffer hearing loss after having had normal hearing well into adult life. The theory is that it is psychologically more difficult to lose one's hearing after having experienced a number of years of normal hearing than it is to be without hearing for all one's life. It should be emphasized, however, that there are many psychologists who disagree with this notion.

Ramsdell[5] refers to three levels of hearing, loss of any one of which would cause some psychological difficulty to the adult who has previously enjoyed normal hearing. The three levels are the *symbolic* level, the *warning* or *signal* level, and the *primitive* level. The *symbolic* level refers to the function of the hearing mechanism in the process of oral communication. Naturally, loss of the ability to communicate will cause the hearing-impaired individual psychological difficulties. Not being able to talk easily with people leads to a tendency to withdraw from conversations, and eventually to withdraw from more and more social contacts. The hard-of-hearing person finds it difficult to enjoy meetings, to attend plays or lectures, or to follow a sermon in church. Thus, loss of hearing on the symbolic level may result in increasing withdrawal, which in turn leads to feelings of depression, because the individual is cut off from normal social life.

The *warning* or *signal* level of hearing refers to the function of the hearing mechanism in making us aware of dangers in the environment. For exam-

[5] Donald A. Ramsdell, "The Psychology of the Hard-of-Hearing and the Deafened Adult," in *Hearing and Deafness*, 4th ed., eds. Davis and Silverman, chap. 19.

ple, we hear the scream of a siren and are immediately alerted to look for an emergency vehicle. The growl of a dog warns us to beware of patting it. The honk of an automobile horn tells us to be careful in crossing the street. Loss of the ability to utilize danger signals means that we must be more alert with other senses. Thus, loss of hearing on the warning or signal level causes an individual to be more hesitant and increases feelings of insecurity. In turn, increased feelings of insecurity tend to add to the feeling of depression.

In many respects, according to Ramsdell, loss of hearing on the *primitive* level creates more serious psychological problems than loss of hearing on the other two levels. The person with normal hearing is always situated in an environment of sound. Although we may not be conscious of the familiar daily sounds that surround us, they form an important part of our environment. If we are suddenly deprived of the background of noises around us, we are aware of a feeling of discomfort and unease. It is awareness on the unconscious level of the environment of sounds surrounding us that is the *primitive* level of hearing.

From a study of the psychological problems of servicemen who had been deafened during World War II, Ramsdell felt that loss of hearing on the primitive level was primarily responsible for the vague feelings of unrest and depression that were characteristic of this group. Many servicemen reported that they felt they were living in a "dead" world. Because the individual was no longer receiving the auditory sensations that had always been associated with his environment, he had the feeling that his environment was lost. Ramsdell thought that it was most important to explain to the deafened individual why he had these feelings of "aloneness" and restlessness because, with the understanding that they stemmed from loss of hearing on the primitive level, the serviceman was better able to accept his feelings of depression and isolation.

Another frequently mentioned psychological characteristic of the adult who becomes hard of hearing is the exaggeration of any tendency to be paranoiac. It is difficult to communicate with a person who has a severe hearing impairment. One must speak carefully to the individual and frequently repeat what one says before the hard-of-hearing person can understand the conversation. It is perfectly natural for the members of the family of a hard-of-hearing person to talk among themselves in a normal manner without taking the trouble to explain what they are talking about. The hearing-impaired person then feels left out of the conversation and may even feel that the other members of the family are making disparaging remarks.

Another psychological characteristic of the hard-of-hearing adult is the reluctance to admit that a sensory handicap exists. To some extent, of course, all handicapped persons have a natural aversion to advertising their handicap. The hard-of-hearing individual, however, manifests this tendency to a greater extent than is true of other handicapped people. The explanation is simple. The person with a hearing handicap has no visible evidence of it. In other words, the part of the auditory system that can be seen looks just the same as that of a normal-hearing individual. Therefore, to the casual observer, the person with a hearing handicap appears to be the same as anyone else.

Further, the hard-of-hearing person exhibits merely exaggerated responses of the sort of which all of us are guilty. When we are listening to an anecdote but fail to appreciate the punch line because of missing an important word or two, our usual reaction is to laugh with the others instead of admitting that we did not get the point of the story. We apparently feel that such an admission would reveal to others that we are stupid. Thus, we try to make the others believe that we, too, heard and understood everything. The hard-of-hearing person, who is in this position much more often and to a much greater extent, will attempt to bluff and give a response that is hoped to be appropriate, rather than admit that a statement or a question was misunderstood. It is not unusual for a hard-of-hearing individual's friends to notice the hearing impairment, although the victim believes firmly that no one is aware of it. For example, it is not uncommon for older schoolteachers to develop sufficient hearing loss to cause them difficulty and embarrassment on many occasions. The students of such a teacher are sure to notice and to take advantage of the hearing handicap long before the teacher suspects that anyone else knows.

An individual who has a serious visual defect cannot successfully bluff through situations where good vision is required. Sooner or later spectacles will be a necessary part of everyday life, and so prevalent are they in our society that the person who must wear them is not penalized by others. On the other hand, hearing aids are a relatively new development when compared with spectacles. Hearing aids are still sufficiently unusual to most people that they attract some attention. It is much more difficult to persuade a hard-of-hearing person to accept a hearing aid than it is to persuade a visually handicapped person to accept spectacles. Almost universally, the hard-of-hearing adult will resist wearing a hearing aid until driven to it through despair.

Very young children with hearing impairments do not have the psychological problems of older children and adults. Audiologists are aware that it is easier to persuade a child of five years of age to accept a hearing aid than it is to secure the acceptance of a child of eight or nine. Girls particularly are reluctant to wear hearing aids because they feel that they will be less attractive to the opposite sex. Boys tend to resist wearing an aid because it sets them off as being different from the rest of the "crowd." Of course, children who are in the "sensitive" period of their lives are prone to shy away from anything that marks them as different from their peers. Unfortunately, children are often cruel to one another, and any difference tends to become the focal point for ridicule. Thus, it is especially difficult to persuade children to accept a hearing aid when they are in the period of conformity. The child's psychological problems, therefore, stem largely from a dislike of admitting a difference from friends and schoolmates.

There are other reasons, of course, why the child may become maladjusted. Difficulty in communication leads to trouble with schoolwork and misunderstandings with family and friends. Thus, the hearing problem heightens tensions within the child. As a result, the hard-of-hearing child is seldom perfectly adjusted. Usually, the child reacts to frustrations either by withdrawing from situations that are difficult or by becoming overly aggressive in behavior. The parents of a hearing-handicapped child face the difficult task of helping their child make an adequate personal adjustment to the disability.

GENERAL CONSIDERATIONS IN REHABILITATION

Adults who have hearing problems generally can achieve a satisfactory adjustment to them through participation in a rehabilitation program. Children who are born with hearing impairments can be trained to get along with a minimum of handicap. Such training is not properly termed *rehabilitation* because these children have never been "habilitated." Children who lose their hearing at some time after they have acquired language can be handled in the same sort of rehabilitation program that is appropriate for adults.

Rehabilitative work with the hard of hearing involves five primary steps. These are a fitting for the hearing aid, speechreading (lipreading), auditory training, speech training, and counseling. Whether the hard-of-hearing individual is a child or an adult, all these basic rehabilitative approaches will be needed to some degree. For the child who is born deaf or severely hard of hearing, a special education program that involves teaching *language* rather than correcting disabilities in oral communication is indicated throughout the child's school life. The remainder of this chapter will be concerned with the five primary facets of an aural rehabilitation program for the hard of hearing. Succeeding chapters will discuss in more detail programs of rehabilitation for children and for adults.

Hearing Aids

No discussion of the rehabilitative needs of the hard of hearing would be complete without some information on hearing aids. The modern hearing aid is the descendant of such preelectronic devices as the speaking tube or horn, which the hard-of-hearing individual held. The speaking tube provided "amplification" by concentrating or focusing the sound waves into the ear canal. The same effect can be achieved less efficiently by cupping the hand behind the auricle. The invention of the carbon microphone and amplifier revolutionized hearing aids. Actually, it was Alexander Graham Bell's search for a means of amplifying speech for the deaf that led to his invention of the telephone. For many years after their development, hearing aids were made with carbon microphones and sometimes carbon amplifiers. The development of the vacuum-tube amplifier, however, again revolutionized hearing aids, and when vacuum tubes were miniaturized, so that a small battery-powered amplifier could be built, the vacuum-tube hearing aid quickly replaced the less-efficient carbon type. Transistors superseded vacuum tubes in hearing-aid designs, resulting in increased efficiency and decreased size. Integrated circuits have allowed the miniaturization process to continue. Aids are designed to be worn on the body, in the frames of spectacles, behind the auricle, and some are so tiny that they fit entirely into the ear canal.

All wearable, electric hearing aids, from the carbon type to the transistor model, are made of the following components: a microphone to change acoustic energy into electricity, a battery-powered amplifier to build up the strength of the signal coming from the microphone, and a receiver to change the amplified electric signal back to acoustic power. The receiver may be of the air-conduction or the bone-conduction type. An air-conduction receiver is connected to an individually molded earpiece, which is inserted in the patient's ear canal.

The amount of amplification, or "acoustic gain," of the instrument depends on many factors. Most companies make several models of varying gain, suitable for different degrees of hearing loss. *Gain* is measured by determining the difference in decibels between the level of the input at the microphone and the level of the output at the receiver.

Hearing aids have built-in limiters of the maximum gain of the amplifier, so that regardless of the level of the input, the output can never exceed a certain predetermined intensity. The typical hearing aid has a volume control to enable the wearer to adjust the output of the amplifier. Some aids contain a telephone circuit. By flicking a switch, the user can disconnect the microphone and connect an induction coil that sends the signals from a telephone to the hearing-aid amplifier, thus bypassing the microphone of the hearing aid. Such an arrangement permits the listener to hear only the signal from the telephone, and unwanted sounds in the listener's environment do not interfere. When using the telephone, the patient switches on the telephone circuit and places the telephone instrument next to the case of the hearing aid. With head-worn aids, the telephone is held in the usual upright position but with the receiver next to the hearing aid—not over the earpiece. With body-worn aids, the telephone instrument may need to be reversed, that is, held so the receiver of the telephone is close to the case of the hearing aid. The telephone circuit works because of electromagnetic leakage from the telephone receiver. In the early 1970s, the Bell System introduced an "improved" receiver with insufficient electromagnetic leakage to be usable with the telephone circuit of a hearing aid. The new receiver unit is being installed in pay telephones and in certain new telephones for home use. In time, the new, more efficient receiver probably will replace all the older types, on whose electromagnetic leakage the hearing-aid telephone circuit depends. In 1974, the Bell System made available for hearing-aid users on a cost basis a battery-powered adapter unit that can be fastened over the receiver of any telephone. The unit generates a magnetic field sufficient to operate the hearing-aid telephone circuit. The adapter unit is available through local telephone company business offices. In addition, the telephone company is mounting a special device inside the handset of new pay telephones that will generate a magnetic field. These modified phones can be identified by a blue grommet where the wire enters the handset.

The air-conduction type of hearing-aid receiver connects to an earpiece fabricated of acrylic or of a flexible plastic from an impression taken of the patient's ear. Amplified sound is delivered to the ear canal through a hole drilled through the earpiece. Earpieces may be of several types, from "canal" molds that consist of only the canal insert, to "skeleton" molds that have a canal insert and a concha ring, to a "receiver" mold that completely fills the concha and has a locking piece that fits in the helix. One purpose of the earpiece is to provide a tight seal at the ear, so that the amplified sound cannot "leak out" around the earpiece and reach the microphone of the aid, thus producing a "squeal," which is called *acoustic feedback*. With head-worn aids containing the receiver within the case of the instrument, the receiver is connected to the earpiece by a short length of plastic tubing. With body-worn aids, the receiver, which is connected to the amplifier with a fine wire, snaps on to a bushing imbedded in the earpiece.

Traditionally, a hearing aid would not be recommended for a patient unless the speech-reception threshold in the better ear exceeded 30 dB. It was assumed that if a patient had one ear that was normal no benefit would be derived from amplification. Such an assumption was based on the observation in the audiology clinic that a patient's sound-field SRT and discrimination score tended to agree closely with the SRT and discrimination score of the better ear. Patients with unilateral impairments complain that they are handicapped in certain situations, however, particularly when people speak on the side of the impaired ear. In 1965, Harford and Barry reported their experience in providing patients with unilateral losses with specially designed head-worn aids that picked up signals through a microphone mounted on the side of the poor ear and transmitted them electrically to a receiver connected with the good ear. The receiver was coupled to the good ear by plastic tubing that was held in place in the outer part of the external canal by an "open" earpiece fitted to the concha. Because the earpiece did not occlude the canal, the good ear could still function normally while also receiving amplified signals from the side of the poor ear. Harford and Barry called their arrangement CROS for *contralateral routing of signals*.[6] Although Harford and Barry utilized a head-

---

[6] Earl Harford and Joseph Barry, "A Rehabilitative Approach to the Problem of Unilateral Hearing Impairment: the Contralateral Routing of Signals (CROS)," *Journal of Speech and Hearing Disorders* 30 (May 1965):121–38.

band for mounting the hearing aid and receiver on opposite sides of the head, the principle of their CROS arrangement was essentially the same as the eyeglass aid with microphone and receiver on opposite sides, as described by Wullstein and Wigand.[7] Harford and Barry reported that although it was not possible to demonstrate in the clinical testing of most of their experimental subjects that the use of a CROS fitting resulted in measurable improvement over the unaided sound-field listening situation, 85 percent of their subjects "reported benefit from CROS hearing-aid use in their daily life activities after a minimum trial of CROS for one week."[8]

The CROS fitting resulted in an unexpected benefit to another group of hearing-impaired individuals for whom hearing aids had rarely been recommended. These are individuals whose hearing for the lower frequencies is excellent but whose sensitivity for the higher speech frequencies drops off abruptly. Patients with sloping audiograms above 1000 Hz generally have speech-reception thresholds close to normal but poor speech-discrimination ability. Hearing aids amplify all frequencies through the speech range, and thus these people generally could not use amplification successfully because the amplified low frequencies tend to mask the weaker, high-frequency sounds. Dodds and Harford, noting that patients with unilateral impairments were able to benefit from CROS fittings even though their good ears had high-frequency losses, decided to experiment with CROS fittings and open ear-pieces with patients who had bilateral high-frequency losses. They hypothesized that the open earpiece would suppress low frequencies and thus result in less masking effect on the higher frequencies and improved speech discrimination. The CROS fitting—separating the microphone from the receiver—should prevent acoustic feedback from the open earpiece. Their results indicated that patients with high-frequency loss using open ear molds in CROS fittings were able to improve their speech-discrimination scores significantly over the scores obtained in routine speech audiometry.[9] Green and Ross, utilizing sound-field Békésy audiometry, compared a subject's aided audiograms when using a standard earpiece and when using an open, or nonoccluding, earpiece with a CROS arrangement. The audiograms clearly indicate that the nonoccluding earpiece suppresses the lower speech frequencies while allowing the higher speech frequencies to be amplified to the same extent as with the standard earpiece. Further, Green and Ross demonstrated that the length of tubing connecting the receiver with the earpiece had a negligible effect on the frequency response of the aid, so that CROS fittings

[7] H. L. Wullstein and M. E. Wigand, "A Hearing Aid for Single Ear Deafness and Its Requirements," *Acta Otolaryngologica* 54 (1962):136–42.

[8] Harford and Barry, "Rehabilitative Approach," p. 134.

[9] Elizabeth Dodds and Earl Harford, "Modified Earpieces and CROS for High Frequency Hearing Losses," *Journal of Speech and Hearing Research* 11 (March 1968):204–18.

could be accomplished as efficiently by running the tubing across the head as by running an electrical wire, thus requiring less modification of a hearing aid.[10] There are now available "wireless" CROS aids that consist of a microphone and FM transmitter on one side of the head and an FM receiver on the other.

The experimental successes of the CROS fitting for unilateral impairments and for patients with bilateral high-frequency losses resulted in the enthusiastic acceptance of this method of fitting. Modifications of the CROS principle have been introduced that provide great flexibility in fitting a variety of patients that heretofore were difficult or impossible to fit. One modification is the BICROS aid, which employs two microphones feeding a single amplifier and receiver mounted in a standard (occluding) earpiece in the better ear. The BICROS is useful for patients with bilateral hearing loss whose poorer ear is not suitable for amplification, so signals from both sides of the head are routed to the better ear. As Green and Ross suggest, the use of microphones of differing frequency-response characteristics should enable the wearer to obtain localization information from a BICROS fitting.[11] Dunlavy believes that the CROS fitting and its various modifications will almost double the number of individuals who can be helped with hearing aids. His preference is to use the CROS principle in an eyeglass fitting with a short length of preformed polyvinyl tubing extending into the ear canal without the need for an open earpiece. Dunlavy reports that the amount of low-frequency suppression can be adjusted by varying the degree of penetration of the tubing into the canal.[12]

With the advent of head-worn aids, the behind-the-ear or in-the-ear type, the use of "true" binaural, that is, stereophonic, hearing became practical. Although binaural aids are almost double the cost of monaural aids, there are many hard-of-hearing individuals who believe that the improved hearing abilities they obtain with stereophonic amplification are well worth the additional expense. In theory, binaural hearing aids should provide many advantages, such as improved localization of sound sources, better discrimination of speech in the presence of noise, and improved "quality" of sound. Many audiologists enthusiastically welcomed the appearance of binaural aids on the market and consistently recommended them to patients who presented problems in hearing-aid fittings. Although standard methods of testing the performance of patients with hearing aids usually did not reflect an advantage of a binaural instrument over a monaural one, the assumption was made that new

[10] David S. Green and Mark Ross, "The Effect of a Conventional Versus a Nonoccluding (CROS-type) Earmold upon the Frequency Response of a Hearing Aid," *Journal of Speech and Hearing Research* 11 (September 1968):638–47.

[11] Ibid., p. 646.

[12] Alfred R. Dunlavy, "CROS: the New Miracle Worker," *Audecibel* 19 (Fall 1970):141–48.

testing techniques needed to be developed for clinical use, and that such new techniques would demonstrate the advantage of binaural instruments.[13] Binaural aids were recommended frequently for young children with severe or profound impairments.

A number of studies compared the performance of hearing-impaired patients with monaural and binaural hearing aids. Generally, these investigations failed to demonstrate that patients perform appreciably better with binaural fittings.[14] Many patients who have purchased binaural aids after having owned monaural instruments report that they obtain superior benefit from the binaural aids, but it is difficult to determine whether they really are deriving acoustic advantages or are simply rationalizing their investment in more expensive equipment.[15] It seems important that audiologists continue their investigations of binaural hearing-aid performance. It is quite possible that the tests used to evaluate the performance of patients with binaural aids are not the most efficient in identifying differences.

Hearing-aid receivers may be of the bone-conduction type. These are small vibrators that fit on the mastoid process. When used with a body-worn aid, they are usually held in place by a narrow metal band that goes across the top of the head. A bone-conduction vibrator may also be built into the tip of the temple of a spectacles frame so that it makes contact with the mastoid process. In this way, bone-conduction hearing may be provided with the glasses type of hearing aid. In the early days of hearing aids, it was thought that any person with a conductive impairment should be provided with a bone-conduction receiver in preference to an air-conduction one. The reasoning was that because the audiogram showed a loss by air but normal hearing by bone, the "better" of the two hearing methods should be improved. In theory this makes sense, but practically it does not work out. In the first place, the bone-conduction vibrator is a less efficient transducer than the air-conduction receiver. Second, because of the impedance of skin and bone, a considerable amount of power is required at the vibrator to produce an audible signal. If the same amount of power is applied to an air-conduction receiver, it is possible to "break through" the conductive block, and the signal that reaches the cochlea is a more faithful reproduction of the original stimulus. Hence, any patient who can successfully utilize a bone-conduction vibrator can usually make even more effective use of an air-conduction receiver, provided that the outer ear

[13] Raymond Carhart, "The Usefulness of the Binaural Hearing Aid," *Journal of Speech and Hearing Disorders* 23 (February 1958):42–51.

[14] Louis M. DiCarlo and William J. Brown, "The Effectiveness of Binaural Hearing for Adults with Hearing Impairments," *Journal of Auditory Research* 1 (September 1960):35–76; James Jerger and Donald Dirks, "Binaural Hearing Aids. An Enigma," *Journal of the Acoustical Society of America* 33 (April 1961):537–38; James Jerger, Raymond Carhart, and Donald Dirks, "Binaural Hearing Aids and Speech Intelligibility," *Journal of Speech and Hearing Research* 4 (June 1961):137–48.

[15] Donald Dirks and Raymond Carhart, "A Survey of Reactions from Users of Binaural and Monaural Hearing Aids," *Journal of Speech and Hearing Disorders* 27 (November 1962):321.

can accommodate an earpiece. The only patients who are given bone-conduction vibrators today are those who have permanently occluded canals, or who, for one reason or another, cannot tolerate an earpiece. Many older patients, most of them otosclerotics, have had bone-conduction vibrators since the early days of hearing aids, and through years of practice they have learned to make effective use of them. Thus, some of these people now refuse to try an air-conduction receiver with their aid, even though its frequency response is greatly superior and they could hear "more" with it. Apparently, having become accustomed after many years to the distortion of the bone-conduction vibrator, these people are disturbed by the fuller range of amplification that the air-conduction receiver delivers to the inner ear. Because bone-conduction vibrators are seldom recommended now, the remainder of this chapter will be concerned only with the air-conduction type of hearing-aid receiver.

Among users of body-worn hearing aids, one of the most frequent complaints is that when the aid is worn under clothing, the noise from the movement of the clothing over the microphone is almost unbearable. Fortunately, most hearing aid users are able to utilize head-worn aids, and so clothing noise does not constitute a problem. Reporting on the sales of aids from July 1, 1975 to July 1, 1976, the editors of the *Hearing Aid Journal* stated that less than 5 percent of the 646,145 aids sold were of the body type. Behind-the-ear models were the most popular, constituting 61 percent of the sales, of which 2 percent were CROS or BICROS aids. Sixteen percent of the sales were eyeglass aids, of which almost 15 percent were CROS or BICROS fittings. Finally, 18 percent of the sales were all-in-the-ear models. The miniaturization of hearing aids and the consequent development of head-worn instruments have resulted in new markets. By 1983, the relative percentages have changed considerably so that body and spectacle instruments constitute only about 1 percent and 3 percent, respectively, of all aids distributed, whereas the behind-the-ear and in-the-ear models each constitute about 48 percent of those distributed.[16] There are many part-time users today who have learned that a hearing aid can be useful in some listening situations. These people often have only slight losses, but with a hearing aid that can be put on and taken off easily and that is free from clothing noise, they become successful users. Some individuals with very severe or profound impairments must still rely on body-worn instruments for best results, because these aids provide a greater amount of amplification without producing acoustic feedback.

Electroacoustic Characteristics

The electroacoustic performance of hearing aids is determined by providing a known input signal at the microphone of the aid and measuring the output at the receiver, which typically is connected to a hard-walled 2-cc coupler in which is mounted a measuring microphone. The volume of the 2-cc cavity has acoustic characteristics which approximate those of the human ear.

[16] *Hearing Journal* 36 (December 1983):12

The output from the measuring microphone is amplified and graphically recorded. The hearing aid, the coupler, and the loudspeaker that delivers the input signal are all housed in an anechoic chamber or test box. The principal measures normally obtained for a hearing aid are (1) the maximum output of which the aid is capable, referred to as the *saturation sound-pressure level* (SSPL); (2) the *gain* of the instrument—the amount of amplification it provides—expressed as the difference between the sound-pressure levels at the microphone of the instrument and in the coupler; (3) the *frequency response* of the aid, which is the range of frequencies to which it responds and the relative amplification across frequency; and (4) the *harmonic distortion* of the instrument that is in the output as multiples or harmonics of the input frequency that were not present in the input. Manufacturers of hearing aids describe the performance of their products in terms of these parameters. For several years, manufacturers and professional societies have sought to standardize the methodology of evaluating the electroacoustic performance of hearing aids and the presentation of the results of performance measurements, and various standards have been published. The Acoustical Society of America has developed and published a standard approved by the American National Standards Institute in 1976 and revised in 1982.[17] This standard, "like its predecessors, contained measurement and specification procedures, but also contained tolerances for measured characteristics."[18] The electroacoustic characteristics of a hearing aid can be determined rapidly by using one of several commercially available hearing-aid measurement systems, which are computer-based.

Besides expressing allowable tolerances for various electroacoustic parameters, the 1976 standard differed from previous standards in two important respects: (1) The frequencies used for calculating average saturation sound-pressure level and average gain are 1000, 1600, and 2500 Hz in place of the traditional 500, 1000, and 2000 Hz; and (2) there is a "reference test gain" specified for measuring frequency response and harmonic distortion.

Saturation sound-pressure level 90 (SSPL 90).   To measure SSPL 90, an input SPL of 90 dB is used, and with the hearing-aid gain control full on, a curve of coupler sound-pressure level versus frequency is generated for the range 200 to 5000 Hz. The average saturation sound-pressure level is computed by averaging the values for 1000, 1600, and 2500 Hz. To differentiate this average from the ones specified in previous standards, it is referred to as the HFA (high-frequency average) SSPL 90. The tolerance allowed for this measure is ± 4 dB from the manufacturer's specifications.

[17] "Specification of Hearing Aid Characteristics," ASA 7-1982, ANSI S3.22-1982 (New York: Acoustical Society of America, 1982).

[18] Roger N. Kasten, "Electroacoustic Characteristics," in *Hearing Aid Assessment and Use in Audiologic Habilitation*, eds. William R. Hodgson and Paul H. Skinner, (Baltimore: Williams and Wilkins, 1977), chap. 5, p. 75.

Full-on gain.   With the gain control full on, the input sound-pressure level is 60 dB if possible, or 50 dB if necessary to avoid distortion. For automatic gain control (AGC) instruments, the input is specified to be 50 dB. The difference between the input SPL and the coupler SPL is the full-on gain of the instrument, which is expressed as the average of the gain at 1000, 1600, and 2500 Hz (HFA full-on gain). The allowable tolerance for this measure is ± 5 dB from the manufacturer's specifications.

Reference test gain.   This is the gain-control setting used for generating the frequency-response curve. The input SPL is 60 dB. The gain control is then adjusted until the coupler output SPL, averaged over 1000, 1600, and 2500 Hz, is 17 dB (± 1 dB) below the HFA SSPL 90. If there is insufficient gain to permit this measurement, the gain control is set at the full-on position. For instruments with AGC, the full-on setting for the gain control is used.

Frequency response.   A frequency response curve for the range 200 to 5000 Hz (or wider range if the aid is capable of it) is generated with the aid set at the reference test gain and an input SPL of 60 dB, except for AGC aids for which the input SPL is 50 dB. A horizontal line is drawn from a point on the ordinate equal to 20 dB below the average frequency response for 1000, 1600, and 2500 Hz. Where the frequency-response curve intersects this horizontal line at the low frequency end is called f_1, and at the high frequency end f_2. The frequency range of the aid is considered to be between f_1 and f_2. Figure 10–1 illustrates a frequency-response curve and points f_1 and f_2 at the extremes of the

FIGURE 10-1.   A hearing-aid frequency-response curve for a 60 dB input SPL with the hearing aid's gain control in the reference test position. Average at 1000-, 1600-, and 2500-Hz response levels equals 114 dB. The curve intersects the horizontal line drawn 20 dB below this average at points f_1 and f_2. The frequency-response range of this aid is from f_1 to f_2, or from 240 to 4000 Hz.

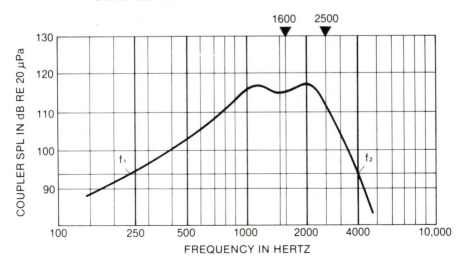

frequency range. The allowable tolerances for a manufacturer's frequency-response curve are ± 4 dB for the "low band" (from 1.25 × f_1 to 2000 Hz) and ± 6 dB for the "high band" (from 2000 Hz to 4000 Hz or 0.8 × f_2, whichever is lower).

Harmonic distortion.   "Harmonic distortion results when new frequencies are generated that are whole number multiples of the original or fundamental frequency and that are not part of the input signal."[19] Harmonic distortion is usually expressed as the percentage of the total amplitude of a test tone due to the presence of harmonics. The formula for computing the percentage of total harmonic distortion (THD) is:

$$100 \sqrt{\frac{p_2^2 + p_3^2 + p_4^2 + p_n^2}{p_1^2 + p_2^2 + p_3^2 + p_n^2}}$$

where p_1 = amplitude of the sound-pressure level of the fundamental frequency, and $p_2, p_3, p_4 \ldots p_n$ = amplitudes of the sound-pressure levels of the higher harmonics.[20] Harmonic distortion is measured in the coupler for input frequencies 500, 800, and 1600 Hz with the aid's gain control set at the reference test position. If the frequency-response curve rises 12 dB or more between any of these test frequencies and its second harmonic, it is not necessary to determine harmonic distortion for that frequency. According to Kasten, the reason for including this provision in the standard was to avoid penalizing an aid that has a sharply rising frequency-response curve.[21] The standard does not provide for any tolerance in respect to harmonic distortion.

Other measures.   The standard makes statements regarding the measurement of the internal noise of a hearing aid, the battery current, and the sound-pressure level that occurs while using the induction coil in the telephone input mode. In addition, two tests designed for use with automatic gain-control hearing aids are described. Automatic gain control is a means of limiting the output of an aid through a feedback circuit that controls the current flow of transistors in the amplifier. The circuit is activated when the signal strength at the microphone reaches a predetermined level, and when the signal strength drops below the predetermined level the full amplification of the aid is restored. The time required for the AGC to function once it is triggered by the signal at the microphone is called the *attack* time, and the time required for full amplification to be restored when the input signal drops below the critical level is called the *release* time. The attack and release times of aids

[19] Michael C. Pollack, "Electroacoustic Characteristics," in *Amplification for the Hearing-Impaired*, 2nd ed., ed. Michael C. Pollack (New York: Grune & Stratton, 1980), chap 2, p. 47.

[20] Kasten, "Electroacoustic Characteristics," p. 84.

[21] Ibid., p. 85.

with AGC are specified by manufacturers in milliseconds. The output of aids without AGC is limited by the amplifying characteristics of the transistor at the output stage and by the mechanical capabilities of the hearing-aid receiver. When these components are "overloaded" by an input that is beyond their ability to handle, *peak clipping* occurs. The elimination of the peaks of the amplified waves causes distortion that can reduce the intelligibility of the amplified signal. The advantage of AGC is that the output can be contained within "safe" limits without the alteration of waveform and resulting distortion that occurs with peak clipping. AGC is also referred to as *compression amplification* and is often recommended for patients who have a very narrow dynamic range.

The first test for AGC aids included in the standard is a measurement of input-output characteristics. The coupler sound-pressure levels are measured for an input of 2000 Hz beginning at an SPL of 50 dB and increasing in 10-dB steps to an SPL of 90 dB. A plot of measured output versus input is then compared with the manufacturer's plot, using the 70-dB input as the matching point. The measured plot and the manufacturer's specified plot must not differ at input SPLs of 50 and 90 dB by more than ± 5 dB.

The second test is a measure of the attack and release times of an AGC aid. The gain control is turned full on and a 2000-Hz input signal is abruptly alternated between SPLs of 55 and 80 dB. Attack and release times can be measured with an oscilloscope. Attack time is the time from the abrupt increase of the input SPL to 80 dB to the stabilization of the output within 2 dB of its steady-state value for an 80-dB input. Release time is the time from the abrupt decrease to 55 dB and the stabilization of the output within 2 dB of its steady-state value for a 55-dB input. The allowable tolerance for both attack and release times is ± 5 msec or ± 50 percent, whichever is larger, of the values specified by the manufacturer.

Limitations of coupler measurements.   The 2-cc coupler does not accurately represent the acoustical characteristics of the human ear, and so one should not place great reliance on electroacoustic data from coupler measurements in selecting a hearing aid for an individual patient. According to Pascoe, coupler measurements underestimate gain in the 1000- to 2000-Hz range and overestimate gain in the region from 2000 to 5000 Hz. Pascoe says, "Aids which are said to reach frequencies as high as 4 kHz (based on coupler measurements . . .) are probably not giving any significant help above 2.5 kHz." Although he agrees that coupler measurements are necessary "as common points of reference between individual functional measurements," Pascoe urges researchers and clinicians to test aids on people in determining gain and frequency response.[22] The use of a computer can help in performing the necessary calculations.

[22] David P. Pascoe, "Frequency Responses of Hearing Aids and Their Effects on the Speech Perception of Hearing-Impaired Subjects," *Annals of Otology, Rhinology, and Laryngology,* supp. 23, vol. 84, no. 5, Part 2 (1975):31.

One attempt to avoid the limitations of the 2-cc coupler but to maintain the repeatability of measurements and objectivity of the measurement procedure is the use of a manikin or artificial head with a built-in Zwislocki coupler—a coupler design that more closely approximates the acoustic characteristics of the human ear. Several clinics and laboratories are now obtaining measurements of hearing-aid performance with a manikin built by Knowles Electronics and called *KEMAR* for *Knowles Electronics Manikin for Acoustic Research.*[23] With KEMAR, evaluations can be made of special performance aids, such as directional and high-pass aids, that are not possible with the 2-cc coupler.[24]

Selection of a Hearing Aid

Assuming that an individual needs a hearing aid and can benefit from it, what are the factors that determine selection? In the order of their importance, as far as the audiologist is concerned, they are acoustic efficiency, ruggedness of design, availability of service, initial cost, operating cost, and attractiveness (size, appearance, and so forth). In the eyes of the purchaser, too often the first consideration is given to attractiveness. Sometimes, of course, it is only the initial cost that influences the decision. Hearing-aid selection services are provided by many audiology clinics or hearing centers. Some centers are more specific in their recommendations than others, but in any event the prospective hearing-aid purchaser is well advised to visit the nearest audiology clinic. If an aid is recommended, it can then be purchased with confidence that it will be of benefit.

At the audiology clinic, the first question that demands an answer is, does the individual have a hearing impairment that will benefit from amplification? The question can be answered by a thorough audiometric evaluation by both pure-tone and speech testing. As stated previously in this chapter, the old rule of thumb that a hearing aid would not be advised until the loss for speech in the better ear exceeds 30 dB is no longer applicable. Each patient's suitability as a candidate for a hearing aid must be individually evaluated, regardless of the degree of impairment demonstrated on hearing tests. Of course, it should be assumed from the outset that the patient has been seen by a physician, who determined that the patient's hearing loss cannot be treated medically or surgically. As stated earlier, the upper limit of hearing loss that can benefit from amplification has yet to be determined. Even though it is not possible to understand speech through hearing alone, at any level of amplification, the profoundly or extremely impaired individual may still benefit from a hearing aid. The amplified sounds provide some clues that

[23] M. D. Burkhard and R. M. Sachs, "Anthropometric Manikin for Acoustic Research," *Journal of the Acoustical Society of America* 58 (July 1975):219–22.

[24] G. Donald Causey, "Current Developments in Hearing Aids," in *Hearing Aids: Current Developments and Concepts,* ed. Martha Rubin (Baltimore: University Park Press, 1976), pp. 9–11.

assist in speechreading, and with the aid, speech production may be better controlled. Also, there is the advantage that the hearing aid does give evidence to other people that a hearing impairment exists, and so they are more careful in speaking.

The person who is likely to benefit most from a hearing aid is one who has a "flat" conductive loss of 30 to 60 dB in extent. This individual hears amplified speech with a minimum of distortion because the loss at each frequency is equal. Also, high levels of amplification can be tolerated because of the protection to the inner ear that the conductive impairment provides and because of the absence of the problem of loudness recruitment. The otosclerotic who is an ideal candidate for surgery is also an ideal candidate for a hearing aid. A poor candidate for a hearing aid is an elderly individual who has a typical sensori-neural impairment with fairly good hearing in the low frequencies, hearing loss that increases by at least 20 dB an octave through the speech frequencies, and a lowered tolerance level, which would limit the amount of acceptable amplification. Because of the uneven response of the hearing mechanism to the various frequencies that are most important to speech, even with amplification the amplified signal will be distorted. This is not to say that all people with sensori-neural losses cannot benefit from a hearing aid; the problem of selecting the aid simply becomes more difficult. Certainly, with such patients the possibility of CROS fittings, or fittings with "high-pass" instruments—aids that amplify only frequencies above 1000, 1500, or even 2000 Hz—should be explored. The use of "open" molds or vented molds will suppress low frequencies and thus in effect cause an emphasis of high frequencies. With the elderly, the problem of hearing-aid selection is complicated by the various physical and psychological concomitants of old age.

At the audiology clinic, hearing-aid selection is based on a number of tests that are conducted with the audiometer in a sound-field situation (testing through the loudspeaker). The benefit of the aid is measured by comparing the results when the patient is tested with and without the aid. The tests with the hearing aid can be compared directly with the patient's unaided speech audiometric scores. In many clinics, the patient is tested with several aids under the same conditions, in order to determine if any one aid is markedly superior. The same measures obtained in standard audiometry are secured also in a hearing-aid evaluation: SRT, MCL, tolerance level, dynamic range, and speech-discrimination ability. In addition, speech discrimination in the presence of noise (recorded background noise) may be measured. The SRT is measured after the volume control of the hearing aid has been set at the point at which the patient feels it is "most comfortable" to listen to running speech, usually at a normal conversation level (50-dB HL). When this setting has been determined, the patient is instructed not to change the volume control throughout the testing of that aid. With each aid to be tested, the patient adjusts the volume control until the running speech of prescribed intensity is "comfortably loud." It is necessary to follow this procedure so that each aid will be tested at a comparable level of amplification. The objective of such an evaluation is to determine whether one particular hearing aid and receiver combination will benefit the patient more than another.

Other things being equal—factors of cost, attractiveness, and so forth—the aid that allows the highest speech-discrimination scores for the patient both in quiet and in noise will be the one selected. However, the "other things" are seldom equal, and frequently different combinations will bring a better score on some tests than on others, so that the selection of the "best" one for the patient may not be easy. Usually, the selection represents a compromise that must take into account, too, the patient's own preferences. If the comparative tests of various hearing aids and receivers reveal no significant differences, the audiologist has the responsibility to tell the patient that any of the combinations can be worn with equal effectiveness. It is the patient's responsibility, then, to make the selection, also taking into consideration the secondary factors of availability of repair service, initial cost, size, and attractiveness of the instrument. In this situation, although the audiologist cannot tell the patient which aid to buy, advice can be given on such matters as the gain requirements of the patient's loss, the type of earpiece, and which ear should be fitted.

If the performance of the patient with the aid is not substantially better than performance without the aid, a hearing aid is probably not indicated, although as we have seen, the advantage of a hearing aid may not always be reflected in improved test scores. Perhaps the decision of whether or not to recommend an aid cannot be made until after the patient has had a trial period of wearing one. Frequently, the value to the patient of a hearing-aid evaluation at an audiology clinic is the discovery that an aid would be of little or no benefit.

Having determined that a patient will benefit from a hearing aid, the audiologist must decide which type of earpiece arrangement provides the most satisfactory results. Generally, an analysis of the patient's monaural speech audiometric scores will yield the information needed to make a selection of the ear to be "fitted,"[25] but sometimes experimentation is required. Other factors being equal, the ear that has the greater SRT, the wider dynamic range, or the better speech discrimination should be chosen in a monaural fitting. Three examples demonstrate the operation of these principles.

	Example 1		Example 2		Example 3	
	Left	Right	Left	Right	Left	Right
SRT	40	50	52	54	60	58
Tolerance	100+	100+	100+	88	96	98
Dynamic Range	60+	50+	48+	34	36	40
Discrimination	84%	84%	78%	80%	82%	54%
Ear to fit	Right		Left		Left	

[25] Unfortunately, the word *fit* implies that a hearing aid may be selected as precisely as a pair of shoes, or with the accuracy with which an eye doctor prescribes

In example 1, the only significant difference between the ears is in the SRT, and so the right ear should be selected for fitting. The logic here is that the patient's better ear can still be of some benefit without amplification, which may not hold true for the poorer ear. In example 2, the only important difference between the ears is in the extent of the dynamic range. The left ear should be fitted, as with this ear the patient can have the advantage of a wider range of amplification. In example 3, it is obvious that the left ear should be the choice because of its greatly superior speech discrimination. A BICROS fitting with the sound delivered to the left ear should be considered, although a head-worn aid might not provide sufficient gain for this patient.

As we have mentioned previously in this chapter, one can argue on a theoretical basis that binaural aids should provide definite advantages over monaural aids, such as improved localization of sound sources and improved discrimination of speech in the presence of background noise. Separate hearing aids on each ear should logically provide more "natural" hearing, because of the stereophonic effect the normal-hearing individual experiences by the separation of the ears. In 1958, Carhart anticipated the development of more refined tests of aided hearing that would reflect the superiority of binaural aids for some patients. Tests of localization involving sounds introduced through more than one loudspeaker and tests of speech discrimination in the presence of recorded background noises and competing speech signals have been attempted in audiology clinics. There still are no tests the audiologist can apply that enable the audiologist with any degree of confidence to tell a patient to wear binaural aids. Some audiologists prefer to recommend a monaural instrument, and after a period of six months or so, when the patient has made a good adjustment to the aid, have the patient try a binaural fitting. Presumably, the difference between binaural and monaural listening might be more evident at this time than at the time of the initial evaluation. In the absence of any test evidence that a binaural fitting is better for a patient, the audiologist must depend on the patient's subjective impressions and preferences.

For more than thirty years, audiologists, hearing scientists, and hearing-aid specialists have been concerned with the issue of "selective" amplification, which refers to "mirroring" the audiogram, or providing the greatest amplification where the audiometric loss is greatest, with the objective of making aided thresholds approach normal thresholds. Generally, hearing-aid manufacturers have espoused the philosophy that there is one combination of microphone, amplifier, and receiver that is best for a given patient, and they have produced several models of aids and receivers with varying electroacoustic characteristics, so that with available internal adjustments, it is possible to provide 100 or more different fittings. Such flexibility enables manufacturers and dealers to advertise that they can "custom fit" an aid to any user's individual requirements. The opposite of selective amplification is

---

glasses. This is not true, but because there is no good substitute the word is sometimes unavoidable.

"uniform" amplification, which holds that regardless of the configuration of a patient's audiogram, performance will be best with an instrument that provides the highest fidelity amplification possible. A research project performed under government sponsorship at the Harvard Psycho-Acoustic Laboratory during World War II measured patients' responses to recorded speech tests with various settings on a "master" hearing aid and concluded that almost all hearing-impaired patients perform best with one of two frequency-response curves: (1) a "flat" response, that is, one that provides equal amplification for all frequencies, so that within the frequency range of the aid there are no peaks or valleys in the response curve; or (2) a pattern that provides increased amplification for higher frequencies at the rate of 6 dB per octave throughout the range of the aid.[26] Subsequent studies performed with commercial aids tended to confirm the findings of the Harvard Report. Pascoe studied the effects of various frequency-response patterns on the speech-discrimination ability of hard-of-hearing subjects, using a master hearing aid with frequency response from 100 to 6300 Hz and a new list of "high-frequency" monosyllabic words. He concluded that most subjects' speech discrimination ability was best when they used a "uniform hearing level" curve individually adjusted to produce an aided threshold curve parallel to the normal curve of audibility, or in other words, a mirroring of the unaided threshold curve to "correct" it to the normal curve. Because of the limitations of coupler measurements as compared to measurements made at the ear, Pascoe believes that previous studies of selective amplification have not been true tests of the concept.[27] One of the results of Pascoe's work is to cast doubt on the common clinical practice of selecting aids based on coupler-generated frequency-response curves. He says, "The frequency responses of hearing aids should be determined by the functional gains they provide. This type of evaluation should include the final configuration in which the aid is used, that is, the earmold and tubing selected."[28]

Hearing-aid evaluations have frequently proved frustrating to clinicians and patients because differences in performance with various aids may be minimal, thus complicating the selection. Because of the difficulties in demonstrating real differences in performance among various aids, some clinics abandoned traditional hearing-aid evaluations with specific recommendations in favor of "consultations," in which the emphasis was on counseling the patient on how to shop for an aid and how to use an aid efficiently. Now, with improved methodology—such as that developed by Pascoe—clinics may be able to do a better job of helping the patient select an aid based on comparative testing.

Another source of frustration to the clinician has been the problem of

[26] Hallowell Davis, S. S. Stevens, R. H. Nichols, Jr., *Hearing Aids: An Experimental Study of Design Objectives* (Cambridge, Mass.: Harvard University Press, 1947).

[27] Pascoe, "Frequency Responses of Hearing Aids."

[28] Ibid., p. 38.

providing the patient with an aid that matches the specifications of the instrument with which performance was best in the clinic. Typically, the clinic's stock of aids is on loan from manufacturers or dealers. When the clinician and the patient agree on the choice of an aid, the clinician directs the patient to a dealer who handles the recommended aid and informs the dealer of the specific model to be supplied to the patient and any internal adjustments to the aid that are to be made. Unless the patient returns to the clinic to be checked out with the new aid, the clinician has no way of knowing whether the dealer has followed the "prescription." Even if the dealer faithfully supplies everything the clinician requested, there is no guarantee that the new aid will perform exactly as the one the patient tried at the clinic. Even with manufacturers' efforts at quality control, there may be some differences among aids of the same model that could be of importance in evaluating a patient's performance.

The Veterans Administration for many years has had a hearing-aid evaluation program that provides the veteran with the very aid with which performance was best in the clinic. The Veterans Administration each year contracts with manufacturers for aids that have scored highest in the electroacoustic tests the National Bureau of Standards conducts for the Veterans Administration. Among these best-performing aids, those with the lowest price are selected for purchase. Veterans Administration clinics are stocked with a wide selection of aids from a central depot, and when a veteran is given an aid the clinic's stock is replenished.

Dissatisfaction with the system of referring patients to dealers led to a movement among some audiologists and clinics to dispense hearing aids to patients directly, so that—as in the Veterans Administration—a patient could be provided with the very instrument with which performance was best. A long-standing prohibition in its Code of Ethics against members' engaging in commercial activities was interpreted by the American Speech and Hearing Association as permitting audiologists to dispense aids at cost, charging patients only for services rendered. Because of a 1978 Supreme Court decision that a professional association cannot limit competition among its members, ASHA removed this prohibition from its Code of Ethics. An ASHA audiologist can now sell aids at a profit, provided that such sales are only part of a total aural rehabilitation program. Many audiologists now dispense aids directly to patients.

Speechreading

Historically, *speechreading,* or *lipreading* as it used to be called, is the oldest of the rehabilitative approaches to some of the problems of impaired hearing. By speechreading is meant the use of visual clues in determining what the speaker says. The newer term *speechreading* is preferred because visual clues come from watching the entire speaker rather than from concentrating solely on the lips. All of us engage in the practice of speechreading, although usually we are not conscious of the fact that our eyes are assisting our ears. It is a common observation, however, that we can more easily understand a lecturer whose face is clearly visible, and we can "hear" better in a well-lighted rather than a dark room. Many hard-of-hearing individuals stoutly maintain that they do not speechread. Nevertheless, they will report that they seem to "hear" better when they can see the speaker. Teaching speechreading is really putting on a conscious level what the patient is already doing to some extent on an unconscious level.

Many people regard speechreading as a mysterious art that can be learned only after years of training and experience. Normal-hearing persons would probably answer a questionnaire by saying that they do not know anything about speechreading. Actually, it is a poor substitute for hearing. At best, it is not possible to speechread 100 percent of what is seen. The reasons are obvious. In English, only about one-third of our speech sounds are clearly visible, that is, are made with articulators involving only the front of the mouth. Sounds such as *k* and *r* are impossible to speechread because the articulators involved in their formation cannot be seen. Even the best speech-reader, therefore, is bound to miss a considerable proportion of what is seen. Moreover, many words that are different in phonetic content and meaning appear alike from the standpoint of the visible movement made in uttering them. The word *mom*, for example, looks to the speechreader almost exactly the same as the words *mop, mob, bob, bomb, palm,* and so forth, because the sounds *p* and *b* and *m* are all made with the lips and are virtually indistinguishable from each other by appearance alone. It is necessary, therefore, for the speechreader to determine from the context of what is seen which particular word of the group the speaker is saying. This is a process that cannot be performed instantaneously; again, therefore, the speechreader is bound to miss a proportion of what is seen. Words that look alike to the speechreader are called *homophenous* words. Almost every textbook on speechreading contains a section devoted to homophenous words.

Training in speechreading consists of the teaching of systematic observation. The patient must be taught how to exercise the powers of observation most efficiently. Naturally, learning speechreading involves a considerable amount of practice. However great the facility the speechreader attains, the person can always learn to become even more effective through increased training and practice. This does not mean that instruction in speechreading requires a number of years. The average hard-of-hearing individual can achieve a working ability in speechreading in a limited number of lessons. Of course, many hard-of-hearing persons do an effective job of speechreading without having had any formal instruction. It is a skill that they develop through necessity because of their inability to follow conversation through hearing alone. Curiously, it is difficult for a normal-hearing person to achieve a high degree of skill in speechreading. Apparently, the motivation of having to depend on speechreading is a necessary prerequisite to proficiency.

As stated, speechreading is a poor substitute for hearing. Most hard-of-hearing individuals have residual hearing on which they can rely to some extent. Speechreading supplements the residual hearing. It enables the individual to comprehend more conversation than would be possible through hearing alone. In fact, the total communication received through a combination of speechreading and hearing is considerably greater than could be obtained through either method alone.

Before hearing aids were invented, speechreading was the only rehabilitative technique available to persons with hearing handicaps. Speechreading classes have been conducted in this country for as many years as educators have been aware of the special needs of those with hearing handicaps. Some teachers of speechreading were resentful toward hearing aids when they first became common. It was as if the teacher considered the hearing aid a threat to the profession. Consequently, many teachers of speechreading refused to allow their pupils to use hearing aids while they were engaged in speechreading lessons. Their attitude was that the pupils were there to learn speechreading, and if they were able to hear at all, they would not be motivated to learn speechreading. Apparently, these teachers believed that learning speechreading for its own sake was a proper goal for a hard-of-hearing person. This attitude toward hearing aids manifested a shortsighted point of view on the part of the teachers toward their function, which must be defined as that of aiding the hard-of-hearing person to communicate more effectively. Because more effective communication can be achieved through combining sight and hearing, the teaching of speechreading should stress the use of both sensory avenues.

Actually, the development of the electronic hearing aid *has* constituted a threat to the old-time teacher of speechreading. With the development of the individual, wearable hearing aid, the patient could combine residual hearing with visual observation. Many people were able to get along satisfactorily by depending primarily on the hearing aid. For them, formal instruction in speechreading was not necessary. Thus, as hearing aids became more popular, schools and individual teachers of speechreading served fewer and fewer hearing-handicapped individuals.

Various methods have been proposed for teaching speechreading. Historically, two of them represent somewhat opposing philosophies. On the one hand, there are the proponents of the *analytic* method, and on the other hand, there are those who believe in the *synthetic* approach. Those who adhere to the analytic school believe that it is necessary to teach a patient, first of all, to recognize individual speech "movements" in isolation. From individual movements, the patient proceeds to words, then phrases, sentences, and finally paragraphs. The synthetic approach operates on the principle that learning is accomplished by starting with wholes. In this method, the speechreader begins by learning to recognize the meaning of whole paragraphs. Theoretically, drilling on individual sounds or movements comes only when a breakdown in the comprehension of paragraphs has occurred. The analytic method was championed by Bruhn, who brought to this country the techniques of Müller-Walle of Germany.[29] The synthetic approach was proposed by Nitchie, who for many years operated a private school of speechreading in New York City.[30] Actually, when the lesson plans proposed by Bruhn and Nitchie are closely examined, it is apparent that there is not so much difference between them as would be presumed from their opposing philosophies.

The Kinzie sisters devised a method that attempted to incorporate the best of the Müller-Walle and the Nitchie systems.[31] Cora Elsie Kinzie herself was hard-of-hearing and had studied with both Bruhn and Nitchie. In addition to these two basic methods of teaching speechreading—the Müller-Walle and the Nitchie methods—a third method was proposed in Jena, Germany, by Karl Brauckmann. The Jena method, so called from its place of origin, was brought to the United States by Bunger.[32] Departing from the usual techniques of working with individual sounds or with paragraphs of running speech, the Jena method proposes drill work on the rhythm patterns of English.

Auditory Training

As stated previously, there are very few individuals who have no hearing. Even those who are educationally classified as "deaf" usually have some measurable residual hearing. The purpose of auditory training, with the deaf as with the hard of hearing, is to teach the hearing-handicapped patient to make the most effective use of the remaining hearing. Auditory training is usually given with the aid of amplification.

Before World War II, auditory training had been confined, for the most part, to teaching pupils in schools for the deaf to be aware of gross sound stimuli. Goldstein, founder of Central Institute for the Deaf in St. Louis, has described techniques for stimulating the hearing of such children.[33] Not until World War II, however, was much attention paid to the problems of teaching the hard of hearing how to make the most of their residual hearing. This is difficult to understand, because the person who is hard of hearing has a greater potential for drawing on residual hearing effectively than has the person who

---

[29] Martha E. Bruhn, *The Müller-Walle Method of Lip-Reading for the Deaf* (Lynn, Mass.: Thos. P. Nichols, 1920).

[30] Edward B. Nitchie, *Lip-Reading Principles and Practise* (New York: Stokes, 1919).

[31] Cora Elsie Kinzie and Rose Kinzie, *Lip-Reading for the Deafened Adult* (Chicago: John C. Winston Co., 1931).

[32] Anna M. Bunger, *Speech Reading—Jena Method* (Danville, Ill.: Interstate, 1944).

[33] Max Goldstein, *The Acoustic Method for the Training of the Deaf and Hard-of-Hearing Child* (St. Louis: Laryngoscope Press, 1937).

is deaf. To a considerable extent, however, the development of interest in auditory training of the hard of hearing followed the development of the wearable hearing aid. Hearing aids were not sold extensively, nor were they common, before World War II.

Actually, then, the origin of auditory training as a rehabilitative technique was in the aural rehabilitation centers operated by the armed services in World War II. Here, for the first time, specialists from many fields were drawn together with a common purpose: to plan and to administer a rehabilitative program that would enable the hearing-impaired serviceman to return to duty or to civilian life with a minimum of handicap. In these military centers, it was found that the fitting of a hearing aid was only one step in the rehabilitation of the hard-of-hearing patient. After the selection of a hearing aid, it was necessary to give the individual training in its proper adjustment for all situations and how to interpret correctly what was heard with it. In addition to classes in speechreading and in "speech conservation," a class of auditory training was developed at each of the military centers. Some included in their program a "listening hour"; at that time, patients would get informal practice in a variety of listening situations, thus supplementing on their own the formal instruction they received in class.

In Chapter 6, we discussed the measures in speech audiometry to evaluate a patient's loss of hearing for speech. One of them is an estimate of the patient's speech-discrimination ability, which is obtained by having the person listen to phonetically balanced (PB) words at above-threshold levels. We have seen that some patients have excellent speech-discrimination ability, whereas other patients do poorly on the PB words, regardless of how loudly they hear them. The results of speech-discrimination tests determine the emphasis to be placed on auditory training in the rehabilitation program. The patient with good understanding of the speech that can be heard requires relatively little auditory training to learn to make effective use of a hearing aid. On the other hand, the patient who does poorly on the PB words may be able to improve speech-discrimination ability by means of a concentrated program in auditory training. An analysis of the specific sounds that the patient confuses in the PB test will determine the training materials needed. Thus, if a patient consistently misses words with high-frequency voiceless consonant sounds in them, such as *s, th, f, k, t, p, sh, ch, wh, h,* the auditory training program should be designed to include practice in differentiating words containing these sounds. It should not be assumed that auditory training can teach the individual with a speech-discrimination problem to make 100 percent discrimination through hearing alone, but any improvement in the ability to recognize words by ear would be beneficial in terms of the total communication that the individual can receive.

For a child or an adult who has not heard for some time, it may be necessary to institute a program of auditory training leading up to the application of a wearable hearing aid. In other words, if the patient has not been accustomed to hearing or having to interpret auditory stimuli, the person must be taught how to *listen* and taught that sounds convey meanings. This kind of training can be accomplished with an *auditory training unit,* a specially designed, high-fidelity, high-output amplifier that directs an auditory signal from a disc recording or microphone to high-quality earphones, the output of which is separately adjustable. These units optimize the signal-to-noise ratio compared to that obtained with a standard hearing aid. Several models of auditory training units are commercially available. Some can be operated with several sets of earphones, so that a group of patients may receive auditory training simultaneously. Some models can be equipped with hearing-aid types of receivers, thus providing an easy transition to an individual hearing aid. Many auditory training units are of the stereophonic type, that is, have two microphones and two amplifiers, so that each earphone receives a separate signal. Such systems provide more "natural" hearing and a "depth perception" that is not possible with a unit that feeds the same signal to each earphone. Some educators of the hearing handicapped use auditory training instrumentation of the "loop-induction" type. In this case, the signal from the amplifier is transferred to the telephone coil of an individual wearable hearing aid through a magnetic field. This arrangement has the advantage of permitting a child to move about the classroom freely without being hampered by wires from the auditory training unit. Another type of wireless unit consists of a transmitter worn by the teacher that broadcasts on an FM radio frequency or via infrared light to receivers worn by the children. The receivers may be combined with one or two microphones and appropriate circuitry so that the units can also function as monaural or binaural hearing aids. The wireless systems offer the maximum flexibility and will probably replace the group "hard-wire" auditory trainers and the loop-induction type.[34]

Speech Training

Most individuals with severe or profound impairments will require some speech training in addition to other rehabilitation. It is obvious that a child born with defective hearing will have considerable difficulty developing intelligible speech because it is a well-known fact that speech is learned largely by hearing. It is not so obvious why an older individual who incurs a hearing impairment after the acquisition of language should need speech training. Generally, the onset of a hearing impairment is not sudden; rather, the progression from normal to profoundly impaired hearing is gradual over a period of years. Those of us who have normal hearing are able to monitor our own speech, to regulate the intensity of our voices to suit the noise conditions in which we are speaking and to correct defects in articulation that arise from

[34] Mark Ross, "Classroom Amplification," in *Hearing Aid Assessment and Use in Audiologic Habilitation,* 2nd ed., eds. William R. Hodgson and Paul H. Skinner (Baltimore: Williams & Wilkins, 1981), chap. 13. pp. 245–47.

misuse of our articulators. The person with a profound or extreme hearing impairment is unable to do this. Thus, it is common, as hearing loss progresses, for a person's voice and speech to show the effect of the hearing impairment.

As was stated in Chapter 3, a person with a conductive impairment may tend to speak too softly or with too little vocal intensity. The reason is that a person with a conductive loss may have bone-conduction sensitivity that is better than normal. Because our own speech is heard to some extent through the mechanism of bone conduction, the conductively impaired individuals may hear their speech at higher than normal levels. They then lower their speech to compensate. On the other hand, the patient with a sensori-neural loss of hearing may tend to speak too loudly because bone-conduction sensitivity is affected along with air conduction. Any person with a profound or extreme hearing impairment will likely have some difficulty regulating voice levels to suit unusual conditions of sound environment. Thus, training is needed to teach these individuals how to regulate their voices by nonaural clues that they can perceive.

Many individual sounds of English require a rather delicate adjustment of the articulators in order to produce the correct acoustic effect. In the presence of a severe, profound, or extreme hearing impairment, these sounds may deteriorate, because we usually depend on our auditory monitoring to tell us whether or not a change in articulator adjustment is necessary. In other words, we tend to make a more-or-less automatic adjustment of our articulators in accordance with what our ears tell us. Two sounds most commonly affected by a hearing impairment are the *s* and the *r*. In both, the articulator adjustment is critical, and without a refined sense of auditory discrimination it is difficult to form these sounds in the correct manner. Generally, the sounds that require a precise adjustment of the tongue blade or the tongue tip will be affected most by a hearing impairment.

Deterioration of speech can occur without the awareness of the patient. Others are much more conscious of a patient's speech deficiencies. Because the deterioration of speech patterns, which have previously been well established, occurs gradually, the ideal time to commence speech training for the hard-of-hearing patient is before a marked deterioration has occurred. In the military aural rehabilitation centers in World War II, the term *speech conservation* was coined to refer to preventive speech therapy given to newly deafened individuals in order to keep their speech and voice disturbances to a minimum. In other words, the speech training was started before any marked changes in speech and voice patterns had occurred, in the hope that through such training the hard-of-hearing individual could maintain good speech.

When the hearing loss makes it impossible to monitor speech through the ear, the patient must be taught how to regulate speech production by other means. The usual method is to teach the patient to perform tactile monitoring, that is, to learn to control speech and voice production through motor-kinesthetic sensations. Because persons with profound or extreme hearing impairment cannot hear the *s*, for example, they must be taught the correct articulator placement for it so that they can get the "feel" of the correct position while speaking. In speech-correction practice, there are two general methods of teaching the correct production of a sound. The preferred technique is the so-called *stimulus* or *acoustic* method, which is based on the fact that the individual can learn correct articulator placement by residual hearing. The other technique is the *phonetic-placement* method, which involves teaching speech sounds by instructing the patient how to place the articulators and how to utilize kinesthetic sensations.

Psychological Counseling

Because the greatest handicap of a hearing loss is frequently the psychological problems that it produces in a patient, a rehabilitation program for the hard of hearing should provide for psychological counseling as needed. Frequently, such counseling may well be the most important part of the rehabilitation program.

The requirements of a counseling program for children differ from those of a program for adults. With a hard-of-hearing child, frequently the counseling must be directed toward the child's parents because an improper attitude on their part will influence the child's point of view. As stated earlier in this chapter, children whose training begins after the age of eight or nine have more problems in learning to accept their disability. Then it may be helpful to approach the child's problems to some extent by counseling associates and teachers. An interested and skilled teacher can accomplish a great deal in determining the attitude of other children in the class toward the handicapped pupil.

The adult who incurs a handicapping hearing impairment faces a number of problems with which the counselor must cope. In the first place, the person may have to be persuaded to accept the hearing loss as a problem. Once it has been admitted that a sensory deficit exists, the patient can be guided to an intelligent approach to the problem. The person can accept wearing a hearing aid without feeling a sense of shame and can advise others that they will have to take care how they speak.

It is likely that the hard-of-hearing adult will feel misunderstood by family members. As a matter of fact, the husband or wife and children do often behave in an inconsiderate fashion in regard to the hearing-handicapped individual. Not infrequently, it is necessary for psychological counseling to extend to others in the family, so that they may be made to realize the patient's limitations and learn ways in which they can help.

Vocational counseling should be offered whenever the hearing impairment poses a problem in the work of the patient. Although hard-of-hearing individuals function effectively in countless professional and vocational activities, there are certain types of positions that cannot be filled properly by a person with faulty hearing. Sometimes, then, a hearing loss will make it impossible for a patient to continue in a position. Naturally, the longer a patient has been employed in a given job, the harder it will be to accept the need for changing to a different type of employment. The vocational counselor can help considerably in the psychological adjustment of the hard-of-hearing adult by correct guidance in the selection of a vocation or in a change from one type of position to another.

We all need to feel liked and wanted by others. The adult who incurs a hearing loss that limits the ability to communicate is likely to become withdrawn and antisocial. Even with proper family acceptance and handling of the handicapped patient in the home, it is necessary that the patient have contacts outside the home and participate in other activities. It frequently requires considerable "pushing" in a delicate way by the patient's family and counselor, but the maintenance of old social contacts and the development of new ones is necessary to a patient's mental health.

REFERENCES

BERGER, KENNETH W. *Speechreading Principles and Methods*. Baltimore: National Educational Press, 1972.

———. *The Hearing Aid: Its Operation and Development*, 2nd ed. Livonia, Mich.: The National Hearing Aid Society, 1974.

BESS, FRED H., ed. *Childhood Deafness: Causation, Assessment and Management*. Chaps. 18, 19, 20, and 21. New York: Grune & Stratton, 1977.

DONNELLY, KENNETH, ed. *Interpreting Hearing Aid Technology*. Springfield, Ill.: Charles C Thomas, 1974.

HODGSON, WILLIAM R., and SKINNER, PAUL H., eds. *Hearing Aid Assessment and Use in Audiologic Habilitation*, 2nd ed. Baltimore: Williams & Wilkins, 1981.

O'NEILL, JOHN J., and OYER, HERBERT J. *Visual Communication for the Hard of Hearing: History, Research & Methods*, 2nd ed. Englewood Cliffs, N.J.: Prentice-Hall, 1981.

OYER, HERBERT J., and FRANKMANN, JUDITH P. *The Aural Rehabilitation Process*. New York: Holt, Rinehart and Winston, 1975.

POLLACK, MICHAEL C., ed. *Amplification for the Hearing-Impaired*, 2nd ed. New York: Grune & Stratton, 1980.

RUBIN, MARTHA, ed. *Hearing Aids: Current Developments and Concepts*. Baltimore: University Park Press, 1976.

SANDERS, DEREK A. *Aural Rehabilitation*, 2nd ed. Englewood Cliffs, N.J.: Prentice-Hall, 1982.

CHAPTER ELEVEN
TRAINING THE
HEARING-IMPAIRED CHILD

The purpose of this chapter is to set forth a general approach to the training of children who have impaired hearing. For the most part, the emphasis will be on the hard-of-hearing child, not on the deaf child. There will be some mention, however, of the educational problems of the deaf, and special attention will be directed to the training of the preschool deaf child. There will be no attempt to give detailed information regarding the planning of lessons for hearing-impaired children. The reader who desires this kind of information is referred to the list of references at the end of this chapter.

The child with a hearing impairment almost always has some degree of language handicap, the extent of the handicap depending on such factors as the degree of loss, the time of onset of the loss, and so forth, as discussed in Chapter 10. The audiologist is concerned with the child's problems in communication, the ability to speak and to understand speech. Further, the audiologist has the responsibility of helping the parents to understand the problems of their hearing-handicapped child and teaching them how they can be of most assistance. Included in this chapter are discussions of the communicative skills that the child must develop. Although these skills are discussed separately, it must be understood that they operate in combination with each other and should be taught together.

SPEECHREADING

Speechreading is the one skill that has universal application to individuals with hearing problems, regardless of the patient's age or the extent of the hearing impairment. Whenever one sensory pathway is impaired, an individual compensates for it by developing an increased capacity to utilize the other senses. Thus, a blind person develops an increased ability to use hearing sensitivity. By the same token, the hard-of-hearing patient must learn to rely more on visual sensations than is necessary for the person with normal hearing. The child who has a hearing loss naturally learns to concentrate on visual clues, even without special training. In fact, one of the diagnostic indications of an auditory impairment is the fact that a child watches speakers' faces with an intentness and concentration that signify dependence on visual clues. The purpose of speechreading training for hard-of-hearing children is to develop their natural capacity for learning through the eyes to the maximum extent. Training in speechreading can succeed in quickening the child's powers of visual observation and systematizing the ability to comprehend speech through visual clues.

As stated previously, speechreading alone is not a perfect substitute for hearing. Because of the relatively large proportion of English sounds that are partially or completely invisible, it is impossible for any speechreader, no matter how skillful, to comprehend 100 percent of what is said. Speechreading training, given in combination with auditory training, can usually yield better results in the total communication the child receives than can either type of training alone.

Educators of the deaf stress the importance of teaching the young child how to "match." Initially, this training consists of teaching the child to match one object to another that is exactly like it. Then the child is taught to match one object to another object that is similar although not exactly the same. The next step is to teach matching of an object to a picture of the object, and then the matching of one picture to another picture. The aim of these matching procedures is to teach the child to be observant of similarities and differences and to realize that symbols (pictures) relate to objects and may be substituted for the objects they represent. This is the first rung on the ladder of abstraction. Finally, the child is taught to match words, as seen on the lips of the therapist or in printed form, with the objects for which the words stand, with the pictures of objects, and with other words. This is the next higher rung on the ladder of abstraction. Thus, through a series of matching experiences, beginning simply and becoming progressively more complex, the child is taught that things have names and that these names may be interpreted as movements of the articulators in a speaker or as combinations of written letters. Initially, the matching is on a concrete basis; that is, symbols that name objects are taught first. Eventually, of course, the child must realize that ideas in the abstract can be conveyed through spoken or written language, and the child must learn to think with symbols—to "match" thoughts and concepts and to express thoughts to others in spoken and written form. This is the ultimate goal of procedures starting with the very simple matching of object to object.

With the hard-of-hearing child who can learn some language through the ear, it is not necessary to follow such a detailed step-by-step procedure in teaching speechreading. How closely the program for the hard-of-hearing child corresponds to procedures pursued with deaf children depends on the language abilities of the child, which in turn are affected by the severity of the loss, the time of its occurrence, and of course the intelligence of the child.

To be effective, a program of speechreading for children must be geared to their interests. As in any kind of teaching of young children, speechreading lessons must be made entertaining and appealing by means of inherently interesting materials. Various games may be devised to give the child the opportunity to practice speechreading without the stiffness and inflexibility of the formal lesson. For example, a lesson could be built around the theme of animals, which most children love. Attractive pictures of animals can be found in children's books or in magazine advertisements, and these pictures can be mounted on colorful construction paper or cardboard. The child can be instructed to "find the cow" or to "place the horse in front of the sheep" and so forth.

In general, the object of speechreading lessons should be to provide experience that will better equip the child to get along in daily life. In the beginning, lessons should be restricted to the vocabulary with which the child is already familiar. As this vocabulary is utilized in speechreading, new words can be introduced. Lessons should be planned to move from the familiar to the unfamiliar, so that the child is motivated to learn by proceeding from what is known to fields of new information and experience. For the school-age child, lessons can be planned around the subject matter of school studies.

Regardless of the subject matter on which the lesson is built, the therapist should observe certain principles in teaching speechreading. These principles follow:

1. Sit or stand so that the lighting is favorable for the child. The light should be on your face and not in the eyes of the child.
2. Talk naturally. Do not exaggerate your articulation, and do not speak carelessly or too rapidly.
3. Do not "talk over the child's head." Phrase your thoughts in simple, easy-to-understand language, but always speak in complete sentences.
4. Because of the additional movements involved and the consequently greater opportunity for the child to observe, longer words or phrases are sometimes better than shorter ones. Thus, it is better to say "It is lunch time, and we must go eat our lunch," rather than "Time to eat."

5. Repeat what you say, still without exaggeration, until the child comprehends, or if necessary rephrase what you have said.

6. Spend little or no time in drill involving movements or nonsense syllables. Conduct the necessary drill work with phrases or sentences. In other words, adopt a synthetic rather than an analytic approach to the teaching of speechreading.

7. Make your speechreading lessons happy and enjoyable experiences for the child with the aid of materials that are bright, gay, and interesting. Collect and organize your own materials; do not depend solely on lesson plans found in books.

8. Integrate speechreading work with auditory training and speech training. For the most part, your speechreading work should be done with a natural voice, although on occasion, to sharpen the child's attention, a low-intensity voice or a whisper may be desirable.

9. Always insist on the child's *watching* you while you speak, so that the importance of visual clues may be learned. Do not speak until you have the child's attention.

10. Be lavish with praise and reward for successful performances.

AUDITORY TRAINING

The kind and type of auditory training that a hard-of-hearing child needs depends on the degree and type of hearing impairment. Naturally, before a child is placed in a training program a careful analysis should be made of the hearing loss. The way in which a child responds to speech audiometric tests will give an indication of what the auditory training needs are. As a result of the evaluation of a child's hearing, a decision can be made about whether or not a hearing aid should be considered and what kind of earpiece arrangement would do best. If the loss is sufficient to warrant a hearing aid, the aid should be fitted at the earliest possible date. However, a period of some auditory training may be necessary before the child can make effective use of an aid. Whether the auditory training precedes or follows the fitting will have to be determined individually for each child. Some children will have hearing that is too good to necessitate an aid but still have poor listening habits. What is more likely is that a child may have good hearing for the low frequencies but poor hearing for the higher speech frequencies and thus would need auditory training even though it may not be possible to use a hearing aid to good effect. The auditory training needs of these categories of children will now be discussed.

Training Before Getting an Aid

Generally, this type of child is one who has a profound loss and without amplification does not hear the ordinary sounds of life sufficiently well to pay attention to them. Such a child needs to be taught, first of all, that sound vibrations can be meaningful. At the start, it will be necessary to make the child aware of the different sounds that exist in the environment and the differences among these sounds that enable us to identify them. Carhart has described this process as the teaching of gross sound discrimination.[1] Thus, the child should be taught that a bell and a horn make different sounds, and that these objects can be differentiated on the basis of their sounds. In the beginning, at least, this training will require amplification, that is, an auditory training unit. A good technique is to show two noisemakers, for example, a bell and a horn. While the child wears the earphones, ring the bell and blow the horn alternately, so that it can be seen which noisemaker is making the sound each time. Then face the child away from you, and sound one of the toys in front of the microphone. Have the child turn around and indicate whether it was the bell or the horn that was heard. When this task is mastered, add a third, then a fourth, and finally a fifth noisemaker. When the child learns to identify consistently which of five noisemakers was activated, progress has been made in teaching gross sound discrimination. Once the child learns to pay attention to sound, it may be possible to teach some gross sound discrimination without amplification.

As soon as the child has learned that sounds may give information about the environment, an individual hearing-aid fitting can be considered. Some audiologists feel that as soon as it has been established that the child has a profound loss of hearing, an aid should be provided in preference to waiting until some training in recognizing and differentiating gross sounds has been received. Their argument is that the child should be exposed to the sound environment throughout the waking hours and not just at the time of the auditory training lesson. They say that it is not fair to the child to deprive amplification until some training has been received in differentiating gross sounds. Certainly, it is important to supply the child with a hearing aid at the earliest opportunity. Nevertheless, when you give it to the child, you want it to be a pleasurable experience. Without any notion of what is being heard, or previous experience with amplified sound, the child may reject the hearing aid. It would be better to prepare the child for it by providing carefully planned and controlled listening experiences with an auditory training unit. The child who has been introduced to amplification in this manner is much more likely to accept a hearing aid from the start than if the aid had to be worn without any preparation at all.

After the child has learned to distinguish gross sounds, the next step in auditory training is to recognize the elements of speech. Preferably, this training should be based on whole words. If the child is able to associate the word *ball* with the object for which it stands, there is no need to spend time on the

---

[1] Raymond Carhart, "Auditory Training," in *Hearing and Deafness*, 2nd ed., eds. Hallowell Davis and S. Richard Silverman (New York: Holt, Rinehart and Winston, 1960), chap. 13, pp. 374–76.

recognition of the separate sounds that make up the word. If, however, the child confuses the word *ball* with the word *bell*, it may be necessary to teach the acoustic differences between the vowels *ah* and *eh*. If work on sounds is necessary, auditory training should start with the vowels, which are acoustically more easily distinguished than are the consonants. Before auditory training on meaningful words is possible, it may be necessary to spend time on the combination of sounds in nonsense syllables. Thus, *baw* and *beh* must be differentiated before the words *ball* and *bell* have recognizable differences. Learning the difference between dissimilar speech sounds is referred to as *gross speech discrimination,* whereas learning the difference between similar speech sounds, such as *f* and *th*, for example, is known as *fine speech discrimination.*[2] A reasonably good mastery of fine speech discrimination is a prerequisite to the understanding of speech.

Training with the Aid

Seldom is it sufficient to give a child a hearing aid without providing some training in its operation. This is true for the child who has received the kind of preparation for an aid referred to previously. It may require considerable adjustment for a child to transfer from an auditory training unit to an individual hearing aid. The problem of adjustment is even greater for the child who has never experienced amplification previously.

Teachers and parents are frequently frustrated in their attempts to get children to wear hearing aids. If a clinician has told a family that they should obtain a hearing aid for the child, the parents quite naturally expect that the least the child can do is to make use of the instrument on which they have spent a considerable sum of money. Frequently, the child will be sent to school with the hearing aid and a note to the teacher explaining that the child is to wear the aid throughout school. If the teacher has had no previous experience with children who wear hearing aids, there is a tendency to regard the instrument with awe and to feel a responsibility to see that the parents' instructions are followed. The child is thus badgered by both parents and teacher to wear an aid that may be unacceptable at this time. If sufficient pressure is brought to bear, parents and teachers can force children to wear hearing aids, but they cannot compel them to enjoy the process. What happens then is that the child takes off the hearing aid at the first opportunity and learns to hate it because it is associated with the authority that insists that it be worn. The usual outcome is that the child does not benefit from it and may be so conditioned against it that even with professional guidance, it will take considerable time to persuade the child to accept it. It is far better to avoid this unpleasantness from the start by placing the child with a new hearing aid under the professional guidance of an audiologist. The audiologist will explain to the parents and teacher the difficulties in adjusting to the aid. The audiologist will instruct the

[2] Ibid., p. 376.

parents and teacher not to force the aid upon the child but to help the child want to wear it by giving praise and approval.

Perhaps the first step in training the child to make effective use of the aid is to explain the instrument's controls and how to wear the aid most comfortably. The child should be shown how the controls function, how to change the battery, how to connect the aid to the earpiece, and how to insert and remove the earpiece. For the aid to be effective, it is fundamental that the mechanics of operating it be learned thoroughly. A body-worn aid generally can be worn most comfortably in a harness secured around the neck and chest. Adjustable harnesses may be purchased from hearing-aid dealers. The harness can be worn either under or outside the clothing. From an acoustic point of view, of course, it would be preferable to wear the aid outside. A child's auricles may be too small to support a behind-the-ear type aid. Such aids can be mounted on headbands similar to those used with bone-conduction vibrators, however. If very much gain is required in the aid, a head-worn type may not be feasible, because of the problem of acoustic feedback. Incidentally, the child will require a new earpiece at regular intervals, because of the growth of the external ears. Even with a body-worn aid, it is necessary to have the earpiece fit snugly so that it effectively seals off the canal. Otherwise, sound leaking around the earpiece will reach the microphone and result in acoustic feedback.

A word of caution is in order regarding the setting of the volume control. The inner ear may be susceptible to additional loss from excessively high sound levels. The inner ear can incur damage from sound levels that are not high enough to produce pain or even physiological discomfort. Further deterioration of hearing sensitivity can be caused by too high a volume-control setting. The audiologist must assume the responsibility for showing the child where the volume control should be set.

The same procedures that are suitable for an auditory training unit may be applied in training the child with a hearing aid. Where to begin the auditory training program with the aid depends, of course, on the capabilities of the child. If the suggestions in the previous section of this chapter are followed, the child will already have some awareness of sound and be able at least to differentiate various dissimilar sounds. Again, the child would be asked to listen to various noisemakers and to select the one that the teacher sounds. In the event that the child is able to recognize and understand certain words, and perhaps phrases or sentences, training with the aid would consist of vocabulary building and work with more difficult words and sentences.

The objectives of the auditory training program are, first of all, to persuade the child to accept the hearing aid, and then to learn to operate it effectively. As in any kind of educational training, the procedure is from the known to the unknown, from the simple to the complex. Although to force the child to attend to auditory signals it may be desirable for training purposes to limit visual cues, the long-range objective is the development of the child's communicative abilities to their ultimate extent. Therefore, auditory training should usually be combined with speechreading, and while the comprehension of speech is being taught emphasis must also be placed on helping the child to improve speech production.

Training Without an Aid

Two groups of children do not need hearing aids and yet would benefit from auditory training. One group includes the children who have losses less than the minimum loss for which a hearing aid is indicated. The other group consists of children who have sensori-neural impairments characterized by good hearing through 500 or possibly 1000 Hz and severe drop in hearing sensitivity at higher frequencies. Of course, some hearing-impaired children have such profound losses that even with a hearing aid it is not possible for them to respond to sound. In this chapter, however, we are concerned with the needs of the hard of hearing, as contrasted with those of the deaf. Another group that might be mentioned, but with which we shall not be concerned, consists of children whose hearing sensitivity as measured on the audiometer is normal but who have poor listening habits. In Chapter 3, mention was made of the fact that some children seem to have considerable difficulty in comprehending auditory verbal stimuli, even though their hearing sensitivity is normal. This group is not dealt with in the present chapter because here we are concerned only with children who have hearing losses.

In the first group of children, the loss for speech as measured with the speech audiometer would be something less than 20 to 25 dB in the better ear. Such loss may be temporary in nature, or it may be permanent. In either event, the loss is not severe enough to warrant constant amplification, yet many situations arise in which the child with this mild loss is handicapped. For such children, auditory training should be directed toward the occasions that cause difficulty. For example, if the child consistently has trouble hearing in the classroom, the audiologist should help the child analyze why there is this problem and try to plan a program that will minimize the difficulties in these circumstances. As part of the attack on the problem, the child may be advised to experiment with different seating in the classroom. Of course, the classroom teacher's cooperation would have to be secured in order to permit such experimentation. The child may find a desk-type hearing aid or portable auditory training unit helpful at least some of the time. Many schools provide such instruments for hearing-impaired pupils.

Instruction in speechreading may be all that the child with a mild loss requires. Some auditory training procedures may prove helpful, however, as an adjunct to speechreading. The emphasis is on teaching the child to pay close attention to speech that can barely be heard. When we are in difficult listening situations, the temptation is to let our attention wander and give up the attempt to listen. The child with a mild loss has the same tendency and may learn to listen more effectively by participating in listening games. For example, the therapist can play a game of lotto with the child, who is not permitted to watch the therapist's face. Each time the child makes the correct response in the lotto game, the therapist speaks a little more softly. Thus, as the game nears the finish, the child has to "strain" to listen, but because the game is almost over, motivation for listening carefully is excellent.

The child with a mild loss should be encouraged to ask for repetitions when speech is not understood. This is easy to say but difficult for the child actually to practice. It is embarrassing to draw attention to oneself by confessing that something was not heard. The line of least resistance is to act as if it was heard, which requires considerable "bluffing," and usually leads to even more embarrassing situations in the long run. Teachers and parents should be advised to speak a little more loudly and carefully to children with mild losses; yet the child still has a responsibility to let them know when something is not understood.

The child with a sloping audiogram through the higher speech frequencies may be considerably handicapped. In some ways, this is a more difficult situation than that of the child with a loss that requires a hearing aid. The hearing aid does advertise to all that the child has an impairment. There is nothing about the appearance of the child with a high-frequency loss that sets the child apart from anyone else. Thus, people tend to expect the same type of behavior as from a child who is normal in all respects.

The child with a loss for the higher speech frequencies has difficulty in understanding speech, yet because of good hearing for the low frequencies, voices can be heard perfectly well. The child may appear to be stupid because of a failure to comprehend what people are saying. Difficulty in comprehension comes from an inability to differentiate words with the same vowel but different consonants. Thus, *think* and *sink* may sound the same. The voiceless consonants, *s, th, f, k, t, p, sh, ch, h,* and *wh,* are the sounds most frequently missed by the child with a hearing loss for the higher speech frequencies. In addition to their being high-frequency consonants, they are voiceless and have very little phonetic power. The combination of high-frequency characteristics and low phonetic power makes these sounds particularly difficult. An example of how a child with this kind of loss might hear running speech demonstrates how difficult is the job of comprehending what is heard. For this example, we shall assume that the child hears vowels and voiced consonants in normal fashion, although in an actual case of a high-frequency hearing loss many other consonants would be heard with considerable distortion. The question, "What time is it?" might be heard by the child as "–a– –ime i– i–?" Is it any wonder that the child says "Huh?" or "What?" Even if the speaker repeats the question in a louder voice, the distortion of speech is still present. The child will simply hear the lower-frequency sounds with greater power. Such a child must depend to a large extent on speechreading as a solution to making the most of what is heard.

Working with paired words that differ only in the consonants present is a good technique for the child with a loss for the higher speech frequencies. A child who can read is able to point to the correct words in print. Pictures of objects can be used with the child who cannot read. A few examples of the type of paired words possible for this exercise follow:

stand	hand
tea	sea
mouse	house
tree	three
nose	toes

At the start, the therapist may have to say each word while pointing to the printed word or to the picture that the word represents and while the child watches for speechreading cues. After extensive practice, however, the child can learn to make many distinctions on the basis of hearing alone. It is not known accurately by what mechanism the child with a severe loss for the higher speech frequencies learns to distinguish similar-sounding words. Some research has indicated that vowel sounds are affected differently by different consonants, so that careful attention to the vowel will reveal subtle changes, which in turn point to the specific consonant preceding or following the vowel.[3] If that is so, certainly there is good reason for presenting auditory training work in terms of complete words, rather than trying to drill on the consonant sounds for which the hearing is defective.

Hearing aids may be of little or no value to these children for the same reason it is useless to shout at them. They do not need amplification in order to hear voices or the low-frequency speech sounds. A hearing aid should not be ruled out, however, without extensive experimentation, particularly with the CROS type of fitting with an open or nonoccluding earpiece that attenuates amplification of the low frequencies. This type of fitting is described in Chapter 10. Also, aids that are designed for high-frequency emphasis may prove to be useful, perhaps in combination with a vented earpiece.

SPEECH TRAINING

A hearing loss of greater than mild degree is almost always reflected in the child's own speech and voice patterns. For this reason, speech training is an important facet of the training program. Speech disorders associated with a hearing loss may range from complete lack of oral language to the presence of

---

[3] Arthur S. House and Grant Fairbanks, "The Influence of Consonant Environment upon the Secondary Acoustical Characteristics of Vowels," *Journal of the Acoustical Society of America* 25 (January 1953):105–13.

only a single articulatory error. A frequent cause for the condition described by speech pathologists as "delayed speech" is a severe hearing disorder. The child with delayed speech will be slow in starting to use words and may not begin to speak until reaching three to four years of age. Vocabulary will be meager, and grammar greatly simplified. The child will omit many sounds and make substitutions for others and will rely greatly on gestures for purposes of communication.[4] All these symptoms may be explained by a hearing impairment, although there are other causes for delayed speech. If the child's hearing for speech is faulty, however, speech production will be faulty because learning to speak is achieved through imitation of the speech that is heard.

Often, indeed, no one suspects that a child's hearing is not normal until adequate oral language fails to develop at the time when other children are learning to speak. Certainly, in every case of delayed speech the hearing of the child should be thoroughly studied. For a hearing loss that can be helped with amplification, a hearing aid should be tried at the earliest opportunity. Sometimes the introduction of amplification is all that is required to produce an immediate improvement in speech development. The authors observed an almost miraculous development of oral language in a four-year-old boy with bilateral atresia of the external canal after being fitted with a bone-conduction hearing aid. Usually, however, it is necessary to give extensive speech training to children even after they are fitted with aids.

With a severe hearing loss, the child's voice will be affected. The most noticeable vocal characteristic is a marked deviation from normal voice quality to what can be described as a dull and lifeless quality. Pitch is usually monotonous, and it may be somewhat higher than desirable. There may be rapid and extensive changes in vocal intensity while the child is speaking, the effect being one of uncontrollable intensity. With lesser degrees of hearing loss, the vocal characteristics of the child are less noticeable. A mild or moderate hearing loss may have no noticeable effect on the voice.

Where vocal symptoms do occur, the therapist must cope with them and strive to achieve as normal a vocal usage as possible. It is easier to effect changes in pitch and intensity than it is to produce improvement in vocal quality. Pitch and intensity can be controlled through kinesthetic sensations, but apparently vocal quality is almost entirely dependent on auditory monitoring. Variations in pitch, or inflections, may be taught by fairly mechanical means and through drill. For example, the child can be taught to vary pitch upward or downward as the therapist raises or lowers a finger. Thus the therapist, in the manner of an orchestra leader, can direct the child's pitch so that expression becomes more natural.

Control over intensity of voice requires an awareness of environment. In noisy surroundings, for example, a room crowded with talking people, in-

[4]Virgil A. Anderson and Hayes A. Newby, *Improving the Child's Speech* (New York: Oxford University Press, 1973), pp. 93–95.

dividuals with normal hearing unconsciously increase the intensity of their voices to make themselves audible over the background noise. On the other hand, when they are in a quiet environment, people tend to speak with decreased intensity. The child with a severe loss of hearing is not able to judge the proper intensity of voice for a given situation, except by a process of trial and error, and will have to depend largely on the reactions of other people. It is advisable, therefore, for the therapist to teach the child to be sensitive to the reactions of those around him, so that if they seem to have difficulty hearing, somewhat greater effort in voice production should occur. Because it is more difficult to judge when one is talking too loudly, it is better to teach the child to decrease voice intensity until it is apparent that others are having difficulty in hearing and then to speak at a slightly higher level, which should be just right.

Equipment has been designed and manufactured for the vocal training of the hard of hearing and the deaf. One such piece of equipment is a vertical bank of lights, which represents the intensity of the voice—the louder the voice, the more lights are illuminated. Another device consists of a vertical bank of lights behind different-colored panes of glass. With this, it is possible to obtain a visual pattern of a single speech sound, usually a vowel. The therapist demonstrates a speech sound while the patient observes the particular color pattern and the intensity of the colors produced on the instrument. The patient then attempts to produce a speech sound that will cause an identical pattern of lights to appear. Although such training devices have some clinical value, they do not by any means take the place of a qualified therapist. Some therapists even object to such training "aids," feeling that they serve to distract rather than to assist the patient.

Errors in articulation (sound formation) are commonly found in children who have even mild-to-moderate hearing losses. As was explained in the preceding chapter, certain English consonants require very delicate adjustments of the articulators. Sounds that involve the precise placement of the blade or the tip of the tongue in relation to other articulators are particularly likely to be defective, for example, *s, r, l, sh,* and *ch.* Generally, it can be said that the sounds that are less visible, are more complex in their formation, and have important high-frequency characteristics are those most likely to be affected by a hearing loss. Sounds with these characteristics are also the last sounds to be mastered in the speech development of the normal-hearing child. As would be expected, sounds that the child hears least well because of a hearing loss would most likely be defective. Thus, the voiceless consonants, which are both weak in phonetic power and contain important high-frequency components, are often defective, especially those that are also relatively invisible and complex in their formation.

The correction of defective articulation of hearing-impaired children requires an approach by the therapist that is largely visual and tactile. Depending on the extent of the hearing loss, an auditory approach is also possible, perhaps with amplification of an auditory training unit. With a severe or profound loss, however, primary dependence would have to be placed on nonauditory techniques. The therapist then resorts to a phonetic placement method, whereby an attempt is made to show the child where the articulators should be placed to produce a given sound. If the sound is at all visible, the therapist can demonstrate correct placement of articulators and encourage the child to be imitative. When the sounds are invisible, the therapist can show a cross-sectional drawing of the articulator placement and try to get the child to duplicate this placement.

It is frequently difficult to demonstrate to the severely impaired child the difference between voiced and unvoiced consonants that have the same articulator position, for example, *t* and *d*. The therapist can place the child's hand on the therapist's larynx and show that with the *d* there is vibration in the larynx, whereas for the *t* no vibration is felt. Plosives, that is, sounds that require the building up of breath pressure and then its sudden expulsion, as in *p, b, t, d, k,* and *g,* can be taught if the therapist places the child's hand in front of the therapist's mouth, so that the child can feel the puff of air that results each time. Nasal consonants, *m, n,* and *ng,* can be demonstrated by having the child feel the vibration in the therapist's nose. Each time the sound that the therapist has produced has been felt, the child should try to imitate it and receive the same feeling. When the same tactile sensations are felt while imitating what can be seen of the therapist's articulator placement, the child will be producing the correct acoustic effect for whatever speech sound is being attempted. Even with children who do not have such severe impairments of hearing, tactile methods can be helpful in teaching correct sound production. At the end of this chapter, the reader will find references containing specific directions for speech-correction work with hard-of-hearing children. The child with impaired hearing has enough difficulty in communication and is sufficiently handicapped without being saddled with a speech handicap also. By teaching proper speech production, the therapist can do much to ease the way for the hard-of-hearing child.

THE HEARING-IMPAIRED PRESCHOOL CHILD

The audiologist is concerned with the hard-of-hearing child. The child who is deaf requires full-time special education, and generally the audiologist is not responsible for this training. An exception to this statement is that of the deaf child of preschool age. Public-school education for deaf children usually is not available until the children are at least three years old, and most of them are not actually enrolled until they are three-and-a-half to four years old. If the child of preschool age is to receive any training before entering school, it becomes the audiologist's responsibility. It is certainly desirable for the training of a deaf child to begin when the hearing handicap is first diagnosed. Normal-hearing children start to develop speech at twelve to eighteen months of age. At this age, their nervous systems have developed to the point that they are "ready" for the unfolding of language concepts. Ideally, the training of the deaf child should commence when the neurological and physiological system is "ready" for this development. If no training whatsoever is given until the child becomes eligible for a public-school special education program, much valuable time will have been lost during which the child might have made a good start on the acquisition of language.

The needs of the preschool deaf child were brought to the attention of otologists, audiologists, and educators most forcefully by Mrs. Spencer Tracy, the wife of the late movie actor. Mr. and Mrs. Tracy's son John was deaf. They had a number of disappointing and discouraging experiences in their attempts to secure the advice and assistance they so desperately needed. Because of their unfortunate experiences, Mrs. Tracy determined to do all she could to help the parents of other deaf children. Originally, she started a discussion group for parents of young children. Teachers of the deaf were enlisted to explain to the parents techniques that were feasible for stimulating the development of language. The next step was the establishment of a nursery school for deaf children, where teachers of the deaf could demonstrate these techniques. As the work of the school became known, parents from all over the country wrote to Mrs. Tracy, asking how they could learn to become better parents of their deaf children. The outcome of these inquiries was a correspondence course, sent free of charge to parents of deaf children anywhere in the world. From the modest beginnings of a parents' discussion group, the John Tracy Clinic, as it is called today, has developed into an outstanding institution in Los Angeles, dedicated to helping parents of deaf children of preschool age, and thereby, of course, helping the children themselves.

Although work with deaf children of preschool age was not entirely unknown before the opening of the John Tracy Clinic, its influence is largely responsible for the development of most of the training programs for the preschool deaf that today are to be found in scores of cities in the United States. Most such programs follow the Tracy Clinic policy of concentrating on parent education, because it is realized that parents have the responsibility of training the preschool child. Although the children can work in groups for a limited time, they are the parents' responsibility for the greatest part of each day. The parents, therefore, must learn how to become teachers in order to help the child develop language.

In addition to training parents to become teachers of their children, the training programs for preschool deaf serve another, equally important function: that of helping the parents to accept and understand their hearing-handicapped children. It is frightening to parents to find that they have a handicapped child, and their reactions are likely to be extreme in one direction or another. They may reject the child completely, or at the other extreme, they may be inclined to overindulge the child. Either way, of course, the effect is unfortunate. By observing a group of hearing-handicapped preschool children under the direction of a competent teacher, parents can learn that the children are first of all *children,* and only secondarily are they *deaf* children. It reassures parents to see that other children are behaving in the same way as their own child. When the parents meet in discussion groups, they can share their fears and frustrations and their awakening awareness of their child's assets, with the result that they all benefit.

Some preschool programs operate a nursery school, which to outward appearances is the same as any other nursery school. A trained nursery-school teacher supervises the children's play and socializing experiences. Language-stimulating activities are provided at every opportunity. There is an audiologist or sometimes a teacher of the deaf on the staff who is responsible for supervising the language stimulation of the children. The audiologist takes them singly and in groups for auditory training and determines when each child is ready for a personal individual hearing aid. The audiologist also explains to the parents what is being done and the reasons for doing it. In addition to the audiologist and/or teacher of the deaf, the nursery-school staff may consist of a clinical psychologist, a child psychologist, or a medical or psychiatric social worker. The function of this staff member is to teach the parents about child development and to help them better understand their own children's periods of development. Also, within the limitations of training and capabilities, this staff member can serve as a general counselor to the parents in their personal and family problems, which the parents of handicapped children frequently have. The counselor can serve as a liaison between the parents and whatever professional people are involved, for example, psychiatrists. The counselor should be familiar with various sources of referral for the kinds of additional help that the parents need.

The parents of the children participate cooperatively with the nursery-school teacher and the audiologist in all phases of nursery-school activities. In this way, the parents become familiar with methods of handling children, their own included, and they learn at first hand how to administer auditory training and other language-stimulating activities so that they can apply these techniques at home.

The children in this kind of program benefit tremendously. They learn to play with other children, to share, and to discipline themselves, and they are in an atmosphere in which oral language is used and encouraged. They learn to accept their hearing aids gracefully, because others in the group wear them. By the time these children reach school age, they already have a substantial background in some aspects of the schoolwork that they will perform during their first year. Teachers of the deaf in public-school systems are quick to praise the work of the preschool programs for the results that are evident in the "graduates." More and more school systems are assuming responsibilities for hearing-handicapped preschool children through tax-supported parent-child programs. Children who have had the advantage of preschool training develop their capabilities in school much more quickly than do other children.

Teachers of the deaf will supervise the training of the child for all the school years. The audiologist can take pride, however, in what has been accomplished through the preschool training program—in sending these children to school with an excellent preparation.

COUNSELING FOR PARENT AND CHILD

As stated in the preceding chapter, the bulk of the counseling required with the hearing-impaired child should be directed to the parents, as the attitudes of the parents toward the handicap are most important in influencing the child's own attitudes. The audiologist has the duty of counseling the parents, and to some extent the child, about the best ways of coping with the problems associated with hearing loss. The audiologist must take care, however, not to undertake more counseling than the situation calls for and not to attempt to handle problems of deep-seated psychological maladjustment. It is the audiologist's responsibility to establish the limits of counseling and to refer to appropriate professional people the cases that require help. In other words, the audiologist must guard against the temptation to assume the role of a psychiatrist or clinical psychologist. The final section of this chapter will deal with the most important areas in which the audiologist's counseling is required.

Acceptance of the Child

Parents of a handicapped child frequently find it difficult to accept the child as a handicapped child. It is the hope of all parents that their children will be perfect in all respects. A handicap means that the parents' hopes have not been realized, and the parents may feel bitter and antagonistic toward the child. Usually, the feelings are submerged, and the parents do not admit even to themselves that they have difficulty in accepting the child. As a matter of fact, their unconscious rejection of the child may result in their protesting vigorously that they want to do everything possible to help realize the child's full potential. Because it is not socially acceptable to reject one's children, the parents may be motivated in their actions by deep-seated feelings of guilt. Those who protest too loudly that they love and accept their children may be expressing only surface feelings. It is a blow to the ego to produce an imperfect child, and many parents blame the child, albeit unconsciously, for being imperfect. On the other hand, some parents feel that their having produced a handicapped child is punishment for their "sins," and their relations with the child are colored by their own feelings of guilt.

Although the audiologist has no business psychoanalyzing the parents or trying to interpret their feelings or motivations, encouragement can be given for a proper acceptance of the hearing-handicapped child through positive actions and statements. Perhaps the most important contribution is that of adopting an optimistic and encouraging attitude toward the child's problems. The audiologist should emphasize the assets and minimize the liabilities of the child. It can be explained to the parents that it is possible to educate deaf children. If it is likely that the child will be able to utilize a hearing aid, the audiologist can emphasize the positive connotations of this fact. What must be avoided in dealing with parents is the attitude that their child has a problem for which nothing can be done. Diagnosticians are too prone to pass on their findings to parents without any mention of what can be done in the way of overcoming or minimizing the handicapping condition. We know today that the hearing-handicapped child can usually be taught to speak and understand speech, be educated, and vocationally trained. By pointing out the positive aspects of the situation, the audiologist may be answering some questions that the parents have been afraid to ask even themselves.

The audiologist can help allay fears and guilt feelings by explaining everything to the parents about the nature of the hearing loss and its cause. For information concerning the diagnosis and etiology, the audiologist will have to rely, of course, on the otological findings. Usually, the otologist will have explained the findings to the parents, but even so the audiologist's repetition and explanation will be helpful to them. Frequently, they are in such a state of shock upon first discovering they have a handicapped child that they cannot comprehend what the otologist is saying to them. Also, some otologists, unfortunately, do not take the time needed to explain fully to the parents just what the child's situation is. By interpreting the otological findings, the audiologist can do the otologist, as well as the parents, a service.

Frequently, hearing loss or deafness is a complete mystery to parents. In that event, the audiologist can help the parents better understand their child's problems by explaining how we hear and what can happen to cause interference with the normal hearing process. The difference between the hard of hearing and the deaf should be explained and the child placed in his proper classification, so far as it is possible to determine it at that time. Parents can be referred to books on the subject of hearing loss and deafness, which will also contribute to their better understanding of their child's problems and what can be done about them.[5]

The audiologist can perform a considerable service to parents by informing them of the existence of the John Tracy Clinic correspondence course and by putting them in touch with the nearest preschool training program. The audiologist can also refer them to other parents of hearing-handicapped children, who have "been through the mill" and who can help and guide these parents from their own experiences.

The dangers of overprotection are almost as great as those of rejection.

[5] Helmer R. Myklebust, *Your Deaf Child: A Guide for Parents* (Springfield, Ill.: Charles C Thomas, 1970).

The healthiest home environment for the hearing-impaired child is one in which the child is treated the same as other children in the family, with appropriate allowances, of course, for communicative difficulties. Above all, the environment should be an *oral* one. The parents and other children in the family should talk with the child at all times and also encourage the child to talk. It is only through constant exposure to speech that the child is motivated to want to understand what is said and to use speech. The child may be receiving the best possible school training in oral language, but if no opportunity is given at home to exercise communicative skills, the school training will be to little avail.

The child who acquires a hearing loss some time after birth requires acceptance just as much as does the child with a congenital hearing problem. Frequently, the problem of fitting a hearing aid to a child with an acquired loss is based on the parents' refusal to accept the situation. Some feel that a hearing aid advertises to others that their child is defective, and they will go to any lengths to avoid this stigma. With such parents, the audiologist must demonstrate, by whatever means, the help that the hearing aid gives the child. Parents of other children who wear hearing aids can be of considerable assistance at this point. If the parents can be brought to accept the aid, with a sensible attitude toward it, it is much easier to convince the child. At the same time, as mentioned in an earlier section, parents must be cautioned against exerting too much pressure on the child to wear a hearing aid when the child is not yet convinced to do so. They must realize that it usually takes time for a child to adjust to a hearing aid. They must be patient and understanding in order to be helpful.

Some parents feel that a hearing aid will restore their child's hearing to normal. Naturally, they are bitter and disappointed when they learn that the child still is handicapped, even with the hearing aid. Thus, the audiologist has the responsibility of explaining to them how hearing aids work and what they can and cannot do. A realistic notion of hearing aids must be given to parents.

Not only must the parents be realistic about what a hearing aid can accomplish; they must also be realistic about the extent of their child's handicap. Some parents do know the difference between the deaf and the hard of hearing but refuse to admit to themselves that their child is deaf. They nurse the hope that with proper instruction and the use of a hearing aid, the child will be able to function in a regular classroom. When the child has difficulty in trying to keep up with the other children, the parents blame the teacher for not giving their child "special attention." The authors remember one such example very vividly. At the age of four, a little girl whom we shall call Ruth was found to have a profound impairment of hearing. She gave no indication of responding to sounds of high intensity when they were presented close to her ear. Ruth was enrolled in the Stanford Speech and Hearing Clinic for experimental therapy to see whether with training she would give any indication of responding to sound. Instruction in speechreading and other techniques of language stimulation were started. Ruth's parents were urged to enroll her in a special class for the deaf conducted in a county school. This the parents refused to do; instead, they enrolled Ruth in a regular kindergarten. Because of the character of kindergarten activities, Ruth was able to get along reasonably well during her first year. No demands were made on her to respond to speech or to speak, and she was able to color, to handle scissors, and to engage in most kindergarten activities. Meanwhile, the parents kept Ruth enrolled at the Speech and Hearing Clinic. They were sure that with the special help Ruth was receiving at the clinic, she would be able to make her way successfully at regular school.

The next fall, Ruth was enrolled in the first grade at the school she had previously attended, although both the kindergarten teacher and the principal of the school recommended her enrollment in the county class for the deaf. Within a few weeks after the beginning of the fall term, in the first grade, it was clear to the teacher that Ruth was wholly unable to profit from the instruction given. In this grade, Ruth was competing with about thirty youngsters whose hearing was normal, and day by day she became more withdrawn and sullen. Finally, everyone concerned with the case cooperated in insisting that Ruth attend the special class for the deaf. The principal of the school that she had been attending refused to let her continue, and the directors of the Speech and Hearing Clinic refused to continue work with her because as long as Ruth attended the clinic two or three times a week, the mother could continue to maintain that Ruth was receiving all the language-training instruction she needed. It was obviously unfair to Ruth, to the teacher, and to the other children in the class to have her continue any longer in the first grade. Thus, Ruth's parents were finally forced to face the true extent of their child's handicap. It can be added that in the county classes for the deaf Ruth made excellent progress and a good psychological adjustment. How much better for her it would have been had her parents faced squarely the true extent of her handicap and permitted her enrollment in a class for the deaf in the first place.

Educational Counseling

Parents need the audiologist's guidance in planning the proper educational program for their hearing-handicapped child. The advice is limited usually to the types of educational programs that are available to the parents in the communities in which they live. It goes without saying that the audiologist must be thoroughly familiar with all the educational facilities for hearing-impaired children that are available.

For hard-of-hearing children, the emphasis today is on "mainstreaming," that is, educating them with normal-hearing children in regular classrooms. Actually, except for some of the most populous school districts in the country, hard-of-hearing children have by necessity had to remain in regular classrooms. Today, this practice is not only condoned but also recommended by educators as having special advantages to those with hearing and other handicaps over segregation with other handicapped children. Unfortunately, most truly deaf children—those who cannot utilize hearing as the primary avenue of communication—cannot be educated properly in the same classes with normal-hearing children, as was demonstrated with Ruth. Possible school placements for deaf children, depending on the area, include a city school for the deaf, a county school with classes for the deaf, a state-supported residential school, and private residential schools. The city and county schools are *day* schools, in contrast with the state-supported and private residential schools. The advantage of the day school is that the children live at home, which is desirable from the standpoint of maintaining the child's security in family relationships. The advantage of the residential schools is that the children enrolled there obtain a more concentrated program of special education that continues throughout their waking hours.

Although it is not the purpose of this book to discuss and evaluate methods of training the deaf, some mention should be made of the educational conflict that has persisted for centuries between the *oralists* and the *manualists*. The oralists maintain that with proper teaching methods the deaf can be taught to produce and understand speech, so that it is possible for them to communicate with normal-hearing people in the usual fashion. On the other hand, the manualists maintain that the results of oral teaching do not justify the tremendous effort required on the part of the child and the teachers. They say that it is unrealistic to expect the deaf to be able to compete on equal terms with people with normal hearing and that little advantage is therefore gained from the time and effort required to teach them speech. The manual method of communication, by means of finger spelling and conventional signs, is relatively easy to teach. By this means, the deaf can communicate easily with each other and with their teachers. Thus, more school time is available for subject matter. The manualists admit that without speech the deaf adult is limited in vocational opportunities and in contacts with normal-hearing people. They stress vocational training, therefore, in such fields as baking, shoe repair, carpentry, machine work, and so forth, where the need for communication is minimal. Their attitude is that the deaf are going to have to look primarily to other deaf people for companionship anyway; thus it does not matter if they cannot communicate readily with those who have normal hearing.

Some schools teach what they call *total communication*, which is supposed to consist of both oral and manual methods. Unfortunately, however, the manual system is easier to learn and use, and in schools where any students are permitted this system, most prefer it to speech. Graduates of the total-communication schools are usually able to do some speechreading, but rarely are they able to speak with real intelligibility. Generally speaking, the city and county schools, the "day" schools, have adopted the oral approach in education, whereas the state-supported residential schools cling to the manual or total-communication methods. It was in protest against the manual method that the private residential schools for the deaf were founded. The accomplishments of the graduates of such private schools as Central Institute for the Deaf in St. Louis, Clarke School in Northampton, Massachusetts, and Lexington School in New York in establishing themselves in professions and business are a tribute to the oralists' belief that with proper training the handicap imposed by deafness can be minimized and the deaf can make their way in a hearing world.

Quite apart from educational differences of opinion, there is a good reason why deaf children should attend day schools rather than residential ones—the genetic implications of segregating the deaf. Some cases of deafness are due to heredity, and if the social contacts of the deaf are limited to others who are deaf, the problem of hereditary deafness will not only be perpetuated but also increase as the deaf intermarry. Thus, from the geneticist's point of view, it is a mistake for deaf children to attend residential schools. It would be much more sensible from the standpoint of the future of the race if deaf children could be educated in public schools where they would mingle with hearing children both on the school playgrounds and at home.

The parents of deaf children must plan for their children's education, and in this they will need the help of the audiologist and otologist. For the reasons just stated, the audiologist and otologist are prejudiced in favor of day schools and the oral method. All factors in a given case must be carefully weighed and evaluated, however. A day school is to be preferred if there are enough deaf children to constitute several classes, each with a narrow age range. In some sparsely settled communities, day-school classes have been established in which there is an age range of six or seven years. It is not possible for a teacher to do effective work with deaf children under these circumstances, even though there may be only six children in the class. Deaf children require such concentrated work in language, in addition to the subject matter, that all members of a class should be of about the same age and in the same stage of development. Faced with a choice between this day-school situation and sending their child to the state residential school, parents may well decide that it is better to send the child to the state school. The alternatives would be to move to a community that does have a strong day-school program or to send their child to a private residential school.

The educational opportunities for the hard of hearing are in some ways more extensive, and in others more limiting, than the opportunties for the deaf. Because by definition the hard of hearing have hearing that is functional with or without a hearing aid, presumably they should be able to profit from the same kind of instruction that normal-hearing students receive. This assumption is basic to the philosophy of mainstreaming. Within the category of hard of hearing, however, there is a wide range of mental abilities as well. Even though classified educationally as hard of hearing, a child may not necessarily be able to function in regular classes. In the larger cities, and in some populous counties, there are special education programs for the hard of hearing as well as for the deaf. There may be special "contact" classes for the hard of hearing, in which the children are given instruction in speechreading, auditory training, and speech for part of the day, while they attend classes with normal-hearing children the rest of the time. In most public schools, however, the child would have to attend regular classes all the time. The school system may employ speech and hearing therapists who travel from school to school and provide special oral language instruction two or three times a week outside the classroom. By and large, therefore, the hard-of-hearing child must get along as best as possible in the regular classroom. If this is the situation, the help parents can give to the child assumes tremendous importance.

Parents cannot expect that every teacher their child has will be familiar with the problems of the hard of hearing, and so they must assume the responsibility for "educating" the teachers about their child's needs. At the beginning of each school year, the child's parents should meet with the teacher and discuss the child's abilities and disabilities. The experience of previous teachers should also be helpful in guiding the new teacher to an understanding of the child's problems. If the child wears a hearing aid, the parents should explain to the teacher how the aid operates and what its limitations are. If the child is embarrassed at wearing an aid, the parents can give helpful suggestions about how the teacher can help the child overcome self-consciousness and make a better adjustment to the situation. The teacher, of course, can do a great deal to determine the attitudes of the other students toward the hearing-handicapped child and particularly toward the hearing aid. Throughout the school year, the parents should keep in close touch with the child's teacher; any problems arising can then be handled promptly through the cooperative action of the parents and teacher. It goes without saying, of course, that in these parent-teacher conferences the child's mother and father must exercise tact and understanding, so that it does not appear that they are dictating to the teacher what can and cannot be done. Teachers most naturally resist overbearing and oversolicitious parents, and the parents must tread a narrow path between showing too much concern on the one hand and failing to give the teacher enough help and support on the other.

For the child's sake, too, the parents must beware of becoming too solicitous, lest the child be "overprotected." Some parents find an emotional "release" in crusading for the betterment of hard-of-hearing children. This is fine as long as the child does not become a pampered, spoiled, incompetent "victim" of the parents' zeal. The audiologist can help the parents keep their "crusading" activities in proper focus. Of course, the better informed the parents are on hearing problems in general, and the situation of their own child in particular, the better able they are to assist the child's teachers in proper handling of the child in school and to help the child in and out of school in a better adjustment.

Children with hearing impairments and their parents must give careful consideration to the choice of a vocation. The effect of the hearing impairment must be placed in proper perspective. The child's intelligence, aptitudes, and abilities must be considered, as well as the limitations imposed by the hearing problem. One important factor in the choice of a vocation is whether or not a college education is feasible or possible. The hard-of-hearing child who has been able to function successfully in public-school programs can certainly continue to function educationally in college, provided that the intelligence and the motivation to do acceptable academic work exist. There are very few deaf individuals, however, who can do college work successfully, because of the tremendous emphasis on communication skills at the college level. Even the deaf person with excellent intellectual equipment finds it almost impossible to compete in college with normal-hearing students without an assistant to take notes in lectures. A good background in oral education is a prerequisite to attending regular college, of course. There is only one liberal arts college in the United States exclusively for deaf students, Gallaudet College in Washington, D.C. Gallaudet College is supported by the federal government, and it is the only liberal arts college that graduates of manual systems of education can attend without being faced with a virtually insurmountable communicative handicap. The federal government also supports the National Technical Institute for the Deaf in Rochester, New York, which is affiliated with the Rochester Institute of Technology and which awards baccalaureate degrees.

Deaf or hard-of-hearing college graduates naturally have a wider vocational choice than do hearing-handicapped individuals who cannot attend college. So in planning for the future, parents of hearing-impaired children must consider whether or not a college education is a possibility. For children who cannot attend college, some kind of vocational training must be planned. There are countless occupations in which a hearing impairment is of secondary importance. The choice of vocation, therefore, should depend primarily on the child's aptitudes and abilities, always keeping in mind, of course, the limitations imposed by the hearing handicap. The parents should be advised to consult with a competent vocational counselor at least by the time the child reaches high-school age. In the matter of vocation, the parents must be willing to accept the child and the handicap just as they must accept the child wholeheartedly when the hearing impairment is first discovered.

REFERENCES

BENDER, RUTH E. *The Conquest of Deafness.* 3rd ed. Danville, Ill.: Interstate Publishers, 1981.

BERG, FREDERICK S. *Educational Audiology: Hearing and Speech Management.* New York: Grune & Stratton, 1976.

BERG, FREDERICK S., and FLETCHER, SAMUEL G., eds. *The Hard of Hearing Child.* New York: Grune & Stratton, 1970.

BESS, FRED H., ed. *Childhood Deafness: Causation, Assessment and Management.* Chaps. 22, 23, 24, and 25. New York: Grune & Stratton, 1977.

BESS, FRED H.; FREEMAN, BARRY A.; and SINCLAIR, J. STEPHEN, eds. *Amplification in Education.* Washington, D.C.: The Alexander Graham Bell Association for the Deaf, 1981.

BESS, FRED H., and McCONNELL, FREEMAN, eds. *Audiology, Education, and the Hearing Impaired Child.* St. Louis: C. V. Mosby, 1981.

CALVERT, DONALD R., and SILVERMAN, S. RICHARD. rev. ed. *Speech and Deafness.* Washington, D.C.: The Alexander Graham Bell Association for the Deaf, 1983.

DAVIS, HALLOWELL, and SILVERMAN, S. RICHARD, eds. *Hearing and Deafness,* 4th ed. Chaps. 12, 13, 14, and 17. New York: Holt, Rinehart and Winston, 1978.

ERBER, NORMAN P. *Auditory Training.* Washington, D.C.: The Alexander Graham Bell Association for the Deaf, 1982.

HARRIS, GRACE M. *Language for the Preschool Deaf Child.* New York: Grune & Stratton, 1971.

HOCHBERG, IRVING; LEVITT, HARRY; and OSBERGER, MARY JOE, eds. *Speech of the Hearing Impaired: Research, Training, and Personnel Preparation.* Baltimore: University Park Press, 1983.

JAFFE, BURTON F., ed. *Hearing Loss in Children.* Chaps. 42–52. Baltimore: University Park Press, 1977.

LING, DANIEL. *Speech and the Hearing-Impaired Child: Theory and Practice.* Washington, D.C.: The Alexander Graham Bell Association for the Deaf, 1976.

McCONNELL, FREEMAN, and WARD, PAUL H., eds. *Deafness in Childhood.* Chaps. 16, 17, 18, and 19. Nashville, Tenn.: Vanderbilt University Press, 1967.

MARTIN, FREDERICK N., ed. *Pediatric Audiology.* Chaps. 9, 10, and 12. Englewood Cliffs, N.J.: Prentice-Hall, 1978.

OGDEN, PAUL W., and LIPSETT, SUZANNE, eds. *The Silent Garden: Understanding the Hearing Impaired Child.* New York: St. Martin's Press, 1982.

SANDERS, DEREK A. *Aural Rehabilitation.* 2nd ed. Englewood Cliffs, N.J.: Prentice-Hall, 1982.

STARK, RACHEL E., ed. *Sensory Capabilities of Hearing-Impaired Children.* Baltimore: University Park Press, 1974.

TRAVIS, LEE EDWARD, ed. *Handbook of Speech Pathology and Audiology.* Chaps. 15 and 16. Englewood Cliffs, N.J.: Prentice-Hall, 1971.

CHAPTER TWELVE
REHABILITATING THE HARD-OF-HEARING ADULT

The therapeutic problems presented by the adult who develops a hearing impairment are in most respects simpler than those of children. The principal difference is that the adult has well-developed language concepts and presumably throughout life has been "auditorily minded." Thus, the therapist can assume that the adult has a memory for sounds, and vocabulary building is not a necessary part of the rehabilitation process. In the area of psychological adjustment, however, the adult presents a more challenging problem. As stated in Chapter 10, it may be more difficult to adjust to a hearing disorder after having had normal hearing for a number of years than it is when there is no memory or knowledge of normal hearing. Counseling, therefore, is a necessary and important part of the rehabilitation of the hard-of-hearing adult. Not infrequently, counseling must precede all other aspects of rehabilitation. Before benefit from instruction in speechreading, auditory training, or speech training can occur, the individual must be motivated. Accepting a hearing aid, for example, may be a trying ordeal for the patient, the patient's family, and the therapist. Rehabilitative work with an adult is rewarding, however, for once the patient has accepted the situation and decided to make an effort, rapid progress can be made.

As in the previous chapter, no attempt will be made here to develop specific lesson plans for the adult. Rather, a general view will be taken of ways to meet the patient's rehabilitative needs. Again, the reader seeking more specific information is referred to the bibliographic listing at the end of the chapter.

SPEECHREADING

Regardless of the extent of hearing loss or whether or not the patient can profit from a hearing aid, instruction in speechreading will be beneficial. As a matter of fact, those of us with normal hearing can improve our communicative abilities through understanding and practicing the skill of speechreading. One of the first tasks of the therapist is to convince the patient that speechreading is not an esoteric art which requires years of training. It is advisable in the beginning to build up the patient's confidence by demonstrating that even without instruction a capacity exists for some speechreading. This can be done by asking the patient a number of questions—questions of the type that would be asked in many common situations, such as applying for a driver's license, a marriage certificate, or a passport. To make the demonstration more convincing, the therapist should use no voice, that is, the normal rate, rhythm, and articulation of speech should be maintained without audible speech, so that the patient cannot claim that auditory clues were present.

The questions should be on the order of the following:

What is your name?
How do you spell your name?
Where do you live?
What is your telephone number?
Are you married?
What is your wife's (or husband's) name?
Do you have any children?
What are their names?
How old are they?

It is easier for the patient to understand when each question follows logically from the preceding one. It may be necessary to ask a particular question two or three times before the patient comprehends it, and on occasion the therapist may have to rephrase the question. For example, it may be easier for the patient to understand the question "What is your address?" than the question "Where do you live?" With skill, the therapist can make this question-and-answer game a rewarding and motivating experience for the patient. Moreover, the way in which the patient responds to this kind of questioning can yield valuable information for the therapist in planning the program of speechreading instruction. If the patient answers quickly and easily, the therapist knows that the speechreading lessons can progress rapidly. On the other hand, if the patient has difficulty with these simple questions, the prognosis for rapid progress in the training program is not too good. In any event, personal questions of the type referred to can be helpful in establishing a friendly working relationship between the therapist and the patient. Besides the insight into facility in speechreading, the therapist can quickly learn a great deal about the patient from the factual answers that are given the questions.

It is well in the beginning to explain to the patient what the object of speechreading instruction is and to give some specific suggestions for becoming an effective speechreader. The purpose of the training in speechreading is, of course, to quicken the patient's powers of visual observation; it does not teach a new skill so much as it systematizes what is already done on a more or less unconscious level. The patient should be informed at the outset that speechreading is not a perfect substitute for hearing. The patient will realize after the initial practice work that it is not possible to speechread all that is seen. The therapist must stress the fact that the patient should not attempt to get every word but should keep up with the pace of the person's speech. While dwelling on a particular word that was not comprehended, the patient loses out on what the speaker is presently saying; thus, at all costs the speechreader must keep pace with the speaker. Another important suggestion concerns the development of a flexible mind. To be an effective speechreader, one must not have too firmly set, preconceived notions of how things should be said. The speechreader should realize that there is more than one way of expressing a thought and should keep alert to what the speaker is saying instead of trying to put words into the speaker's mouth.

It is our feeling that a synthetic method of teaching speechreading is preferable for adults. At least it should be given first choice. As long as the patient is able to do a reasonably good job of speechreading sentences and paragraphs, there seems little point in spending time on an analysis of individual sounds. It has been our experience that the adult who cannot do well with a synthetic approach will likewise have difficulty with analytic procedures. The only time that work on individual sounds is justified is when it becomes clear that a particular sound is causing the patient difficulty. Even then, the sound usually can be demonstrated in words or phrases more effectively than in isolation.

As in working with children, speechreading for the adult should be approached as one of several related communicative skills which are combined to compensate for a hearing loss. The therapist must keep the overall objectives of the rehabilitative program in mind and not succumb to the temptation to regard ability in speechreading as a goal in itself. While receiving instruction in speechreading, the patient should be encouraged to utilize hearing as well. The therapist then should strive to teach the adult to combine speechreading with whatever auditory ability exists. Some voice should be employed during the speechreading lessons, so that the patient can make use of hearing as well as of vision. If, however, the therapist speaks in such a manner that the patient can understand every word by hearing alone, he or she will develop little or no ability in speechreading per se. It is preferable, therefore, for the therapist to speak in a voice that is barely audible to the patient and that presents a difficult listening situation. This is the kind of practical, everyday communicative condition in which the patient will have trouble. The therapist can vary the difficulty of the speechreading lessons on occasion with whispered voice or some of the time with no voice at all. These techniques should be applied sparingly. By and large, the patient should be given experience in meeting situations that will be confronted in the normal course of events.

Numbers are a good way to start speechreading instruction. They are important to all of us in our daily living. We live by the numbers on the clock and the calendar, and we pay for our living with the numbers on money. It is easy to plan lessons around them. For example, a patient may be asked to set the hands of a clock to the time that the therapist designates. To start, the therapist should talk about the various ways of stating times: *Twenty minutes before ten* is the same as *nine-forty; twelve o'clock* may be *noon* or *midnight*; and so forth. Then the therapist should give practice to the patient in speechreading numbers from one to sixty. This ability can then be put to the test by asking the patient to set the hands of the clock.

Working on dates provides an opportunity for the patient to learn the days of the week and the months of the year as well as both ordinal and cardinal numbers. In the first place, the patient should be given an opportunity to learn the days of the week as the therapist goes over them in sequence. The months of the year can be practiced and learned in the same way. Then dates in the form of the day of the week and the day of the month can be practiced, for example, *Tuesday, September 9.* Finally, the days of the week and the month should be combined with the four digits of a year, for example, *Friday, February 22, 1985.* Holidays that occur every year provide interesting ways of practicing dates. Thus, the therapist can give a date, such as *December 25*, and ask the patient to reply what holiday it is. If the patient is at all proficient in history, the dates of famous historical events can be employed in the same way, as a test of the patient's ability to speechread months, days, and years.

Further practice on numbers is possible by planning lessons around money. As with time, there are various ways of talking about money. A dime may be spoken of as *ten cents*; a quarter as *twenty-five cents* or *two bits*; and a dollar may be referred to as a *buck* or any of several additional slang terms. The prices of articles in the grocery store can be practiced in numbers from one cent to ten dollars. Items of clothing permit practice on prices from a few dollars to several hundred dollars, and other commodities from washing machines to yachts provide the opportunity to practice on the higher-numbered prices. In dealing with prices, the therapist must point out to the patient that *two ninety-eight* is the same as *two dollars and ninety-eight cents,* or, depending on the commodity being discussed, *two hundred and ninety-eight dollars.*

Certain numbers will consistently give difficulty. *Eight* and *nine* are almost indistinguishable from each other in speechreading. Numbers such as *thirteen* and *thirty, fifteen* and *fifty,* and so forth, are frequently confused. The patient cannot always rely on speechreading with these numbers. In a "real" situation, the hearing-impaired person should always repeat the number in order to check it. Thus, if, in reply to a question about train or bus schedules, the ticket agent says something that the patient reads as 9:17, the patient should ask the agent, "Did you say 9:17?" It might just as well have been 8:17, and without asking, the patient can never be sure.

Speechreading instruction can be made interesting to adult patients by planning lessons around so-called life situations. In the preceding paragraph, mention was made of a conversation between a patient and a ticket agent. The therapist can prepare a dialogue between a hypothetical ticket agent and the patient, involving questions and answers about particular trains or buses, their schedules, and the price of tickets. Again, instead of drill on prices alone, a dialogue could be prepared on a shopping visit to the grocery or a visit to the shoe store or any of dozens of situations that involve the pricing of objects. Situations in which the patient is most likely to be involved should be selected for these dialogues. After explaining what the situation is, the therapist should proceed with the complete dialogue between the two characters involved, while the patient speechreads both parts of the conversation. With this kind of material, the therapist should first go through the complete dialogue without stopping, and then ask the patient questions about what was said. After the questions, which will disclose how much of the dialogue the patient is able to speechread on the first attempt, the therapist should go back over the dialogue on a sentence-by-sentence basis, asking the patient to repeat each sentence. It may be necessary at this point for the therapist to repeat a given sentence two or three times or perhaps to rephrase the sentence before the patient can comprehend it. The therapist should accept the patient's version of a sentence, even if it should not be word-perfect, if the patient has succeeded in understanding the thought. As a final step, the therapist should then repeat the whole dialogue without stopping, in order to give the patient an opportunity to synthesize on a sentence-by-sentence basis.

These should be fairly easy speechreading experiences for the beginner. As the patient develops facility in this kind of situation, the therapist should provide more difficult speechreading experiences. Short anecdotes, such as those that appear in the *Reader's Digest,* provide good material for speechreading lessons. Because they are written for the silent reader, it is usually desirable for the therapist to rewrite the story in an oral style. Anecdotes usually contain a "punch line" at the end. The test of the patient's speechreading ability is whether the point of the story is understood on the first attempt. The same procedure should be followed as with the life-situation dialogues. The therapist should give the story as a whole to begin with, ask questions about it, repeat it on a sentence-by-sentence basis, and finally give the story in its complete form again.

It is helpful and stimulating for patients to obtain some experience in a group. Ideally, groups should be organized so that all members have similar interests and similar speechreading abilities. Group speechreading experiences help the patient to realize that other hard-of-hearing individuals have difficulties of the same type. Group work may stimulate the individual to greater effort because of the spirit of competition. Finally, the members of the group may help each other to achieve a better speechreading ability and also a healthier attitude toward their hearing handicaps. In group work, each member should take a turn being a speaker, so that the members of the group may have practice in speechreading a number of different speakers. As the members of the group become more proficient, more difficult experiences may be provided, like setting up actual dialogues so that the speechreaders must shift their attention from one speaker to another, and giving the speechreaders the opportunity to view speakers from various distances and angles. Group work does not take the place of individual instruction in speechreading, but it can supply an interesting and profitable means of putting speechreading ability to practical use.

AUDITORY TRAINING

The hard-of-hearing adult does not require as extensive auditory training as does the child because of previous experience as a normal-hearing individual. Thus, with the adult it is not necessary to start with gross auditory discriminations or even with gross speech-sound discriminations unless, of course, the person has suffered almost a complete loss of hearing. Generally, it is with the consonant sounds that the adult has difficulty, and usually it is the high-frequency, low-powered voiceless consonants that give the most trouble. Whether or not the adult will require any auditory training depends, of course, on the severity of the loss, the length of time that the person has been hard of hearing, and also the audiometric configuration of the loss. The adult with a hearing impairment that is easily compensated for by a hearing aid may require no auditory training, whereas an individual with a typical sensori-neural impairment, who has considerably better hearing in the low frequencies than in the high ones, will probably benefit from auditory training whether or not the person wears a hearing aid. The test of whether or not auditory training is indicated is the individual's ability to *understand* speech with or without amplification. The candidate for a hearing aid may profit from auditory training administered with amplification, such as that provided by an auditory training unit. The person who cannot successfully utilize a hearing aid should receive auditory training without amplification, for the most part, although on occasion an auditory training unit may be employed for the purpose of focusing attention.

As with speechreading instruction, a worthwhile starting technique in auditory training is the use of numbers. The therapist starts with two-digit numbers, such as *four-six,* and asks the patient to repeat them or to write them down. As the patient gains facility in recognizing two-digit numbers, three-digit numbers can be introduced, and eventually four- and five-digit numbers.[1] Numbers are good because the choices that the patient has to make are limited; and because many numbers can be differentiated on the basis of vowels alone, the patient can do well with a minimum of auditory clues.

As was suggested in auditory training for children, practice with paired words that differ only in their initial or final consonant is a good technique. The therapist gives the patient a written list of paired words and then says one word in each pair while the patient checks the word that the therapist said. This can be extended to as many as five words, all of which are similar, such as *fear, dear, near, cheer, beer.* The therapist says one word, and the patient must check which of the five possible words it was. This type of auditory training material is available in recorded form.

The word lists customary in speech audiometry for obtaining thresholds (spondees) and speech-discrimination scores (phonetically balanced words) are useful also for auditory training. The spondee words, being easier, should be practiced first. Whenever the patient misses a spondee word, it should be noted and put on a list, which will then serve for extensive drill. The phonetically balanced words are more difficult, because they are monosyllables and thus contain a minimum of auditory clues. As was suggested with spondee words, lists should be kept of the PB words that are consistently missed by the patient, and they can serve also for drill. Because of the difficulty of the words in the phonetically balanced lists, it cannot be expected that the patient will be able to understand 100 percent of them, no matter how extensive the training. In other words, an individual who has a loss for the higher speech frequencies is bound to make some mistakes on the PB word lists, and it is advisable not to set too high standards of performance for the patient on these words. Other tests for speech discrimination described in Chapter 6, such as the Rhyme Test, the Modified Rhyme Test, and the CNC word lists, are useful for auditory training.

From single words, the therapist should progress to sentences and paragraphs. Davis and Silverman reproduce several sentence tests that have been used at various times for testing intelligibility.[2] In one test, prepared at

---

[1] J. C. Kelly, *Clinician's Handbook for Auditory Training* (Dubuque, Iowa: Wm. C. Brown, 1953).

[2] Hallowell Davis and S. Richard Silverman, eds., *Hearing and Deafness,* 4th ed. (New York: Holt, Rinehart and Winston, 1978), pp. 534–38.

the Harvard Psycho-Acoustic Laboratory, each sentence contains five key words. The patient is asked to repeat the sentence or to write it down. Each of the five key words must be heard correctly for the sentence to be scored correct. An example of the sentences is the following one, in which the key words are italicized: "The *birch canoe slid* on the *smooth planks*." The sentences may be repeated a number of times for the sake of practice, but once the patient becomes familiar with them they lose their value for auditory training.

The therapist may prepare paragraphs that deal with simple subjects such as "how to sew on a button." For each paragraph, a number of questions should be prepared that test the patient's ability to follow the running-speech material. The therapist can also adapt for auditory training the materials that are suitable for speechreading practice. Although it is frequently necessary to spend time drilling on words in auditory training, the object should be to increase the patient's ability to understand running speech.

One of the objectives of an auditory training program for adults may be to increase the patient's tolerance for speech of high intensity. In conditions of sensori-neural loss characterized by recruitment, there may be such a narrow range between the threshold of speech reception and the threshold of discomfort that a hearing aid is contraindicated. With training, it is possible to increase the patient's tolerance level and thus make a hearing aid feasible. Such training requires equipment with amplification that can be carefully controlled, such as an auditory training unit. Recorded speech materials are possible, with the auditory training unit set at a volume level that corresponds with the patient's present ability to tolerate intense speech. The person is permitted to increase the volume and to discontinue the listening whenever the process becomes unbearably annoying. With many patients, very little practice in listening to intense speech enables them to accept more amplification. With some patients, a low tolerance level is the result of living for years without hearing very intense speech. In the beginning, they are unable to tolerate amplification because having gradually become accustomed to their defective hearing, they are disturbed at hearing speech loudly again. As they become more familiar with amplified speech, they are gradually able to accept higher and higher levels of amplification. The only purpose of training to increase the usable range of hearing for speech is to enable the patient to benefit from a hearing aid.

HEARING-AID ORIENTATION

Even the patient who does not require auditory training will frequently benefit from a program of instruction after being fitted with a hearing aid. Hearing-aid orientation consists both of instruction in the mechanics of operating the instrument and psychological strengthening of the individual's resolve. A large proportion of hearing aids sold directly to patients without preparation or orientation end up in the proverbial dresser drawer. The military aural rehabilitation programs demonstrated that with proper selection procedures and a period of orientation, patients fitted with hearing aids would continue to wear them. Therefore, it is certainly worth a few dollars of the patient's money and a few hours to effectively master an aid.

Before an aid is purchased, the patient should be made to realize that any hearing aid has limitations. Too many patients expect that the hearing aid will be the answer to all their hearing problems and that once they start wearing the aid they will be able to hear just as well as they did when their hearing was normal. Unfortunately, this is not true. As we have seen in Chapter 10, a hearing aid is an amplifier system, and not a very high-fidelity one. The patient who has speech-discrimination problems, as demonstrated by poor scores on the discrimination tests in speech audiometry, may still have discrimination problems with the hearing aid. However, if the patient needs amplification in order to hear speech, the hearing aid will be of assistance. Therefore, the first step in a hearing-aid orientation program is to discuss with the patient the limitations related to the hearing loss and the limitations of the benefit that can be expected from the hearing aid.

Most patients will be disappointed with the comparatively poor quality of the speech reproduction that they receive with the hearing aid. If the patient is told what can be expected in the way of quality of reproduction, the person is prepared for the ensuing disappointment. It should be pointed out to the patient, however, that the quality of reproduction of the hearing aid is sufficient to cover the principal speech frequencies, so that with the aid it will be possible to understand speech even though it may not sound natural. We are all accustomed to the limited frequency response of the telephone and the way in which it distorts voice quality. Yet with the telephone we are able to achieve extensive comprehension, and excellent communication is possible. The hearing-impaired individual can learn to communicate successfully with the limited frequency response and distortion of the hearing aid also.

The patient must be told that it will take time to become accustomed to hearing with the aid, and that for the first several days, or even several weeks, there may be discouraging experiences. In the beginning, the patient should not attempt to wear the aid throughout the day but should start by wearing it only a few minutes at a time. Each day, the time can be increased as the individual becomes used to the amplification received. The goal eventually, of course, is for the patient to reach the point of wearing the aid throughout the day, just as the person would wear spectacles if vision were impaired. Some adults find it difficult to adjust to bifocals or to false teeth. A hearing aid is a prosthetic device also, and it requires time to become used to wearing it. When an individual has gone for a number of years without hearing normally, the sudden introduction of amplification can be a startling experience.

A common complaint of hearing-aid users is the amount of noise that the aid delivers to the ear. The noise may be from two sources: the environment of the individual, and then it is heard by everyone else as well; or the instrument itself, for example, in the case of a body-worn aid, from the movement of clothing across the microphone grill. Patients must learn to accept the noise, whether it is external or internal in nature, and to ignore it while concentrating on what they want to hear. Those of us who have normal hearing must go through this process of selecting what we want to hear from the surrounding noise, which is undesirable but which we have to tolerate. The person with a long-standing hearing loss may have forgotten that our environment is so noisy, and it will take time to adjust to background noises.

The new hearing-aid user must not expect to obtain good results with an aid in difficult listening situations. Examples of difficult situations are a play, a lecture, a church service, a meeting in which many people are speaking at a distance from the listener, and conversation outdoors in loud traffic noises. Generally, a situation that is difficult for people with normal hearing will be one in which a hard-of-hearing patient will have special difficulty in using the aid to good effect. A play on the legitimate stage is an extremely difficult listening situation, because of the fact that a number of people with unfamiliar voices are speaking rapidly and perhaps not too carefully, and the listener is seated in an auditorium filled with people coughing, moving their feet, rustling their programs, and otherwise making noise that tends to mask out the words of the actors. At the movies, the listener's problem is further complicated by the presence of people who enjoy eating popcorn and other "noisy" food. The individual with a hearing aid in any of these circumstances may be getting excellent reception of the sounds that are close by, that is, the noises made by members of the audience, and will have considerable difficulty "tuning in" the dialogue on the stage or the screen. What the hearing-aid user frequently does not realize is that in these difficult listening situations the person with normal hearing also may be missing a considerable amount of what is said. It is not advisable for the hearing-aid wearer to attempt to use the aid in difficult listening situations until becoming thoroughly accustomed to it in easier situations. In any event, the individual should be warned that the results in these situations are likely to be very disappointing. The reason that the aid should not be worn out of doors at the outset is that loud traffic noises will cause extreme annoyance and may discourage further attempts with the aid. Again, once the person has learned to make effective use of the aid indoors and in easy listening situations, the aid then can be worn outdoors. The easiest situations are those in which there is a minimum of background noise and a limited number of speakers. Thus, even the beginning hearing-aid user should be successful with the aid at home with family members.

An important part of the hearing-aid orientation program is to teach the patient how to wear the aid most effectively and how to take proper care of it. Some patients will accept the hearing aid only if they can effectively conceal it. Some are able to conceal hearing aids effectively by employing appropriate hair styling. The therapist must understand the problems of adjustment faced by the patient when first wearing a hearing aid and be patient and sympathetic. It is to be hoped, however, that as the patient becomes adjusted to the idea of wearing the aid, the person will accept the wearing of it in the most efficient manner. The therapist has the responsibility at least to inform the patient how to obtain the best possible service from the aid.

Adult patients frequently are timid about turning the amplification to the degree desirable. Some patients constantly adjust the volume control, turning it up when they cannot hear well and down if someone speaks a bit too loudly. It is difficult for a patient to benefit from the hearing aid when constantly fiddling with the controls. The therapist should encourage the patient, therefore, to select a volume-control setting that is adequate and to leave the control at that setting regardless of changes in the levels of voices. People with normal hearing must adjust to varying levels of loudness, and the person with a hearing aid can learn to do the same. The patient should learn to insert and remove the earpiece with facility and also how to change the battery in the instrument. The person should be instructed to carry extra batteries at all times, so that in the event of a battery failure the aid is not put out of commission.

A part of the hearing-aid orientation program should be instructing the patient how to locate the source of difficulty when the aid is not functioning properly. The commonest cause of difficulty is a dead battery. Unless the aid has been dropped, it is not likely that it will develop faults. Sometimes the canal piece of the ear insert becomes clogged with wax, which of course interferes with the transmission of sound from the receiver to the ear. The patient should be instructed to keep the earpiece clean by washing it in soap and water and by running a pipe cleaner through the hole at frequent intervals.

The patient needs instruction in manipulating the aid with the telephone. If the aid has a telephone circuit, the individual can be shown how to operate the switch and how to hold the telephone next to the aid. Patients sometimes complain that their hearing aids are not functioning correctly, when the difficulty proves to be that the microphone has been switched off and the telephone circuit switched on. Patients should be reminded, therefore, that after a telephone conversation they must return the switch on the aid to the microphone position. When no telephone circuit is contained in the aid, the patient may still use it with the telephone by placing the receiver next to the microphone of the hearing aid. It is sometimes difficult for hearing-aid users to realize that their "ear" is the microphone of the hearing aid. Some patients who wear hearing aids are able to hear over the telephone successfully with the unaided ear. For people who prefer to use the telephone without their hearing aid, the telephone company has available a special phone with a built-in amplifier that can be adjusted for intensity. Also, amplifiers are available on the market that clamp onto the receiver of the telephone. The hard-of-hearing person can carry this kind of amplifier and have it ready for a conversation over any telephone.

The patient who has had the limitations of the hearing loss explained and demonstrated, who has been guided through a series of graded experiences with the hearing aid, and who has thoroughly learned the mechanics of operating it is in a position to become a good hearing-aid user. The first few weeks with it are the difficult ones. Assistance in the form of hearing-aid orientation at this point can be of untold benefit to the patient in a lifelong "career" as a hearing-aid user.

SPEECH TRAINING

The adult who has a mild-to-moderate hearing loss, who has no problems of speech discrimination, and who can derive benefit from a hearing aid will probably have no observable speech symptoms of hearing impairment. On the other hand, the individual who has a severe, profound, or extreme degree of hearing loss and who does have speech-discrimination problems will usually demonstrate through voice quality and articulation the effects of the hearing impairment. Because the quality of our speech depends largely on auditory monitoring, our speech production may deteriorate if our auditory monitoring becomes faulty. A hearing aid assists in the monitoring process, particularly in helping the individual to achieve proper voice control, but when there is a severe, profound, or extreme loss, even a hearing aid cannot wholly prevent some deterioration of speech. The therapist must keep in mind, therefore, that in addition to whatever speechreading instruction and auditory training the individual needs, some work on speech will frequently be indicated.

In the military aural rehabilitation centers of World War II, one of the rehabilitative services provided was termed *speech conservation,* as has been previously mentioned. Here, hearing-impaired service personnel were made aware of the danger that their speech might deteriorate because of the hearing loss and were taught techniques that, it was hoped, would prevent serious speech deterioration. In other words, the work in speech conservation was a kind of "insurance" for the future. Speech conservation, as it was taught in the military centers, is probably not a practical procedure for a civilian population. Although the hard-of-hearing adult may be convinced of a need for speechreading and training with a hearing aid, it is difficult to persuade the person that time and money should be spent working on speech when currently no speech problems exist.

The effects of a profound or extreme loss are usually reflected in the patient's lack of proper voice control and in a general "mushiness" of articulation. The voice-control problem consists of an inability to judge the proper intensity of voice needed in a given speaking situation. The commonest example of the effect of a hearing loss on the voice is the hard-of-hearing individual who shouts. It was explained in Chapter 3 that the hard-of-hearing person who shouts or speaks too loudly is probably evidencing one symptom of a sensorineural hearing loss. If the hearing loss is of long duration and is profound or extreme, vocal quality will be affected. The voice will lose its vitality and tend to develop a "deadness" of quality, such as we find in the congenitally deaf individual. In an adult with this marked an impairment of long duration, monotony of pitch will probably also be present. The first sounds to deteriorate are those that require the most delicate adjustment of the articulators and the greatest amount of auditory monitoring. As with the child, referred to in the preceding chapter, these sounds include most prominently the *s, r, l, sh,* and *ch* consonants.

The correction of the voice and of articulation disorders, which the adult demonstrates as a result of hearing impairment, is based on principles discussed in the preceding chapter dealing with hearing-impaired children. The therapist can teach the adult patient to control voice intensity by being conscious of the muscle tensions in the larynx. Carhart suggests that the individual learn to speak at each of four to five levels of intensity, judging by the kinesthetic sensations in the larynx. The individual will then have to judge by the reactions of other people whether or not the proper level of laryngeal tension meets the needs of the situation.[3] Difficulties of inflections can be handled in the same manner as was suggested for children in the preceding chapter. The correction of articulatory difficulties is based on an analysis for the patient of the way in which faulty sounds can be corrected, relying on knowledge of phonetic placement and learning to utilize kinesthetic sensations. Sometimes, the patient's attention can be focused on correct articulation by means of an auditory training unit. As mentioned previously, the hard-of-hearing adult's hearing aid also will be of benefit in regulating speech and voice usage.

For the most part, instruction in speech should be integrated with instruction in speechreading and the auditory training program. The therapist must be alert to seize every opportunity to correct speech difficulties in the patient as they occur.

COUNSELING

In Chapter 10, the psychological problems of the hard-of-hearing individual were discussed, and the need for counseling the patient was stressed. There is little that can be added here to what has already been covered in Chapter 10, except to emphasize again the fundamental principle that the hearing-impaired individual must be willing to accept and admit the handicap before profit can be realized from the rehabilitative procedures discussed.

The hard-of-hearing adult who presents the greatest challenge to the

[3] Raymond Carhart, "Development and Conservation of Speech," in *Hearing and Deafness*, 3rd ed., eds. Hallowell Davis and S. Richard Silverman (New York: Holt, Rinehart and Winston, 1970), chap. 14, p. 370.

therapist is the person with a typical sensori-neural impairment, who has such good hearing in the low frequencies that even a CROS-type hearing aid may not be utilized successfully, but whose hearing for the higher speech frequencies is so impaired that severe speech-discrimination problems exist. This is the person who says, "I can hear you, but I don't understand what you are saying." The individual can usually benefit little from auditory training but will have to rely primarily on speechreading. This individual, for whom so little can be done in the way of compensating for hearing impairment, may be bitter toward the therapist and the otologist, who are relatively powerless to help. The person observes other hard-of-hearing people deriving satisfactory results from hearing aids and resents the inability to secure similar assistance. Because the person does not wear a hearing aid, there is no outward sign of being handicapped, and so other people do not realize that they must take special pains in speaking.

The therapist can only hope that such a patient will eventually arrive at an acceptance of the disability and a thankfulness that at least some hearing exists. The only salvation for this type of individual is to admit freely to all that hearing is faulty. It is necessary to develop a "thick skin" and to take the initiative by telling other people how they can most effectively communicate.

As was mentioned in Chapter 10, there is a tendency for the hard-of-hearing adult to become withdrawn and psychologically depressed. The therapist must make every effort through counseling the patient and, if necessary, through counseling the patient's family, to keep the person from withdrawing from social contacts. Somehow, the individual must be brought to the realization that although hearing loss is an inconvenience, it is not a tragedy. The person is the same individual as before the hearing problem developed, and there is no need to abandon former activities and interests because of the change in hearing ability. Some adjustments may be necessary in vocational and avocational pursuits, but they are usually of a minor character and need cause no great concern. Patients who have major problems of psychological adjustment should be referred for psychiatric or psychological guidance, and those who are faced with difficult vocational problems should be directed to a vocational counselor.

It is helpful to individuals who become handicapped to be reminded of others who were able to surmount their handicaps and live happy and useful lives. There are several inspiring autobiographies to which the hearing-handicapped person can be referred.[4] The best cure for persons who feel sorry for themselves is to realize that others even more severely handicapped have succeeded in spite of their handicaps. The supreme example, of course, is the late Helen Keller, who was able to rise above the double handicap of deafness and blindness.

[4] Examples of such autobiographies are Marie Hays Heiner, *Hearing Is Believing* (Cleveland: World, 1949); Frances Warfield, *Cotton in My Ears* (New York: Viking, 1948); and George W. Frankel, *Let's Hear It!* (New York: Stratford House, 1952).

REFERENCES

ALPINER, JEROME G., ed. *Handbook of Adult Rehabilitative Audiology,* 2nd ed. Baltimore: Williams & Wilkins, 1982.

BERGER, KENNETH W. *Speechreading Principles and Methods.* Baltimore: National Educational Press, 1972.

BROBERG, ROSE FEILBACH. *Over-Fifty Nifties.* Washington, D.C.: The Alexander Graham Bell Association for the Deaf, 1975.

FISHER, MAE. *Lipreading for a More Active Life.* Washington, D.C.: The Alexander Graham Bell Association for the Deaf, 1977.

HENOCH, MIRIAM A. *Aural Rehabilitation for the Elderly.* New York: Grune & Stratton, 1979.

HULL, RAYMOND H. *Rehabilitative Audiology.* New York: Grune & Stratton, 1982.

JEFFERS, JANET, and BARLEY, MARGARET. *Speech Reading.* Springfield, Ill.: Charles C Thomas, 1971.

O'NEILL, JOHN J. *The Hard of Hearing.* Englewood Cliffs, N.J.: Prentice-Hall, 1964.

O'NEILL, JOHN J., and OYER, HERBERT J. *Visual Communication for the Hard of Hearing,* 2nd ed. Englewood Cliffs, N.J.: Prentice-Hall, 1981.

ORDMAN, KATHRYN A., and RALLI, MARY P. *What People Say,* 5th ed. Washington, D.C.: The Alexander Graham Bell Association for the Deaf, 1976.

OYER, HERBERT J. *Auditory Communication for the Hard of Hearing.* Englewood Cliffs, N.J.: Prentice-Hall, 1961.

OYER, HERBERT J., and FRANKMANN, JUDITH P. *The Aural Rehabilitation Process.* New York: Holt, Rinehart and Winston, 1975.

SANDERS, DEREK A. *Aural Rehabilitation,* 2nd ed. Englewood Cliffs, N.J.: Prentice-Hall, 1982.

SCHOW, RONALD L., and CHRISTENSEN, JOHN M. *Communication Disorders of the Aged: A Guide for Health Professionals.* Baltimore: University Park Press, 1978.

SCHOW, RONALD L., and NERBONNE, MICHAEL A., eds. *Introduction to Aural Rehabilitation.* Baltimore: University Park Press, 1980.

SMITH, CLARISSA R., and KARP, ADRIENNE, eds. *A Workbook in Auditory Training for Adults: With a Special Section on the Institutionalized Geriatric Patient.* Springfield, Ill.: Charles C Thomas, 1978.

URBANTSCHITSCH, VICTOR. *Auditory Training for Deaf Mutism and Acquired Deafness.* Translated by S. Richard Silverman from the original German text of 1895. Washington, D.C.: The Alexander Graham Bell Association for the Deaf, 1982.

YANICK, PAUL. *Rehabilitation Strategies for Sensorineural Hearing Loss.* New York: Grune & Stratton, 1979.

CHAPTER THIRTEEN
THE PROFESSION
OF AUDIOLOGY

The previous chapters have been designed to give the reader some acquaintance with the subject matter of the field of audiology. One purpose of this book is to interest students in audiology as a profession. This final chapter, therefore, will be concerned with professional opportunities in audiology and the preparation necessary to become a professional worker in the field. Because the development of the profession of audiology has been closely related to the evolution of professional service programs, and because many of the employment opportunities in audiology are in centers of various sorts, the first section of this chapter will deal with service programs.

THE PROFESSIONAL SERVICE PROGRAM

There are at present approximately 800 professional service programs in the United States.[1] These are variously sponsored and offer a variety of services, but basically their purpose is the same: to provide diagnostic and rehabilitative services for individuals with speech and hearing impairments. The term *hearing center*, as it appears in this chapter, refers to any professional

[1] A *Guide to Professional Services in Speech-Language Pathology and Audiology* (Rockville, MD.: The American Speech-Language-Hearing Association, 1983).

agency, regardless of its name, which offers diagnostic and rehabilitative services to the hearing impaired.

History of the Hearing Center

As indicated in Chapter 1, historically audiology is the progeny of two parents: otology and speech pathology. The two were united in the aural rehabilitation centers of World War II, which were established by the medical departments of the armed forces to provide the medical and rehabilitative services required by servicemen and -women who incurred hearing impairment. The Army established three such centers: Borden General Hospital at Chickasha, Oklahoma; Hoff General Hospital at Santa Barbara, California; and Deshon General Hospital at Butler, Pennsylvania. The Navy established an aural rehabilitation center at the Naval Hospital in Philadelphia. By the end of World War II, all these centers had proved their tremendous value in rehabilitating hard-of-hearing service personnel.

To establish the services necessary to operate an effective program of rehabilitation for the hard of hearing, the military sought help from college and university speech clinics, teachers of lipreading, teachers of the deaf, and psychologists. Because the aural rehabilitation programs were the responsibility of medical departments, they were put under the command of physicians—ear, nose, and throat specialists. The medical and nonmedical specialists together planned a program that would meet the needs of aural casualties. Naturally, the first responsibility of the aural rehabilitation center was to determine whether a given casualty would benefit from medical or surgical care. In evaluating the type and degree of hearing loss that a patient presented, a thorough audiometric examination was required. Some specialists in speech became classified as *acoustic physicists*, charged with the responsibility of developing and administering adequate tests of the hearing function. Today, such specialists would be referred to as *audiologists*. Patients who could not be helped by medicine or whose hearing loss was of a permanent, nonreversible nature, were placed in the rehabilitation program, which included determination of the need for and selection of an individual hearing aid; speechreading, auditory training, and speech training as needed; and psychological and vocational counseling.

The military aural rehabilitation centers were so successful in returning hearing-handicapped service personnel to duty or to civilian life with a minimum of handicap, that all who were concerned with these wartime programs were impressed with their effectiveness. Thus, when the war was over and the various specialists returned to civilian life, many were of the opinion that similar aural rehabilitation programs should be organized for the civilian population. It was primarily the otologists who were responsible for initiating action in their own communities to establish programs for the hearing handicapped. However, although the otologists were the "spark plugs" of the new activities, they did not have the time nor the desire to perform all the services required. Thus, otologists turned for help to the group of specialists who had developed the audiometric techniques and rehabilitative services in war-time—primarily specialists in speech—to administer and perform the clinical work in the newly established civilian centers. Since the war, otologists have assumed more of an advisory than a directive role in the development of hearing centers. To the otologist, however, belongs the credit for the initial interest that prompted the establishment of the first postwar civilian centers.

One of the outstanding contributions of the military aural rehabilitation center was the development of procedures to determine whether or not a patient needed a hearing aid and, if so, to select the hearing aid. An integral part of the hearing-aid selection was training with the aid that the patient received. The military programs established an enviable record in the percentage of hearing aids used by patients who were provided with them. Previous to World War II, studies had revealed that as many as 50 to 60 percent of the hard-of-hearing individuals with hearing aids did not use them after the first week or two. The studies of graduates of the military aural rehabilitation programs revealed that as high as 94 percent of the individuals receiving hearing aids continued to use them several months after their discharge from the center.[2] The civilian hearing centers that began to spring up after the war were usually created primarily for the purpose of bringing systematic hearing-aid selection services to the civilian population. In addition, other services were offered as required, but the major emphasis was on hearing-aid selection. Many civilian centers attempted to establish training programs similar to those that had been in effect during the war. The civilian centers soon discovered, however, that most civilians were not willing to devote several weeks to a training course, and being civilians, they could not be ordered to do so. Thus, the transfer of aural rehabilitation procedures from a military to a civilian setting required many adjustments.

A word of credit should be given here to the Veterans Administration for helping to develop the concept of the civilian hearing center. Immediately after the war, there were thousands of veterans with service-connected hearing impairments who required services of the sort that had been available to them in wartime. Also, of course, veterans of previous wars needed help with hearing problems. The V.A. met the various needs by establishing audiology clinics in some regional offices and veterans hospitals and by contracting for these services elsewhere with college and university speech clinics and with other types of hearing centers. At present, there are relatively few "contract clinics" because the V.A. has greatly expanded its own audiology and speech pathology program. The earlier necessity for handling hearing-handicapped veterans on a contractual basis, however, served as a tremendous impetus to colleges and universities to develop training programs and clinical services in

---

[2] Eris L. Adams, "Adjustment of the Hard of Hearing After Leaving the Service," *Supplement to United States Naval Medical Bulletin* (U.S. Navy Bureau of Medicine and Surgery, March 1946), p. 249.

the field of audiology. Also, the V.A. contracts lightened the burden of financial support for many community hearing centers. Anderman[3] and Newby[4] have described the details of the V.A. audiology program.

Types of Professional Service Programs

Professional service programs are of many types as far as sponsorship and organizational structures are concerned. In point of number, centers sponsored by colleges and universities account for a large percentage. For the most part, colleges and universities merely added aural rehabilitation services to an already existing speech clinic. Before World War II, college speech clinics had been concerned primarily with the speech problems of children and adults, including such disorders as stuttering, aphasia, cleft-palate speech, vocal problems, and articulatory difficulties. Some speech problems handled by the clinic were related to hearing disorders, but the speech clinic, as it existed in prewar days, as a general rule did not offer any services for the hard-of-hearing individual except speech training.

It is interesting to note the influence of center activities on college and university programs. Until 1947, most clinic programs in connection with the training of students in speech pathology were called "speech" clinics. In 1947, the American Speech Correction Association changed its name to the American Speech and Hearing Association and the name of its official publication from the *Journal of Speech Disorders* to the *Journal of Speech and Hearing Disorders*. Concurrently, in colleges and universities around the country, there was a movement to change the name *speech clinic* to *speech and hearing clinic*. By 1950, training programs in audiology were in existence in almost all the colleges and universities where any previous training in the field of speech correction had been offered. Thus, five years after the termination of the war, the importance of audiology as a related but separate discipline from speech correction had been recognized.

The primary purpose of the college- or university-sponsored hearing center is to provide a laboratory in which students of audiology may observe and obtain experience in handling patients. Just as the medical student must learn to diagnose and treat illnesses in patients by obtaining supervised experience in medical clinics, so the embryo audiologist must also "learn by doing." Service to the public is therefore only incidental to the training purpose of the college- or university-sponsored center.

---

[3] Bernard M. Anderman, "The Veterans Administration Audiology Program," in *Hearing and Deafness*, 3rd ed., eds. Hallowell Davis and S. Richard Silverman (New York: Holt, Rinehart and Winston, 1970), chap. 19, pp. 449–56.

[4] Hayes A. Newby, "Veterans Administration," in *Hearing and Hearing Impairment*, eds. Larry J. Bradford and William G. Hardy (New York: Grune & Stratton, 1979), chap. 49, pp. 621–29.

A second type of center is one that operates as part of a hospital or rehabilitation center and serves only the patients referred by physicians connected with that institution. Generally, the audiology program in a hospital is associated with a department of otolaryngology, whereas in a rehabilitation center it may be part of a department of physical medicine. In either event, this kind of center provides a specialized service to only a limited number of physicians and their patients.

In contrast to the two types of centers just discussed, there are activities that we shall designate as "community" hearing centers because they serve the entire community and not just a segment of the hard-of-hearing population. In the community hearing center, the emphasis is on providing professional services to all who need them, provided that they are properly referred through medical channels. Some community hearing centers are affiliated with local chapters of the National Association of Hearing and Speech Action (NAHSA), formerly the American Hearing Society, and some were created as separate, nonprofit, privately sponsored agencies. Most community hearing centers, whether or not they are affiliated with NAHSA or a local hearing society, receive some aid from the community chest or united fund, although they also require a considerable amount of private underwriting. Most such centers also depend somewhat on fees collected from patients. For community hearing centers to be successful in securing the support needed to continue in existence, they must prove themselves through the high quality of professional services that they offer the community.

A fourth type of hearing center is the government-sponsored one, which provides audiological services for personnel of the armed forces and for veterans. The Army maintains audiological services in a number of hospitals in this country and abroad. The Air Force and the Navy have their own audiological facilities, although they are more limited than the Army in number of locations. The Veterans Administration audiology and speech pathology services or clinics are geographically distributed throughout the country. These clinics, together with other hearing centers with which the Veterans Administration contracts, serve the needs of approximately 100,000 veterans who are service-connected for hearing loss and/or otological disease. The Veterans Administration clinics provide hearing aids to eligible veterans and are responsible for conducting the examinations on which compensation for service-connected hearing disabilities is based.

The four types of centers account for the vast majority of clinical audiology programs that are in existence today. There are some miscellaneous programs, however, that do not fit into these categories. For example, a hearing center may be sponsored by a religious organization, by the Junior League or other service organization, or by a school for the deaf. Also, in some cities there are so-called hearing centers that are actually the activities of a single audiologist in private practice.

Services of the Hearing Center

As stated, initially the most important service offered by a hearing center was hearing-aid selection. This service is one that is still fairly universally offered by hearing centers, regardless of their type or sponsorship. With so many makes and models of hearing aids commercially available at a wide range of prices, the hard-of-hearing person in need of a hearing aid is bewildered about how to make a choice. Objective consideration of the problem is required, which the average hearing-aid dealer is not equipped to give. The hearing center is the place where the patient can obtain an objective approach.

The services of a hearing center may generally be divided into two main classifications: diagnostic services and rehabilitative or training services. Under the first classification are such services as diagnostic audiometry, pre- and postoperative audiometry, and hearing-aid selection. *Diagnostic audiometry* refers to the measurement of a patient's hearing and an analysis of the hearing problems to assist the otologist toward a proper diagnosis. Diagnostic audiometry with young children has assumed increasing importance as techniques have been developed to make hearing measurements with very young patients more valid and reliable. With very young children, it is important to discover the hearing impairment at the earliest possible time so that medical attention can be given to the disability and adequate training procedures can be initiated. Evoked response, immittance, and acoustic reflex measurements are important parts of the identification and diagnostic process. The sooner the training of the hard-of-hearing child starts, the better is the prognosis. Thus, diagnostic audiometry with children is a particularly valuable service of the hearing center. Included under this heading also is the differentiation of hearing problems from other types of auditory disorders. Children who do not develop an understanding of oral language or an ability to speak are frequently classified as deaf, when in fact their ability to respond to pure-tone test stimuli may be perfectly normal. The differentiation of hearing impairment from other types of disorders, such as brain injury, mental retardation, and emotional difficulty, is important in order to discover with what problem or problems the physician and therapist are dealing and to permit the planning of an adequate medical and rehabilitation program.

With adults, diagnostic audiometry is concerned with establishing a hearing loss as being organic or functional and in determining the relation between air conduction and bone conduction as an indication of whether the loss is conductive or sensori-neural in nature. As with children, tympanometry and acoustic reflex measurements are important tools in the diagnostic process. If surgery on the middle ear is contemplated, it is important to the otologist to have an accurate assessment of the patient's cochlear reserve. The determination of the site of lesion is an important part of diagnostic audiometry. Hearing centers in medical settings may provide electronystagmography (ENG) measurements in addition to audiometric, evoked response, and immittance data.

The remaining activity—the selection of hearing aids—was discussed in Chapter 10. When the civilian hearing centers were first established, this activity was almost their sole *raison d'être*. In the early postwar days, however, hearing aids were crude and somewhat unreliable. Differences from aid to aid could easily be demonstrated in test situations. However, as hearing aids became more refined and their parts standardized, it became harder to establish differences on this basis. Although some hearing centers still test a patient with six to eight different aids and then recommend which aid to purchase from a dealer, today many centers offer a more general type of hearing-aid selection. Some centers have changed the name of their service from *hearing-aid selection* to *hearing-aid evaluation*, in line with their deemphasis of comparative tests.

The selection of hearing aids continues to be an important service in government-sponsored audiology clinics. At these clinics, the patient who needs a hearing aid is provided with the particular aid with which performance was best in the test. Furnishing the patient with a hearing aid is part of the responsibility that the government assumes for those who are eligible for the services of a military or Veterans Administration audiology clinic. Because so many thousands of patients are involved in these government programs, it is economically more advantageous to the government, and of course eventually to the taxpayer, to contract for hearing aids on a large-lot basis, and to assume the responsibility for dispensing them, than to send each patient to a hearing-aid dealer for an aid of the recommended type. Moreover, with this method, the patient is assured that the instrument selected is the very one with which performance was best. In spite of quality-control measures applied by hearing-aid manufacturers, no hearing aid is exactly like every other aid of the same make and model. Unfortunately (for the patient), it is not possible for most non-government-sponsored hearing centers to make hearing-aid selections in this manner, and so their hearing-aid "consultations" are of necessity "watered-down" varieties. As mentioned in Chapter 10, however, there is a growing tendency for hearing centers to become involved in dispensing hearing aids. In such centers, a patient may be provided with the instrument actually used in the evaluations, as in the government-sponsored clinics.

The rehabilitation services offered by hearing centers usually include the following: group and individual instruction in speechreading, auditory training, speech training, and hearing-aid orientation. In addition, some centers provide special training programs for preschool-age deaf and hard-of-hearing children and their parents. These rehabilitative services have been discussed elsewhere in this book and need no further elaboration here.

Accreditation of Hearing Centers

In 1959, the American Speech and Hearing Association established the American Boards of Examiners in Speech Pathology and Audiology. Since 1980 this group has been called the Council on Professional Standards in

Speech-Language Pathology and Audiology. One of the constituent boards of this organization is the Professional Services Board, which is charged with the responsibility for processing applications regarding the accreditation of those clinical services that have applied. When a clinical service activity is approved, a certificate of approval is issued, and the name of the activity is added to a registry of approved clinical services that is published regularly. A clinical activity may be approved for services in audiology, in speech pathology, or in both areas. A clinical activity must meet high standards in regard to personnel, equipment, organizational structure, range of services, and relations with other agencies and professional personnel in order for approval by the Professional Services Board. Thus, the public and referring physicians and agencies can be assured that they are receiving the best clinical services when they make use of a hearing center that has been so approved.

EMPLOYMENT OPPORTUNITIES FOR AUDIOLOGISTS

As long as there is a demand for trained audiologists, there will be a need for college and university teachers of audiology, and so the field of higher education provides one very important employment opportunity for audiologists. For practical purposes, the doctoral degree is an essential requirement for the audiologist who has academic aspirations. University teaching in the field of audiology is far from being an "ivory-tower" type of existence, however. Audiology can be learned only through a combination of work with patients and academics. Therefore a necessary part of the university training program in audiology consists of clinical practicum. The audiologist in charge of a training program thus becomes a clinic supervisor and administrator while performing a considerable amount of clinical work. The university teacher of audiology must of necessity keep up with new developments in all aspects of the field and ideally should participate to some extent in research. Certainly one of the duties, if involved in a graduate training program, is that of directing the research of students and reading and criticizing theses and dissertations. Thus, a teacher of audiology at the university level will undoubtedly have as busy a day and as fully occupied a work year as any other professional person. The audiologist-teacher receives all the satisfactions of any teacher in vicariously experiencing the professional successes of the students. In addition, of course, the teacher of audiology has ample opportunity for reaping the pleasure of working with patients.

The increasing popularity of the community hearing center presents a stimulating professional challenge to the audiologist who is more interested in clinical work than in teaching. Because most such hearing centers are directed by professional audiologists, they offer the added opportunity of administrative experience. The director of a community hearing center must combine the talents of a successful clinician with the abilities of a public relations expert, a personnel counselor, and a fund raiser. Clinical workers in the community hearing center should have a master's degree in audiology.

Government positions represent another opportunity for professional employment. The Veterans Administration employs many audiologists as clinicians and administrators in its audiology and speech pathology clinics throughout the country. A master's degree is required for employment as a staff audiologist, and directors (chiefs) of V.A. clinics must have doctorates. Civil service appointments in the military audiology clinics compare to the V.A. positions. Individuals with a master's degree and at least the academic requirements for clinical certification in audiology from the American Speech and Hearing Association (as described in the following section) are eligible for commissions in the Medical Service Corps of the Army and the Biomedical Science Corps of the Air Force.[5] As of now, there are no provisions for commissions in the Navy for audiologists. Opportunities for enlisted personnel with some training in audiology exist in all three branches of the armed forces.

Another employment possibility for the audiologist is in a hospital or medical school. Such positions usually constitute appointments in a department of otolaryngology, and the audiologist works closely with ear, nose, and throat physicians. Generally, the qualifications for such a position would be a master's degree in audiology.

At the present time, there is a growth of rehabilitation centers, which consist of various medical and allied medical specialists working as a team. Because a communication disorder represents a handicapping impairment, most rehabilitation centers must deal with problems of speech and hearing. In the setting of a rehabilitation center, the person in charge of the audiology program should have a master's degree.

Public-school work in speech and hearing represents perhaps the area of greatest personnel need. In addition to employment opportunities as audiometrists, public schools need speech and hearing therapists or teachers of special classes for hearing-handicapped children. Because the schools have accepted the responsibility for the "whole" education of their pupils, they must attempt to meet the needs of those who are handicapped in hearing. In most public schools, a credential issued by the state department of education, or for audiometrists, a certificate from the state department of health, is a requirement for employment.

As yet, few opportunities exist for the audiologist in industry, although some companies concerned with the manufacture of hearing aids and audiometers have begun to attract audiologists. It is conceivable that at some time in the future all hearing aids will be dispensed by individuals who have been professionally trained in audiology. At present, hearing-aid dealers are usually not required to have any formal academic training in audiology, and as

[5] Jerry L. Northern and James E. Endicott, "Military Opportunities in Speech Pathology and Audiology," *Asha* 10 (August 1968):325–30.

a result many dealers are merely salespeople, without knowledge of the special problems of the hard-of-hearing people with whom they are dealing.

Another industrial opportunity for audiologists lies in organizing and directing hearing-conservation programs in noisy industries. As our civilization becomes a noisier one, both employers and employees are becoming aware of the hazards to hearing from noise exposure. Claims for noise-induced hearing impairment are becoming more and more common, and insurance carriers and employers alike are alarmed at their increasing frequency. As we saw in Chapter 9, one of the requirements of an industrial hearing-conservation program is that employees be given regular audiometric tests for the purpose of (1) detecting the presence of any hearing loss as soon as it occurs, and (2) preventing further loss of hearing by proper placement of employees within an industry. At present, most routine testing in industries is conducted by nurses under the supervision of the medical director of the company. Hearing-conservation programs in large factories, however, generally require more specialized supervision than the average company physician can provide. It is possible, therefore, that we shall see "industrial audiologists" performing these services in the near future. In any event, the field of industrial audiology presents opportunities for consultation by professionally qualified audiologists, if not full-time employment.

Audiologists are now employed as full-time consultants in departments of health and education in state governments. In these positions, it is the responsibility of the audiologists to consult with local health or school officials on problems of hearing impairment and to organize hearing-conservation programs on the local level. These consultants also confer with other branches of their state departments of health and education in such matters as planning special-education programs in the public schools and health education. This type of position calls for a person with a master's degree in audiology and with a considerable amount of organizational ability.

Finally, there is an opportunity for audiologists to engage in private practice. This vocational possibility is usually implemented in association with one or more otologists under various arrangements. Some otologists with extensive practice engage audiologists to provide diagnostic and rehabilitative services in their offices. Other arrangements include private practice in a group medical practice, or in a free-standing office.

In summary, the requirements of existing positions in the field of audiology demand training through the master's degree. The doctorate is a necessity in many positions, particularly in college and university teaching.

Thus far in this discussion, we have been concerned with employment for audiologists in clinical environments. Career opportunities exist for individuals who have received special preparation in laboratory research methods. In past years, most research in audition and on the ear and its function had been performed by specialists whose training was in fields other than audiology. Now, however, departments that produce clinical audiologists are also graduating research audiologists, who are joining physiologists, physicists, experimental psychologists, and representatives of other scientific disciplines in making important contributions to our knowledge of normal and disordered hearing. As more individuals complete their professional preparation in audiology, which is primarily a clinical discipline, it may be expected that more of them will become interested in pursuing a career in research. Also, if more government and private funds become available for research into audiological problems, and more hearing centers of various sorts expand their facilities to include laboratories, many more opportunities should arise for research-minded audiologists. Thus, in each of the employment possibilities mentioned, there should be opportunities for research audiologists. Because a Ph.D. is a research degree, it is reasonable to assume that a research position should be filled by an audiologist with a doctorate.

CERTIFICATION REQUIREMENTS FOR AUDIOLOGISTS

The professional organization to which audiologists belong, and which provides certification of clinical competence for those who qualify, is the American Speech-Language-Hearing Association. This organization is for the professions of audiology and speech pathology what the American Medical Association is for physicians and what the American Psychological Association is for psychologists. The American Speech-Language-Hearing Association was founded as the American Academy of Speech Correction in 1925. The name American Speech and Hearing Association was adopted in 1947 as a recognition of the importance of work in hearing. The current name was adopted in 1978 in recognition of the work in language (the acronym *ASHA* has been retained), and the organization has had steady growth since then. The purposes of the American Speech-Language-Hearing Association, as stated in its bylaws, are as follows:

> The purposes of this organization shall be to encourage basic scientific study of the process of individual human communication, with special reference to speech, hearing, and language, promote investigation and prevention of disorders of human communication, and foster improvement of clinical procedures with such disorders; to stimulate exchange of information among persons and organizations thus engaged; and to disseminate such information.[6]

To be eligible for full membership in the American Speech-Language-Hearing Association, an individual must hold a master's degree or its equivalent, with major emphasis in speech pathology, audiology, or speech and hear-

[6]By-Laws of the American Speech-Language-Hearing Association, Article II, *Directory of the American Speech-Language-Hearing Association* (1983), p. IX.

ing science, or have a master's degree or its equivalent and present evidence of active research, interest, and performance in the field of human communication. Each year, a selected group of members are chosen as fellows of the association in recognition of their professional or scientific achievements. The association publishes the *Journal of Speech and Hearing Disorders*; *Journal of Speech and Hearing Research*; and *Language, Speech, and Hearing Services in Schools*, all of which appear quarterly, and one monthly publication, *Asha*, which gives news and announcements and carries articles dealing with professional matters. The association's national office is near Washington, D.C.

The American Speech-Language-Hearing Association assumes responsibility for awarding clinical certification to those of its members who meet the published requirements. Clinical certification is granted either in speech-language pathology or in audiology. There is provision for dual certification for those who qualify in both fields. Certification is granted on recommendation of the Clinical Certification Board of the Association upon application and submission of credentials and upon passing an examination. The current requirements for clinical certification may be obtained by writing to the American Speech-Language-Hearing Association, 10801 Rockville Pike, Rockville, Maryland 20852.

Generally, the requirements for clinical certification in audiology are a minimum of sixty semester hours of course work at accredited colleges or universities, including at least twelve semester hours in courses that provide fundamental information applicable to the normal development and use of speech, hearing, and language, and at least forty-eight semester hours in courses that provide information about and training in the management of speech, hearing, and language disorders and supplementary information. The major portion of this course work must be in audiology. Also required for certification are the completion of at least 300 clock hours of supervised, direct clinical experience as part of the training program, and an academic year's full-time "satisfactory" professional employment under supervision following completion of the training program.

The association publishes a Code of Ethics, to which all members must subscribe. The Code of Ethics outlines the professional responsibilities of the person performing clinical work in speech and hearing. It is similar to the code of ethics subscribed to by other professional groups. Although formerly the Code of Ethics prohibited members of the association from engaging in sales or promotional activities of products related to their professional field, that section of the code was changed in 1978, as explained in Chapter 10, so that audiologists may now sell hearing aids as part of a complete aural rehabilitation program.

As the gap between the number of positions to be filled and the number of fully qualified audiologists available for employment has narrowed as a result of increased enrollments in training programs, it is becoming increasingly necessary for an individual seeking employment as an audiologist to hold the ASHA certificate of clinical competence. The best guarantee that the public will receive competent professional services is a strong national organization with the power to determine which individuals are qualified to practice the specialties of audiology and speech pathology. There is a trend now toward state licensing of individuals who wish to practice either as audiologists or speech pathologists. Most states require licensing of professional personnel in audiology and speech pathology, just as of physicians, dentists, clinical psychologists, and so on. The requirements for licensure are generally less than or equal to those for certification.

Since certification by the American Speech-Language-Hearing Association should be the primary goal of every student training in the field of speech and hearing, training institutions must take into account the course requirements that the association has established. The specific course requirements published by the American Speech-Language-Hearing Association may change from time to time, and training programs must be sufficiently flexible to adapt to the changing requirements of a growing professional field.

THE PREPARATION OF AUDIOLOGISTS

In 1982, more than 230 master's-degree programs in speech pathology and audiology were listed by the American Speech-Language-Hearing Association.[7] It is estimated that about half of these programs provide sufficient course work and supervised clinical practice in audiology to qualify graduates for the ASHA certificate of clinical competence in audiology.

Educational programs in audiology are usually found in colleges of arts and sciences, although some programs are situated in colleges of education, and a few are in schools of medicine. In many of the larger universities, separate departments have been established under such titles as *speech pathology and audiology, audiology and speech sciences, communicative disorders, speech and hearing science,* and so forth.

The American Boards of Examiners in Speech Pathology and Audiology of the American Speech-Language-Hearing Association established the Education and Training Board for the purpose of accrediting master's-degree programs in speech pathology and/or audiology. This name was changed to the Educational Standards Board in 1983. The Council on Postsecondary Education and the U.S. Department of Education have recognized the American Speech-Language-Hearing Association as the official accrediting body in this field. As of January 1, 1984, at least seventy-eight university and college programs had received accreditation in audiology.[8] To receive accreditation, a

---

[7] *A Guide to Graduate Education in Speech-Language Pathology and Audiology 1982* (Washington, D.C.: American Speech-Language-Hearing Association, 1982).

[8] "Profile of Educational Programs in Speech-Language Pathology and Audiology," *Asha* 26 (January 1984):43–48.

program must submit an application describing its academic and clinical program in detail. Following a site visit, approved programs are awarded certificates and are appropriately identified in various directories and brochures issued by the American Speech-Language-Hearing Association.

The content of an educational program must depend on the professional job requirements of positions in audiology, as well as on the certification requirements of the American Speech-Language-Hearing Association. No attempt will be made here to specify every course which the audiologist-in-training should take. Rather, suggestions will be made concerning the breadth of knowledge that it is desirable for the audiologist to have in various areas. Naturally, the numbers and types of courses an individual takes would depend on the degree and professional goals. A complete educational program that extends through the doctoral-degree level should cover all the course work indicated in the following areas. No significance should be attached to the order in which these areas are discussed. It is assumed that courses in various areas would be taken concurrently.

Audiology

Naturally, it is necessary for students to have a solid grounding in the theoretical and practical aspects of audiology. In addition to a survey course in audiology, they should take courses in basic and advanced audiometry, hearing aids, experimental audiology, speechreading, auditory and speech training for the hearing handicapped, and methods of teaching the preschool deaf child, as well as seminars to become more thoroughly acquainted with topics that can only be touched on in the formal courses. There should be ample provision for supervised clinical practice, which is equally distributed among all aspects of audiology, that is, not limited to testing, for example. As a minimum, students should obtain the number of clock hours of clinical practice required for certification by the American Speech-Language-Hearing Association.

Speech Pathology

The specialty of audiology is closely related to the field of speech pathology, just as speech and hearing are related communication skills. Both require similar clinical techniques. Audiologists who know nothing of speech disorders other than those directly associated with a hearing impairment are too narrowly specialized to be able to perform their functions as audiologists satisfactorily. The American Speech-Language-Hearing Association recognizes the necessity of receiving some training in speech pathology and correction and requires at least six semester hours of course work and a minimum of thirty-five clock hours of supervised clinical practice in this field for certification in audiology. In our opinion, even more course work and clinical practice in speech pathology should be required. The audiologist-in-training should take courses in speech pathology, organic speech disorders, voice and articulation disorders, language disorders, and a seminar in speech pathology. The student should also have extensive, supervised clinical experience with various types of speech problems.

Speech and Hearing Sciences

In point of chronological order, courses in this field should precede at least the advanced courses in audiology and speech pathology. Just as the medical student must take courses in sciences that are basic to clinical medicine, so the student audiologist should be thoroughly grounded in the sciences that are basic to clinical work in the field of speech and hearing. This includes such courses as descriptive phonetics, experimental phonetics, basic and advanced speech science, language development, linguistics, acoustics, bioacoustics, psychoacoustics, speech and hearing instrumentation, and research methods in speech pathology and audiology. Some of these courses—acoustics, for example—may be taught in other departments within the university.

Psychology

Psychology is the discipline perhaps most closely related to the fields of speech and hearing. The student audiologist should take courses in statistics, child psychology, sensation and perception, physiological psychology, abnormal psychology, experimental psychology, learning, and mental hygiene. Course work and experience in intelligence and personality testing are also highly desirable.

Other Fields

Because audiology is also closely related to medicine, it is to be hoped that the student will have the opportunity to obtain some course work that is taught in a school of medicine. Ideally, there should be close liaison and cooperation between the department in which audiology is taught and the school of medicine, so that courses specifically for students in speech pathology and audiology can be arranged. One of these courses should cover the anatomy, physiology, and neurology of the communicative mechanism. Of course, this could be taught also by the nonmedical specialists in the student's major department, but it would be preferable to have the course taught by specialists in anatomy, physiology, and neurology. Another desirable course is one dealing with the medical backgrounds of speech and hearing disorders, that is, the pathology underlying disorders of the type with which the audiologist and the speech pathologist will be concerned. Such a course should be taught by the medical specialists concerned with particular disorders, for example, a neurologist or neurosurgeon, a pediatrician, a physiatrist, and an otolaryngologist.

The student who is preparing for a career in speech and hearing in the public schools should take a number of courses in general and special education to be prepared to work cooperatively with teachers and other personnel in the school system. For the student preparing to be a clinician in a hearing center of some type, courses in education would not be required.

Clinical Internship

The training of audiologists is not complete without some provision for supervised professional experience. As stated previously, certification by the American Speech-Language-Hearing Association requires an academic year's professional experience. If employers are to be educated to hire only audiologists who have been certified by the association, a dilemma is created. Where can the beginning audiologist secure the experience that is prerequisite to being certified? The solution to this problem lies in the affiliation of training institutions with nonacademic hearing centers. The affiliation serves two purposes: First, it provides the university with an outlet for its products—a chance to put new audiologists into internships; and, second, it enables the hearing center to obtain additional help at a minimum of expense. There is an additional benefit to the hearing center: the prestige attached to an academic connection, tenuous though the connection may be. It is difficult to attract highly trained personnel to work that is purely clinical. If the chance to develop an academic affiliation on a "clinical staff" basis is offered to a promising audiologist, a position at a hearing center becomes more attractive. For many years, a large number of medical schools have obtained the part-time services of a clinical teaching staff merely by granting academic status to practicing physicians who gain only in increased prestige. Clinical audiologists, too, are hungry for the prestige that a university appointment bestows.

Just as no medical school in the country can consider the training of physicians complete without a year's internship, so the departments in which audiologists are trained should consider it necessary to arrange for a year's internship for audiologists before considering their training complete. Such internship, under proper professional supervision, would satisfy the professional experience certification requirement of the American Speech-Language-Hearing Association. With certification, the audiologist can then accept a position with confidence.

APPENDIX
MATERIALS FOR SPEECH AUDIOMETRY

WORD LISTS FOR C.I.D. AUDITORY TEST W-1[1]

List A

1. greyhound	10. duckpond	19. baseball	28. oatmeal
2. schoolboy	11. sidewalk	20. stairway	29. toothbrush
3. inkwell	12. hotdog	21. cowboy	30. farewell
4. whitewash	13. padlock	22. iceberg	31. grandson
5. pancake	14. mushroom	23. northwest	32. drawbridge
6. mousetrap	15. hardware	24. railroad	33. doormat
7. eardrum	16. workshop	25. playground	34. hothouse
8. headlight	17. horseshoe	26. airplane	35. daybreak
9. birthday	18. armchair	27. woodwork	36. sunset

List B

1. playground	10. railroad	19. toothbrush	28. eardrum
2. grandson	11. baseball	20. mushroom	29. greyhound
3. daybreak	12. padlock	21. farewell	30. birthday
4. doormat	13. hardware	22. horseshoe	31. hothouse
5. woodwork	14. whitewash	23. pancake	32. iceberg
6. armchair	15. hotdog	24. inkwell	33. schoolboy
7. stairway	15. sunset	25. mousetrap	34. duckpond
8. cowboy	17. headlight	26. airplane	35. workshop
9. oatmeal	18. drawbridge	27. sidewalk	36. northwest

[1] These word lists are reproduced with the permission of the Veterans Administration and Dr. Ira J. Hirsh of the Central Institute for the Deaf.

List C

1. birthday	10. woodwork	19. farewell	28. sunset
2. hothouse	11. stairway	20. mousetrap	29. cowboy
3. toothbrush	12. daybreak	21. armchair	30. duckpond
4. horseshoe	13. sidewalk	22. drawbridge	31. playground
5. airplane	14. railroad	23. mushroom	32. inkwell
6. northwest	15. oatmeal	24. baseball	33. eardrum
7. whitewash	16. headlight	25. grandson	34. workshop
8. hotdog	17. pancake	26. padlock	35. schoolboy
9. hardware	18. doormat	27. greyhound	36. iceberg

List D

1. hothouse	10. duckpond	19. playground	28. greyhound
2. padlock	11. baseball	20. oatmeal	29. mousetrap
3. eardrum	12. railroad	21. northwest	30. schoolboy
4. sidewalk	13. hardware	22. woodwork	31. whitewash
5. cowboy	14. toothbrush	23. stairway	32. inkwell
6. mushroom	15. airplane	24. hotdog	33. doormat
7. farewell	16. iceberg	25. headlight	34. daybreak
8. horseshoe	17. armchair	26. pancake	35. drawbridge
9. workshop	18. grandson	27. birthday	36. sunset

List E

1. northwest	10. greyhound	19. headlight	28. eardrum
2. doormat	11. cowboy	20. airplane	29. mushroom
3. railroad	12. daybreak	21. inkwell	30. whitewash
4. woodwork	13. drawbridge	22. grandson	31. hothouse
5. hardware	14. duckpond	23. workshop	32. toothbrush
6. stairway	15. horseshoe	24. hotdog	33. playground
7. sidewalk	16. armchair	25. oatmeal	34. baseball
8. birthday	17. padlock	26. sunset	35. iceberg
9. farewell	18. mousetrap	27. pancake	36. schoolboy

List F

1. padlock	10. baseball	19. mousetrap	28. mushroom
2. daybreak	11. woodwork	20. workshop	29. armchair
3. sunset	12. inkwell	21. eardrum	30. whitewash
4. farewell	13. pancake	22. greyhound	31. hotdog
5. northwest	14. toothbrush	23. doormat	32. schoolboy
6. airplane	15. hardware	24. horseshoe	33. headlight
7. playground	16. railroad	25. stairway	34. duckpond
8. iceberg	17. oatmeal	26. cowboy	35. birthday
9. drawbridge	18. grandson	27. sidewalk	36. hothouse

C.I.D. AUDITORY TEST W-22 (PB WORD LISTS)[2]

List 1A

1. an	14. low	27. as	40. jam
2. yard	15. owl	28. wet	41. poor
3. carve	16. it	29. chew	42. him
4. us	17. she	30. see (sea)	43. skin
5. day	18. high	31. deaf	44. east
6. toe	19. there (their)	32. them	45. thing
7. felt	20. earn (urn)	33. give	46. dad
8. stove	21. twins	34. true	47. up
9. hunt	22. could	35. isle (aisle)	48. bells
10. ran	23. what	36. or (oar)	49. wire
11. knees	24. bathe	37. law	50. ache
12. not (knot)	25. ace	38. me	
13. mew	26. you (ewe)	39. none (nun)	

List 2A

1. yore (your)	14. now	27. young	40. off
2. bin (been)	15. jaw	28. cars	41. ill
3. way (weigh)	16. one (won)	29. tree	42. rooms
4. chest	17. hit	30. dumb	43. ham
5. then	18. send	31. that	44. star
6. ease	19. else	32. die (dye)	45. eat
7. smart	20. tare (tear)	33. show	46. thin
8. gave	21. does	34. hurt	47. flat
9. pew	22. too (two, to)	35. own	48. well
10. ice	23. cap	36. key	49. by (buy)
11. odd	24. with	37. oak	50. ail (ale)
12. knee	25. air (heir)	38. new (knew)	
13. move	26. and	39. live (verb)	

List 3A

1. bill	14. oil	27. when	40. on
2. add (ad)	15. king	28. book	41. if
3. west	16. pie	29. tie	42. raw
4. cute	17. he	30. do	43. glove
5. start	18. smooth	31. hand	44. ten
6. ears	19. farm	32. end	45. dull
7. tan	20. this	33. shove	46. though
8. nest	21. done (dun)	34. have	47. chair
9. say	22. use (yews)	35. owes	48. we
10. is	23. camp	36. jar	49. ate (eight)
11. out	24. wool	37. no (know)	50. year
12. lie (lye)	25. are	38. may	
13. three	26. aim	39. knit	

[2] These word lists are reproduced with the permission of the Veterans Administration and Dr. Ira J. Hirsh of the Central Institute for the Deaf.

List 4A

1. all (awl)	13. my	26. darn	39. few
2. wood (would)	14. leave	27. art	40. jump
3. at	15. of	28. will	41. pale (pail)
4. where	16. hang	29. dust	42. go
5. chin	17. save	30. toy	43. stiff
6. they	18. ear	31. aid	44. can
7. dolls	19. tea (tee)	32. than	45. through
8. so (sew)	20. cook	33. eyes (ayes)	(thru)
9. nuts	21. tin	34. shoe	46. clothes
10. ought	22. bread (bred)	35. his	47. who
(aught)	23. why	36. our (hour)	48. bee (be)
11. in (inn)	24. arm	37. men	49. yes
12. net	25. yet	38. near	50. am

List 1B

1. carve	14. twins	27. stove	40. could
2. wire	15. isle (aisle)	28. ache	41. them
3. felt	16. ace	29. us	42. high
4. thing	17. deaf	30. him	43. or (oar)
5. knees	18. she	31. not (knot)	44. low
6. poor	19. none (nun)	32. me	45. jam
7. owl	20. mew	33. it	46. ran
8. law	21. skin	34. see (sea)	47. east
9. there (their)	22. hunt	35. earn (urn)	48. toe
10. give	23. up	36. true	49. bells
11. what	24. day	37. bathe	50. yard
12. chew	25. an	38. you (ewe)	
13. as	26. dad	39. wet	

List 2B

1. way (weigh)	14. air (heir)	27. chest	40. two (two, to)
2. by (buy)	15. that	28. thin	41. flat
3. smart	16. does	29. gave	42. new (knew)
4. eat	17. own	30. rooms	43. key
5. odd	18. hit	31. knee	44. now
6. ill	19. live (verb)	32. send	45. off
7. jaw	20. move	33. one (won)	46. ice
8. oak	21. ham	34. hurt	47. star
9. else	22. pew	35. tare (tear)	48. ease
10. show	23. die (dye)	36. dumb	49. well
11. cap	24. then	37. with	50. bin (been)
12. tree	25. yore (your)	38. and	
13. young	26. ail (ale)	39. cars	

List 3B

1. year	4. hand	7. may	10. this
2. cute	5. raw	8. pie	11. do
3. though	6. lie (lye)	9. have	12. wool

13. aim
14. book
15. use (yews)
16. end
17. smooth
18. jar
19. oil
20. is
21. start
22. on

23. ears
24. we
25. add (ad)
26. west
27. ate (eight)
28. tan
29. dull
30. out
31. if
32. king

33. no (know)
34. farm
35. shove
36. camp
37. tie
38. when
39. are
40. ten
41. done (dun)
42. owes

43. he
44. knit
45. nest
46. glove
47. say
48. chair
49. bill
50. three

List 4B

1. chin
2. all (awl)
3. who
4. few
5. stiff
6. my
7. nuts
8. save
9. his
10. tin
11. aid
12. yet
13. art

14. so (sew)
15. why
16. darn
17. tea (tee)
18. men
19. of
20. pale (pail)
21. our (hour)
22. through
    (thru)
23. dolls
24. yes
25. at

26. wood
    (would)
27. bee (be)
28. they
29. dust
30. ought (aught)
31. jump
32. leave
33. in (inn)
34. ear
35. than
36. bread (bred)
37. will

38. eyes (ayes)
39. arm
40. toy
41. cook
42. shoe
43. hang
44. near
45. go
46. can
47. net
48. clothes
49. where
50. am

List 1C

1. felt
2. bells
3. owl
4. jam
5. what
6. them
7. isle (aisle)
8. bathe
9. none (nun)
10. it
11. up
12. stove
13. an

14. not (knot)
15. skin
16. us
17. earn (urn)
18. deaf
19. wet
20. as
21. or (oar)
22. there (their)
23. east
24. knees
25. carve
26. yard

27. thing
28. ran
29. law
30. high
31. chew
32. me
33. ace
34. see (sea)
35. mew
36. him
37. day
38. ache
39. hunt

40. you (ewe)
41. she
42. dad
43. true
44. could
45. give
46. low
47. poor
48. twins
49. wire
50. toe

List 2C

1. smart
2. well
3. jaw
4. off
5. cap
6. does
7. that
8. with

9. live (verb)
10. one (won)
11. die (dye)
12. gave
13. chest
14. yore (your)
15. knee
16. ham

17. tare (tear)
18. new (knew)
19. cars
20. young
21. key
22. else
23. star
24. odd

25. way (weigh)
26. bin (been)
27. eat
28. ice
29. oak
30. send
31. tree
32. and

33. flat
34. hurt
35. move
36. rooms
37. then

38. ail (ale)
39. thin
40. pew
41. own
42. hit

43. dumb
44. air (heir)
45. too (two, to)
46. show
47. now

48. ill
49. ease
50. by (buy)

List 3C

1. though
2. bill
3. may
4. nest
5. do
6. use (yews)
7. tie
8. done (dun)
9. oil
10. no (know)
11. ears
12. dull
13. ate (eight)

14. if
15. start
16. add (ad)
17. shove
18. are
19. he
20. raw
21. smooth
22. year
23. aim
24. have
25. say
26. three

27. hand
28. glove
29. pie
30. owes
31. wool
32. end
33. jar
34. farm
35. is
36. out
37. we
38. west
39. tan

40. on
41. king
42. when
43. camp
44. book
45. ten
46. knit
47. this
48. lie (lye)
49. chair
50. cute

List 4C

1. wood (would)
2. bee (be)
3. they
4. dust
5. ought (aught)
6. jump
7. leave
8. in (inn)
9. ear
10. than
11. bread (bred)
12. will
13. darn

14. of
15. toy
16. cook
17. shoe
18. hang
19. near
20. go
21. aid
22. net
23. clothes
24. where
25. am
26. chin

27. all (awl)
28. who
29. few
30. stiff
31. my
32. nuts
33. save
34. his
35. tin
36. so (sew)
37. yet
38. art
39. can

40. why
41. eyes (ayes)
42. tea (tee)
43. men
44. arm
45. pale (pail)
46. our (hour)
47. through
    (thru)
48. dolls
49. yes
50. at

List 1D

1. owl
2. wire
3. isle (aisle)
4. give
5. up
6. she
7. wet
8. ace
9. skin
10. day
11. east
12. law
13. thing

14. carve
15. mew
16. earn (urn)
17. chew
18. or (oar)
19. hunt
20. an
21. true
22. none (nun)
23. poor
24. what
25. felt
26. toe

27. jam
28. low
29. bathe
30. dad
31. stove
32. ache
33. us
34. see (sea)
35. as
36. high
37. knees
38. yard
39. ran

40. there (their)
41. you (ewe)
42. deaf
43. him
44. not (knot)
45. me
46. it
47. twins
48. bells
49. could
50. them

List 2D

1. jaw	14. way (weigh)	27. off	40. else
2. ease	15. tree	28. show	41. key
3. that	16. and	29. too (two, to)	42. own
4. die (dye)	17. move	30. hit	43. rooms
5. new (knew)	18. tare (tear)	31. well	44. yore (your)
6. with	19. dumb	32. ail (ale)	45. pew
7. knee	20. live (verb)	33. ham	46. one (won)
8. then	21. now	34. young	47. air (heir)
9. cars	22. cap	35. send	48. flat
10. does	23. smart	36. hurt	49. ill
11. star	24. by (buy)	37. odd	50. gave
12. oak	25. thin	38. bin (been)	
13. eat	26. chest	39. ice	

List 3D

1. may	14. say	27. nest	40. year
2. chair	15. wool	28. knit	41. end
3. tie	16. smooth	29. done (dun)	42. are
4. ears	17. is	30. jar	43. cut
5. king	18. shove	31. dull	44. if
6. ten	19. tan	32. west	45. on
7. start	20. ate (eight)	33. he	46. no (know)
8. we	21. camp	34. farm	47. book
9. add (ad)	22. oil	35. raw	48. use (yews)
10. when	23. this	36. owes	49. lie (lye)
11. aim	24. do	37. have	50. bill
12. pie	25. though	38. three	
13. hand	26. cute	39. glove	

List 4D

1. they	14. my	26. at	39. who
2. yes	15. so (sew)	27. dust	40. net
3. leave	16. am	28. our (hour)	41. hang
4. pale (pail)	17. tin	29. in (inn)	42. aid
5. bread (bred)	18. shoe	30. tea (tee)	43. nuts
6. eyes (ayes)	19. can	31. will	44. arm
7. toy	20. darn	32. art	45. why
8. yet	21. men	33. cook	46. than
9. near	22. ear	34. his	47. of
10. save	23. through	35. go	48. jump
11. clothes	(thru)	36. stiff	49. dolls
12. few	24. ought (aught)	37. where	50. bee (be)
13. all (awl)	25. wood (would)	38. chin	

List 1E

1. them	4. ace	7. yard	10. an
2. give	5. deaf	8. earn (urn)	11. dad
3. it	6. law	9. see (sea)	12. what

13. toe
14. jam
15. none (nun)
16. ache
17. or (oar)
18. high
19. carve
20. there (their)
21. day
22. not (knot)
23. she
24. bells
25. wire
26. owl
27. up
28. twins
29. poor
30. him
31. thing
32. ran
33. chew
34. as
35. true
36. stove
37. felt
38. low
39. bathe
40. skin
41. us
42. hunt
43. knees
44. mew
45. you (ewe)
46. east
47. me
48. wet
49. could
50. isle (aisle)

List 2E

1. that
2. ill
3. knee
4. pew
5. star
6. and
7. tree
8. odd
9. dumb
10. ham
11. smart
12. with
13. off
14. thin
15. gave
16. now
17. send
18. move
19. ice
20. eat
21. rooms
22. cars
23. air (heir)
24. new (knew)
25. jaw
26. well
27. die (dye)
28. one (won)
29. then
30. own
31. bin (been)
32. key
33. oak
34. young
35. live (verb)
36. hit
37. by (buy)
38. chest
39. show
40. cap
41. ail (ale)
42. tare (tear)
43. hurt
44. way (weigh)
45. else
46. does
47. yore (your)
48. too (two, to)
49. flat
50. ease

List 3E

1. add (ad)
2. we
3. ears
4. start
5. is
6. on
7. jar
8. oil
9. smooth
10. end
11. use (yews)
12. book
13. aim
14. wool
15. do
16. this
17. have
18. pie
19. may
20. lie (lye)
21. raw
22. hand
23. though
24. cute
25. year
26. three
27. bill
28. chair
29. say
30. glove
31. nest
32. farm
33. he
34. owes
35. done (dun)
36. ten
37. arc
38. when
39. tie
40. camp
41. shove
42. knit
43. no (know)
44. king
45. if
46. out
47. dull
48. tan
49. ate (eight)
50. west

List 4E

1. ought (aught)
2. wood (would)
3. through
   (thru)
4. ear
5. men
6. darn
7. can
8. shoe
9. tin
10. so (sew)
11. my
12. am
13. few
14. all (awl)
15. clothes
16. save
17. near
18. yet
19. toy
20. eyes (ayes)
21. bread (bred)
22. pale (pail)
23. leave
24. yes
25. they
26. be (bee)
27. dolls
28. jump
29. of
30. than
31. why

32. arm
33. hang
34. nuts
35. aid
36. net

37. who
38. chin
39. where
40. stiff
41. go

42. his
43. cook
44. art
45. will
46. tea (tee)

47. in (inn)
48. our (hour)
49. dust
50. at

List 1F

1. isle (aisle)
2. ace
3. east
4. hunt
5. earn (urn)
6. what
7. jam
8. ache
9. him
10. bells
11. owl
12. twins
13. as

14. there (their)
15. not (knot)
16. ran
17. high
18. stove
19. low
20. poor
21. an
22. mew
23. law
24. wet
25. give
26. it

27. could
28. yard
29. dad
30. us
31. you (ewe)
32. none (nun)
33. felt
34. carve
35. up
36. wire
37. she
38. chew
39. thing

40. day
41. skin
42. true
43. or (oar)
44. bathe
45. toe
46. knees
47. see (sea)
48. me
49. deaf
50. them

List 2F

1. knee
2. flat
3. tree
4. else
5. smart
6. ail (ale)
7. gave
8. by (buy)
9. ice
10. oak
11. air (heir)
12. then
13. die (dye)

14. jaw
15. bin (been)
16. rooms
17. live (verb)
18. send
19. thin
20. off
21. hurt
22. dumb
23. yore (your)
24. star
25. that
26. ease

27. pew
28. does
29. odd
30. tare (tear)
31. with
32. chest
33. now
34. young
35. eat
36. own
37. new (knew)
38. well
39. one (won)

40. cars
41. key
42. move
43. hit
44. show
45. cap
46. ham
47. way (weigh)
48. and
49. too (two, to)
50. ill

List 3F

1. west
2. start
3. farm
4. out
5. book
6. when
7. this
8. oil
9. lie (lye)
10. owes
11. glove
12. cute
13. three

14. chair
15. hand
16. knit
17. pie
18. ten
19. wool
20. camp
21. end
22. king
23. on
24. tan
25. we
26. ears

27. ate (eight)
28. jar
29. if
30. use (yews)
31. shove
32. do
33. are
34. may
35. he
36. though
37. say
38. bill
39. year

40. nest
41. raw
42. done (dun)
43. have
44. tie
45. aim
46. no (know)
47. smooth
48. dull
49. is
50. add (ad)

List 4F

1. our (hour)	14. bee (be)	27. in (inn)	40. of
2. art	15. eyes (ayes)	28. men	41. aid
3. darn	16. than	29. cook	42. nuts
4. ought (aught)	17. save	30. tin	43. clothes
5. stiff	18. toy	31. where	44. who
6. am	19. my	32. all (awl)	45. so (sew)
7. go	20. chin	33. hang	46. net
8. few	21. show	34. near	47. can
9. arm	22. his	35. why	48. will
10. yet	23. ear	36. bread (bred)	49. through
11. jump	24. tea (tee)	37. dolls	(thru)
12. pale (pail)	25. at	38. they	50. dust
13. yes	26. wood (would)	39. leave	

CHILDREN'S SPONDEE LIST[3]

1. sidewalk	20. sunset	39. hopscotch
2. birthday	21. daylight	40. jump rope
3. cupcake	22. footstool	41. shoelace
4. airplane	23. pancake	42. hairbrush
5. headlight	24. hotdog	43. necktie
6. blackboard	25. outside	44. ash tray
7. shotgun	26. scarecrow	45. bedroom
8. eyebrow	27. playmate	46. toy shop
9. railroad	28. rainbow	47. playpen
10. baseball	29. toothbrush	48. dollhouse
11. stairway	30. dishpan	49. highchair
12. armchair	31. bathtub	50. downtown
13. playground	32. jackknife	51. meatball
14. doorstep	33. ice cream	52. sunshine
15. mousetrap	34. schoolroom	53. barnyard
16. cowboy	35. backyard	54. bus stop
17. wigwam	36. doorbell	55. football
18. coughdrop	37. drugstore	56. bluejay
19. churchbell	38. streetcar	57. birdnest

[3] The first eight spondee words are taken from Jean Utley, *What's Its Name* (Urbana: University of Illinois Press, 1951), p. 126; and the second series of eight spondees is from ibid., p. 127.

KINDERGARTEN PB WORD LISTS[4]

List 1

1. please	14. rag	27. bath	40. neck
2. great	15. put	28. slip	41. beef
3. sled	16. fed	29. ride	42. few
4. pants	17. fold	30. end	43. use
5. rat	18. hunt	31. pink	44. did
6. bad	19. no	32. thank	45. hit
7. pinch	20. box	33. take	46. pond
8. such	21. are	34. cart	47. hot
9. bus	22. teach	35. scab	48. own
10. need	23. slice	36. lay	49. bead
11. ways	24. is	37. class	50. shop
12. five	25. tree	38. me	
13. mouth	26. smile	39. dish	

List 2

1. laugh	14. turn	27. feed	40. as
2. falls	15. grab	28. next	41. grew
3. paste	16. rose	29. wreck	42. knee
4. plow	17. lip	30. waste	43. fresh
5. page	18. bee	31. crab	44. tray
6. weed	19. bet	32. peg	45. cat
7. gray	20. his	33. freeze	46. on
8. park	21. sing	34. race	47. camp
9. wait	22. all	35. bud	48. find
10. fat	23. bless	36. darn	49. yes
11. ax	24. suit	37. fair	50. loud
12. cage	25. splash	38. sack	
13. knife	26. path	39. got	

List 3

1. tire	14. else	27. thick	40. frog
2. seed	15. nest	28. if	41. bush
3. purse	16. jay	29. them	42. clown
4. quick	17. raw	30. sheep	43. cab
5. room	18. true	31. air	44. hurt
6. bug	19. had	32. set	45. pass
7. that	20. cost	33. dad	46. grade
8. sell	21. vase	34. ship	47. blind
9. low	22. press	35. case	48. drop
10. rich	23. fit	36. you	49. leave
11. those	24. bounce	37. may	50. nuts
12. ache	25. wide	38. choose	
13. black	26. most	39. white	

[4] These three kindergarten PB word lists were devised by Harriet Haskins Pike as part of her M.A. thesis at Northwestern University and are reproduced here with her permission. A fourth list of these PBK words (the original List 2) was discarded for clinical use because it was found to be too easy (personal communication from Mrs. Pike).

CNC WORD LISTS[5]

List 1

1. jar	14. home	27. dime	40. dead
2. boil	15. cape	28. bean	41. chore
3. tough	16. shore	29. thin	42. boat
4. tooth	17. wreck	30. seize	43. wish
5. goose	18. shirt	31. hate	44. name
6. toad	19. knife	32. wood	45. pick
7. rout	20. hull	33. check	46. ripe
8. mess	21. yearn	34. ditch	47. fall
9. kite	22. sun	35. rose	48. lag
10. jug	23. wheel	36. merge	49. gale
11. pad	24. fit	37. lease	50. sob
12. salve	25. patch	38. loop	
13. van	26. make	39. king	

List 2

1. rail	14. hash	27. choice	40. beam
2. vine	15. lead /lid/	28. met	41. ring
3. root	16. jet	29. red	42. dam
4. fake	17. south	30. goal	43. tire
5. cob	18. dire	31. should	44. tall
6. moon	19. beg	32. car	45. late
7. talk	20. pan	33. pave	46. coat
8. fern	21. much	34. love	47. suck
9. this	22. dodge	35. which	48. choose
10. nose	23. weep	36. bought	49. puff
11. ship	24. wag	37. soul	50. hill
12. leak	25. sap	38. gain	
13. nurse	26. hide	39. germ	

List 3

1. jail	14. kid	27. lake	40. toll
2. rat	15. dike	28. gull	41. joke
3. toss	16. mate	29. rouge	42. head
4. soon	17. well	30. bar	43. with
5. faith	18. rig	31. tone	44. keen
6. sung	19. four	32. chin	45. more
7. keg	20. bush	33. piece	46. leave
8. vote	21. dip	34. purge	47. hut
9. size	22. gap	35. bell	48. noise
10. numb	23. perch	36. work	49. man
11. dab	24. sheep	37. life	50. yam
12. what	25. house	38. pod	
13. room	26. fade	39. shine	

[5] From Gordon E. Peterson and Ilse Lehiste, "Revised CNC Lists for Auditory Tests," *Journal of Speech and Hearing Disorders* 27 (February 1962):62–70. Reproduced by permission of Dr. Ilse Lehiste. Letters enclosed between slant lines are phonetic symbols.

List 4

1. sock	14. thumb	27. cash	40. war
2. pool	15. loan	28. hire	41. mill
3. chief	16. take	29. gas	42. hoof /huf/
4. pause	17. birch	30. phone	43. void
5. give	18. dose	31. can	44. date
6. lap	19. him	32. mop	45. shut
7. write	20. deal	33. rage	46. loud
8. serve	21. net	34. long	47. mirth
9. bone	22. job	35. nice	48. foot
10. said	23. wail	36. till	49. keep
11. tower	24. read /rid/	37. youth	50. bug
12. wig	25. shake	38. when	
13. chum	26. rice	39. pack	

List 5

1. veil	14. boot	27. nag	40. five
2. worm	15. yoke	28. wire	41. myth
3. half	16. tease	29. robe	42. match
4. gaze	17. hot	30. thought	43. cab
5. limb	18. peg	31. beach	44. sing
6. juice	19. then	32. dim	45. sail
7. light	20. rough	33. purse	46. knit
8. zeal	21. raid	34. tell	47. shop
9. town	22. dawn	35. coal	48. lean
10. chalk	23. pull	36. cup	49. hush
11. bathe	24. luck	37. dock	50. back
12. food	25. nudge	38. care	
13. mean	26. good	39. sore	

List 6

1. whip	14. sour	27. niece	40. dig
2. bud	15. bed	28. cat	41. bad
3. shone	16. lawn	29. move	42. live/lɪv/
4. rug	17. sit	30. cool	43. map
5. cheese	18. tube	31. web	44. wife
6. chain	19. veal	32. knock	45. fan
7. look	20. get	33. jot	46. birth
8. dull	21. pace	34. cage	37. team
9. pope	22. night	35. mode	48. howl
10. calf	23. hiss	36. search	49. hike
11. fire	24. shock	37. gone	50. jam
12. turn	25. wing	38. rush	
13. raise	26. door	39. pole	

List 7

1. note	4. hole	7. mouth	10. big
2. doom	5. join	8. sure	11. fan
3. coke	6. third	9. vague	12. gun

13. pearl	23. nap	33. tape	43. wit
14. loot	24. mine	34. sack	44. did
15. save	25. was	35. ridge	45. call
16. side	26. reach	36. cheek	46. neck
17. heat	27. face	37. dumb	47. such
18. bun	28. bet	38. top	48. lose
19. fish	29. caught	39. young	49. gem
20. have	30. laugh	40. led	50. tar
21. mole	31. shall	41. rig	
22. pine	32. geese	42. pass	

List 8

1. moss	14. seek	27. touch	40. dive
2. daze	15. lash	28. calm	41. rain
3. loathe	16. hail	29. gin	42. sad
4. road	17. page	30. some	43. cub
5. muff	18. lock	31. real	44. shoot
6. vowel	19. gear	32. bite	45. den
7. tip	20. hoop /hup/	33. near	46. bag
8. thing	21. learn	34. gag	47. bath
9. week	22. guide	35. cheap	48. there
10. wheat	23. fuss	36. wake	49. cough
11. foam	24. jerk	37. hurl	50. shawl
12. poor	25. pose	38. tin	
13. wet	26. rot	39. noose	

List 9

1. lack	14. pill	27. yes	40. deck
2. watch	15. both	28. sin	41. cut
3. power	16. shade	29. curve	42. need
4. mire	17. jazz	30. haze	43. cheer
5. nail	18. lathe	31. girl	44. soap
6. thine	19. catch	32. time	45. feet
7. word	20. white	33. book	46. tick
8. tool	21. chair	34. reap	47. roof
9. mob	22. loaf	35. fudge	48. dog
10. hen	23. pun	36. voice	49. beat
11. got	24. ham	37. rag	50. dish
12. sane	25. lip	38. mud	
13. shout	26. wrong	39. ball	

List 10

1. sub	9. loose	17. bit	25. pile
2. lot	10. palm	18. nick	26. shack
3. din	11. judge	19. neat	27. cone
4. death	12. wash	20. hair	28. sell
5. chill	13. rob	21. safe	29. your
6. coin	14. fine	22. hit	30. term
7. cause	15. while	23. jade	31. mood
8. burn	16. chat	24. hurt	32. deep

33. meek	38. gore	43. load	48. cave
34. rope	39. fool	44. path	49. thatch
35. witch	40. guess	45. peak	50. towel
36. ride	41. mouse	46. run	
37. bake	42. lung	47. sag	

NAME INDEX

Waardenburg, P. J., 87
Waldron, Daryle L., 253
Walsh, Theodore E., 69, 244
Walton, W., 285
Warburton, Edward A., 202
Ward, Paul H., 98, 262, 413
Ward, W. Dixon, 92, 315–18, 326, 330, 333, 352, 356–57
Warfield, Frances, 427
Warshofsky, Fred, 59
Weaver, Marlin, 88, 95, 286
Weber, Harold J., 286, 289
Webster, John C., 330
Wedenberg, Eric, 262
Wehrs, R., 72
Weiss, Erwin, 144
Welch, Annemarie S., 357
Welch, Bruce L., 333, 357
Westlake, Harold, 127
Wever, Ernest Glen, 56–57, 59
Wheeler, D. E., 349, 351–52
White, Frederick A., 307, 332, 357
Wigand, M. E., 368
Wilber, Laura Ann, 112–13, 115, 174, 189–94, 197–200, 276, 278, 288
Wiley, Terry L., 198
Williams, Carol Troffer, 202
Williams, Charles R., 298, 302, 304
Williams, Frederick, 48, 58
Williams, Henry L., 82
Williams, Peggy S., 195–97
Williston, J., 206
Wilson, W., 285
Winchester, Richard A., 95, 257
Windle, William F., 58
Wishik, Samuel M., 287
Wolfson, Robert J., 95
Work, Walter, P., 255
Wright, H. N., 217
Wullstein, H. L., 73, 368

Yaffe, Charles D., 310, 314–15
Yanick, Paul, 428
Yantis, Phillip A., 222
Yerges, Lyle F., 357
Yost, William, 59

Zemlin, Willard R., 36–39, 45–47, 49, 53–54, 57, 59
Zink, David, 286, 289
Zwislocki, Jozef, 124, 135, 216, 219

SUBJECT INDEX

AAOO method of computing percentage hearing loss, 157–60, 300
Absolute bone conduction, 131–34
Accreditation of hearing centers, 435
Accreditation of training programs, 441
Acoustic reflex, 46
  testing, 110, 113, 197–200, 259, 276–77, 288
Acoustic trauma, 91–92, 295
Acoustical Society of America, 372
Action potential (AP) from VIIIth nerve, 203–7

Acupuncture, 96
Adaptation, 126, 226, 230–31
Adenoids, 67, 74
Adult rehabilitation, 414–28
Adventitiously deaf, defined, 359
Agenesis of the auricle, 63
Aging, effect on hearing, *see* Presbycusis
Agnosia, 99
Air-bone gap, 245–48
Air conduction, hearing by, 45–52
Air-condition testing, 118–27
  masking in, 124
  symbols on audiogram, 145–48
Air Force Biomedical Science Corps, 437
Air Force noise regulation, 311–12, 315
Alternate binaural loudness-balance (ABLB) test, 213–16, 232, 234
A.M.A. (Fowler-Sabine) method of computing percentage hearing loss, 157, 159
American Academy of Occupational Medicine, 349
American Academy of Ophthalmology and Otolaryngology, 148, 263, 287
American Academy of Pediatrics, 263
American Association of Industrial Nurses, 349
American Boards of Examiners in Speech Pathology and Audiology, 435, 441–42
American Council of Otolaryngology, 349
American Industrial Hygiene Association, 349
American Medical Association, 157, 439
American National Standards Institute (ANSI), 18, 137–44, 342, 372
American Psychological Association, 439
American Speech, Language and Hearing Association ASLHA, 148, 176, 263, 283, 349, 435, 439–42, 444
Amplitude, 21–22
Ampulla, 39, 41
Anacusis, 359
Analytic method of speechreading, 383–84
Analyzers, noise, 302–4
Anatomy of the ear, 30–45
Anechoic chamber, 16
Ankylosis of the stapes, 68, 192–93
ANSI, *see* American National Standards Institute
Anthelix, 30
Antitragus, 30
Anvil, *see* Incus
Aphasia, 99
Apportionment of liability, 344
Arachnoid, 39
Army Medical Service Corps, 437
Articulation function, 171–72, 234–35
Articulation index, 328
Artificial ear, 136–42
Artificial mastoid, 144
ASLHA, *see* American Speech, Language and Hearing Association
Atresia of external meatus, 63, 71
Attic, *see* Epitympanic recess
Audibility, area of, 17
Audiogram, pure-tone, 145–61
  as aid to diagnosis, 150–55
  as guide to rehabilitation, 155–61
  reference or base line, 344–48
  symbols on, 145–49